Managing Clinical Risk

ANDERSON 'RI

Violence directed towards others and violence directed towards oneself cause an immense amount of physical and psychological damage – to the harmed and the harmful person alike, to their families, and to the public at large. *Managing Clinical Risk* is an authoritative manual for practitioners working with harmful men, women, and young people, containing up-to-date information and guidance on what to do and how they can assess and manage clinical risk, communicate their concerns about risk, and account for their decisions about risk management to their clients and to the Courts.

This book provides an evidence-based understanding of risk in key areas of practice – violence, sexual violence, firesetting, suicide, and self-harm, working with individuals and organizations alike – and among special groups: women, young people, serving and former military personnel, clients with comorbid presentations, and clients with cognitive impairment. Further, it suggests and describes the skills practitioners need to communicate their concerns to all who need to know about them through coverage of interviewing and risk-formulation skills.

This is a guidebook to effective practice. All its contributors have a record of research, practice, and considered thinking in the area of clinical risk assessment and management. They all have a wide range of knowledge and experience about the notion of risk, conducting risk management in real-world mental health, correctional, and community settings, and about working with clients with a label of high risk. Together, they combine theoretical and research knowledge with a wealth of practical skills in care and management, emphasizing the collaborative and recovery-focused nature of modern risk management.

Caroline Logan is Consultant Forensic Clinical Psychologist in Greater Manchester West Mental Health NHS Foundation Trust and Honorary Research Fellow in the Department of Community Based Medicine at the University of Manchester.

Lorraine Johnstone is Lead Consultant Clinical Forensic Psychologist in a forensic mental health service for children and adolescents. She also holds an honorary position as Research Fellow at the Centre for the Study of Violence, Glasgow Caledonian University.

Issues in Forensic Psychology
Edited by Richard Shuker, HMP Grendon

Issues in Forensic Psychology is a book series which aims to promote forensic psychology to a broad range of forensic practitioners. It aims to provide analysis and debate on current issues and to publish and promote the work of forensic psychologists and other associated professionals.

The views expressed by the authors/editors may not necessarily be those held by the Series Editor or NOMS.

1. **Research in Practice for Forensic Professionals**
   Edited by Kerry Sheldon, Jason Davies and Kevin Howells

2. **Secure Recovery**
   Approaches to recovery in forensic mental health settings
   Edited by Gerard Drennan and Deborah Alred

3. **Managing Clinical Risk**
   A guide to effective practice
   Edited by Caroline Logan and Lorraine Johnstone

Managing Clinical Risk

A guide to effective practice

**Edited by Caroline Logan and
Lorraine Johnstone**

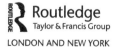
Routledge
Taylor & Francis Group

LONDON AND NEW YORK

First published 2013
by Routledge
2 Park Square, Milton Park, Abingdon, Oxon, OX14 4RN

Simultaneously published in the USA and Canada
by Routledge
711 Third Avenue, New York, NY 10017

*Routledge is an imprint of the Taylor & Francis Group, an informa
business*

British Library Cataloguing in Publication Data
A catalogue record for this book is available from the British Library

Library of Congress Cataloging-in-Publication Data
Managing clinical risk/edited by Caroline Logan and Lorraine Johnstone.
    p. cm. — (Issues in forensic psychology)
  Includes bibliographical references and index.
  1. Forensic psychology. 2. Violent offenders—Care. 3. Violence—
Forecasting. 4. Violence—Prevention. I. Logan, Caroline.
II. Johnstone, Lorraine.
RA1148.M25 2012
614'.15—dc23   2012021532

ISBN: 978-1-84392-854-6 (hbk)
ISBN: 978-1-84392-853-9 (pbk)
ISBN: 978-0-203-10643-3 (ebk)

Typeset in Times New Roman by
by Keystroke, Station Road, Codsall, Wolverhampton

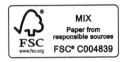

FSC
www.fsc.org
MIX
Paper from
responsible sources
FSC® C004839

Printed and bound by CPI Group (UK) Ltd, Croydon, CR0 4YY

Contents

Notes on contributors

Leena K. Augimeri, PhD, is the Director of the Centre for Children Committing Offences (CCCO) and Program Development at the Child Development Institute, and Adjunct Professor at the University of Toronto, Canada. For the past 25 years, this scientist practitioner's work has focused on the development of a comprehensive crime-prevention strategy for young children engaged in aggressive and antisocial behaviour that focuses on police–community referral protocols, gender-sensitive evidence-based interventions, and clinical-risk need-assessment tools. She is a co-founder of the longest sustained gender-sensitive evidence-based intervention for young children with conduct problems – the SNAP® Model – and co-developer of the EARL-20B and EARL-21G structured professional judgement assessment tools. She is a noted author, trainer, consultant, and presenter, responsible for all the CCCO's national and international development activities. Dr Augimeri is a Fellow of the Academy of Experimental Criminology and the recipient of the Child Welfare League of Canada's inaugural Outstanding Achievement Research and Evaluation award.

Adam J. E. Blanchard is an MA student in the Clinical Forensic Psychology programme at Simon Fraser University in Vancouver, Canada. He completed his Honours BA under the supervision of Dr Kevin Douglas, also at Simon Fraser University. His honours thesis investigated the concurrent validity of the third version of the *Historical-Clinical-Risk Management-20* (HCR-V3), focusing on its relation to previous violence. Most broadly, his research interests include risk assessment and risk management, as well as the perpetration of crime and violence. More specifically, he is interested in the link between risk assessment and risk management, the role of specific risk factors in the occurrence of harmful outcomes, multi-level risk assessment, integrated treatment services, and homelessness. His Master's work is being funded by the Canadian Institute of Health Research and a C. D. Nelson Memorial Graduate Entrance Scholarship.

David J. Cooke is a professor of psychology at Glasgow Caledonian University in Scotland and a visiting professor at Bergen University, Norway. For 23 years, he was head of the forensic clinical psychology service in Glasgow. He is a fellow of the Royal Society of Edinburgh and of the British Psychological Society. He has a longstanding interest in risk assessment and psychopathy.

Rajan Darjee co-founded and co-leads the NHS Lothian Sex Offender Liaison Service, based at the Royal Edinburgh Hospital, which offers consultation, assessment, management advice, and treatment for sexual offenders managed in the community by criminal justice and other agencies, particularly complex cases and those under Multi-Agency Public Protection Arrangements (MAPPA). He is accredited by the Scottish Risk Management Authority (RMA) to assess risk in serious violent and sexual offenders. He has presented on issues related to sexual offending at conferences, and has trained practitioners from various agencies in assessing and managing violent and sexual offenders. He is undertaking research on the clinical characteristics of sexual offenders and implications for management. He was previously Lecturer in Forensic Psychiatry at the University of Edinburgh, and a Consultant Forensic Psychiatrist at the State Hospital, Carstairs and then the Orchard Clinic in Edinburgh, Scotland. He has written over 40 published papers and book chapters, on topics including mental health legislation, mentally disordered offenders, personality disorder, risk assessment, and sexual offending.

Kevin S. Douglas is currently Associate Professor and Coordinator of the Law and Forensic Psychology Program in the Department of Psychology at Simon Fraser University (SFU) in Vancouver, Canada. He has been at SFU since 2004, after having spent three years on faculty at the University of South Florida, Tampa. Dr Douglas received his law degree in 2000 from the University of British Columbia, and his PhD in clinical (forensic) psychology from SFU in 2002. He received a Michael Smith Foundation for Health Research Career Scholar Award (2005–2010), and was the recipient of the Saleem Shah Award for Early Career Excellence in Psychology and Law (2005), awarded jointly by the American Psychology-Law Society and the American Academy of Forensic Psychology. His research has been funded by the National Science Foundation (USA), Canadian Institutes of Health Research, Social Sciences and Humanities Research Council of Canada, and the Michael Smith Foundation for Health Research. His research interests include violence risk assessment and management, the association between various mental and personality disorders (i.e., psychosis, psychopathy) and violence, and dynamic (changeable, treatment-relevant) risk factors. He is co-author of the Historical-Clinical-Risk Management-20 (HCR-20) violence risk assessment measure, which has been translated into 16 languages and is used broadly around the world in correctional, forensic, and psychiatric settings to help guide decisions about violence potential and how to reduce it. Dr Douglas is lead author on the latest (third) revision of the HCR-20, called the HCR-V3. More recently, he has been conducting research on other violence-related adverse experiences, including suicide-related behaviour and being victimized by violence. On these topics, Dr Douglas has authored approximately 100 journal articles, books, and book chapters.

Melissa C. Hendry is a doctoral student in clinical psychology at Simon Fraser University (SFU) in Vancouver, Canada, specializing in law and forensic psychology. She obtained her MA from SFU in 2009 and a BA (Honours) from

Concordia University in 2007. Her research interests include the role of anger, hostility, and persecutory delusions in suicide-related behaviour and violence perpetration, as well as the measurement of short-term changes in dynamic risk factors. Her clinical interests include cognitive behavioural therapy for psychosis and the assessment of sexual and non-sexual violence in civil psychiatric patients and mentally ill offenders.

Lorraine Johnstone is Consultant Clinical Forensic Psychologist at the Forensic Child and Adolescent Mental Health Service, NHSGGC and honorary research fellow at Glasgow Caledonian University in Scotland. Lorraine has a long-standing interest in the assessment, treatment, and management of mentally disordered offenders. Lorraine has collaborated on several research studies related to violence risk assessment and personality disorder. She has examined the relevance of both individual and situational variables in violence risk. Lorraine has published in peer-reviewed journals and edited books, and she regularly provides training on violence risk assessment. Before moving to work with high-risk children and adolescents, she worked across the different levels of security in adult forensic mental health and has extensive experience working as a clinician in these contexts.

Caroline Logan is a Consultant Forensic Clinical Psychologist at the Edenfield Centre, which is an NHS medium secure hospital in Greater Manchester, and an Honorary Research Fellow in the Department of Community Based Medicine at the University of Manchester, England. She has worked as a researcher and a clinician in forensic mental health services in England for many years, working directly in roles with both male and female clients who are at risk to themselves and to others. She has also undertaken various consultancy roles with the multi-disciplinary teams and the local and national health and criminal justice organizations that look after and manage this client group, examining risk assessment and management practice, especially in relation to personality-disordered offenders, and proposing and evaluating developments and change. Dr Logan has ongoing research interests in the areas of personality disorder, psychopathy, and risk, and she has a special interest in gender issues in offending.

John Marham was born in Manchester and joined the Army at the age of 16, where he served for 23 years in the Scots Guards. He served in several theatres of operation during his time in the forces, including the Gulf War (1990–1991), and was attached to 33 Field Hospital, where he worked on a High Dependency Unit. He completed his service at the rank of Colour Sergeant, then went on to train as a mental health nurse in Cambridge. Once qualified, he practised in a medium secure unit, in a psychiatric intensive care unit, and in a variety of acute admission wards. Subsequently, he helped to set up and run one of the first Ministry of Defence units operated by the NHS to provide a range of specialist mental health and substance misuse facilities for Service men and women who were experiencing mental health difficulties and who required an inpatient admission. John is currently working as a Community Psychiatric Nurse for

Combat Stress, the UK's leading charity specializing in the care of Service veterans with mental health problems. His role is to provide evidence-based assessments, including risk assessments, mental health treatment and support for veterans in their own homes, with the primary aim of improving the quality of life for veterans and their families.

Christine Michie has a BSc honours degree (first class) in mathematics from the University of Glasgow. She has been employed as a statistician and mathematician in the Statistics Team at the Marine Laboratory in Aberdeen, the principal institution for fisheries research in the Department of Agriculture and Fisheries for Scotland. Her major areas of interest were population dynamics and growth modelling. Until recently, she was a researcher in the Department of Psychology at Glasgow Caledonian University, working on various research projects with Professor David Cooke. She has investigated the structure and performance of various risk and personality assessment scales using item response theorem and structural equation modelling methods, and has conducted several studies into item and test bias in scales when they are used on different populations from those on which they were developed.

Suzanne O'Rourke, PhD, is a Consultant Forensic Clinical Neuropsychologist at the State Hospital, Carstairs and a Senior Teaching Fellow at the University of Edinburgh, Scotland. She has also worked as a behavioural investigative advisor for the National Policing Improvement Agency in the UK. During her time as lead of the State Hospital's neuropsychology service, she applied the expertise gained from her PhD research in clinical neurosciences to bring an innovative approach to the care and treatment of mentally disordered offenders. Suzanne's areas of interest include the cognitive correlates of both offending behaviour and severe and enduring mental illnesses, along with their implications for the assessment, treatment, and reduction of risk in mentally disordered offenders.

Corine de Ruiter, PhD, is presently Professor of Forensic Psychology at Maastricht University in the Netherlands. From 1999 to 2004, she served as Professor of Forensic Psychology at the University of Amsterdam; from 1995 to 2002, she worked as Head of Research at the Van der Hoeven Kliniek in Utrecht, the Netherlands. She is a licensed clinical psychologist and a Fellow of the Society for Personality Assessment. Her research interests include the relationship between mental disorders and violence, the development of antisocial personality disorder/psychopathy, effective treatment for antisocial behaviour disorders in children and adults, and forensic psychological assessment, including structured risk assessment. She is co-developer of the *Structured Assessment of Protective Factors for violence risk* (SAPROF). Dr de Ruiter has published in national and international peer-reviewed journals and currently serves as Associate Editor for the *International Journal of Forensic Mental Health* and as President of the *International Association of Forensic Mental Health Services*. She provides training workshops on forensic assessment issues and regularly serves as an expert witness in court.

Katharine Russell is a Consultant Forensic Clinical Psychologist based at the Orchard Clinic in Edinburgh, Scotland. She is co-lead and co-founder of the Sex Offender Liaison Service, which offers consultation, assessment, management advice, and treatment for sexual offenders managed in the community by criminal justice and other agencies, particularly for complex cases and those subject to Multi-Agency Public Protection Arrangements (MAPPA). She is involved in various research projects including looking at the clinical characteristics of sexual offenders and implications for community manage-ment. She has presented workshops, seminars, and keynotes on issues related to sex offending, particularly personality disorder, at conferences, and has trained practitioners from various agencies in assessing and managing violent and sexual offenders. She completed her undergraduate degree in psychology at Glasgow University before training in clinical psychology in the same institution. She previously worked as a clinical psychologist at the State Hospital, Carstairs, the high security hospital for Scotland, and the Orchard Clinic, a medium secure unit in Edinburgh. She has published papers and book chapters on fire-raising, sexual offenders, risk assessment, and personality-disordered offenders. She is accredited by the Scottish Risk Management Authority (RMA) to assess risk in serious violent and sexual offenders.

John L. Taylor is Professor of Clinical Psychology, Northumbria University and Consultant Clinical Psychologist and Psychological Services Professional Lead with Northumberland, Tyne and Wear NHS Foundation Trust in the north of England. He is a Past President of the British Association for Behavioural and Cognitive Psychotherapies (BABCP). He has published work related to his clinical research interests on the assessment and treatment of mental health, emotional, and behavioural problems experienced by people with intellectual and developmental disabilities in a range of research journals, books, and professional publications.

Ian Thorne is a Principal Forensic Psychologist with Northumberland, Tyne and Wear NHS Foundation Trust in England. Since qualifying as a forensic psychologist, he has worked for HM Prison Service in young offender and high security dispersal settings in the north-east of England, before transferr-ing to the NHS. His current responsibilities in forensic learning disability services involve the development, coordination, and delivery of group-offending behaviour programmes, which include sex offender and firesetter treatments. Previous published work relates to the assessment and treatment of offenders with developmental disabilities in a range of research and professional journals.

Vivienne de Vogel is a psychologist and head of the Department of Research at the Van der Hoeven Kliniek in Utrecht, the Netherlands. Since 2001, she has been involved in the implementation and study of the structured professional judgement model and is considered to be one of the leading experts in violence risk assessment in the Netherlands. Her current research focuses on protective factors and violence (risk assessment) in women. She is the first author of two risk assessment tools: the SAPROF (*Structured Assessment of Protective Factors for violence risk*) for the assessment of protective factors and the FAM (*Female Additional Manual*), an additional manual to the HCR-20 for violence risk assessment in women. In addition to this, she works as a practitioner, particularly with respect to the assessment and management of violence risk in female forensic psychiatric patients.

Michiel de Vries Robbé is a psychologist in the Department of Research at the Van der Hoeven Kliniek, a forensic psychiatric hospital in Utrecht, the Netherlands. Since 2004, his research focus has been on violence risk assessment in forensic clinical practice. Together with his co-authors, he developed a risk assessment tool for protective factors: the SAPROF (*Structured Assessment of Protective Factors for violence risk*). He coordinates the international SAPROF project, as the tool has now been translated into many different languages and implemented in clinical practice around the world. His near-finished PhD research focuses in particular on protective factors for violence risk. In addition, he is co-author of the recently developed FAM (*Female Additional Manual*), an additional manual to the HCR-20 for assessing risk for violence in women.

Foreword

Managing Clinical Risk: a guide to effective practice is a remarkable work that seamlessly joins the often separate worlds of risk assessment and risk management. Drs Caroline Logan and Lorraine Johnstone and their colleagues articulately argue for the insufficiency of concentrating on risk assessment while ignoring risk management. They believe that an evidence-led and clinically relevant understanding of violence risk must balance answers to two questions: 'What level of risk does this person present?' and 'What can be done to reduce this level of risk?'

In terms of violence risk assessment, almost all scholarly accounts are bottomed on Paul Meehl's canonical distinction between 'clinical' and 'actuarial' prediction. In recent years, however, many approaches to risk assessment have been developed that are not adequately characterized by a simple dichotomy. Rather, contemporary risk assessment practice now exists on a continuum of rule-based structure (or organization), with completely unstructured ('clinical') assessment laying claim to one pole of the continuum, and completely structured ('actuarial') assessment laying claim to the other. Between these two poles lie (at least) three semi-structured approaches to risk assessment.

One of these intermediate approaches to risk assessment might be termed the 'Modified Clinical' approach. Here, a professional performs a violence risk assessment by reference to a standard array ('checklist') of risk factors that either have been found by research to be empirically valid, or are at least part of widespread received clinical wisdom in the field. A standard list identifies which risk factors the clinician should attend to in conducting his or her assessment. But it does not go further and specify how to measure the designated risk factors.

A second intermediate approach – the one that is the focus of *Managing Clinical Risk* – is known as Structured Clinical Judgment. This approach organizes both the identification and the measurement of risk factors, but it does not specify in advance how the individual risk factor scores should be combined in clinical practice to yield a total risk score. This step is believed to require clinical judgement.

The final intermediate approach is a form of 'Modified Actuarial' risk assessment. Approaches to risk assessment under this rubric structure the identification, the measurement, and the combination of violence risk factors, but not the final estimate of the likelihood of violence. Given the possibility that rare factors influence the likelihood of violence in a particular case – and that, precisely because such factors rarely occur, they will never appear on any fully actuarial instrument – a clinical review of the risk estimate produced by the instrument is strongly advised.

Of these various approaches to violence risk assessment, the Structured Professional Judgment approach, has taken most seriously the potential benefits of being able to join risk assessment and risk management. The proponents of other approaches to violence risk assessment have much to learn from the careful and systematic attempts by the contributors to *Managing Clinical Risk* to integrate the considerable challenges of violence risk assessment with the even greater – and to date largely ignored – challenges of violence risk management.

John Monahan, PhD
John S. Shannon Distinguished Professor of Law
Professor of Psychology
Professor of Psychiatric Medicine and Neurobehavioural Sciences
University of Virginia, USA

Preface

Let us be clear from the start, clinical risk assessment and management – the prevention of harm – is not about adding up numbers. Therefore, this book is not about the quantification of risk. Instead, it is about *understanding* risk in order to do something about it, something effective – risk management – which results in the prevention or, at the very least, the limitation of the harmful behaviour thought possible in the person being assessed. The practice of formulation – risk formulation – is fundamental to this task and to this book because we regard this process of understanding the underlying mechanism of risk as the essential link between risk assessment and risk management. Therefore, all the contributors to this book have emphasized this critical skill to help their readers to make sense of the array of risk and protective factors present – or absent – in their clients and to guide them towards individual, and therefore meaningful, strategies for their management. In our view, there is insufficient guidance available that addresses how we might understand risk as a condition of doing something about it with our individual clients. We wish that this book might make a useful contribution to what we hope to be a growing literature addressing this very particular and very striking shortfall.

This book is intended to be an authoritative manual for practitioners working with harmful men, women, and young people, containing up-to-date information and guidance on what to do and how to assess and manage clinical risk, how to communicate their concerns about risk, and how to account for their decisions about risk management to their clients and to the Courts. The book emphasizes the structured professional judgement approach to clinical risk assessment and management because we believe this approach is the most rational and the most clinically relevant way to address risk. All of the contributors to this book have a record of research, practice, and considered thinking in the area of clinical risk assessment and management, and in the use of the structured professional judgement approach. They all have a wide range of knowledge and experience in understanding risk in key areas, working with clients with a label of high risk, and undertaking risk management in real-world mental health, correctional, and community settings. Together, they combine theoretical and research knowledge with a wealth of practical skills in the organization and systematic delivery of care, emphasizing the collaborative and recovery-focused nature of modern risk management. We hope, therefore, that this book might be a useful contribution to the knowledge and understanding of its readers, as well as their practice.

The book begins with a powerful overview of risk assessment by David Cooke and Christine Michie. Their theoretical chapter is a clarion call for a move away from traditional risk prediction approaches to the structured professional judgement approach, within which risk formulation is central. The book then moves on to consider the application of the structured professional judgement approach to key areas of clinical practice, namely risk assessment and management in relation to violence (in chapters authored by Kevin Douglas, Adam Blanchard and Melissa Hendry, and by Lorraine Johnstone), sexual violence (in a chapter authored by Katharine Russell and Rajan Darjee), suicide and self-harm (in a chapter authored by Caroline Logan), and pathological fire setting (in a chapter authored by John L. Taylor and Ian Thorne). Moving away from individuals to the situations in which they are based and managed, David Cooke and Lorraine Johnstone then examine how environments such as prisons and secure hospitals and the ways in which they are organized – or disorganized – contribute to the harm potential of the clients within.

The special considerations required by key clinical populations are then addressed. Suzanne O'Rourke provides practical guidance on assessing and managing risk in clients with cognitive impairment. Corine de Ruiter and Leena Augimeri describe ways of working with young people to prevent harm. Vivienne de Vogel and Michiel de Vries Robbé then discuss issues in working with women who are violent, and John Marham overviews the very particular challenges for practitioners and services when working with military personnel and the veterans of war.

The book draws to a close with consideration of two special areas of practice, namely forensic clinical interviewing (in a chapter authored by Caroline Logan) and the very real necessity of attending to protective factors or strengths in clients and the contribution this makes to our understanding of risk (in a chapter authored by Michiel de Vries Robbé and Vivienne de Vogel). The book concludes with a postscript written by its editors, which is a summary of the key points made in each of the chapters and a proposal for future directions in practice and research.

As editors, we would like to acknowledge the contribution of a number of people to the writing of this book. First and foremost, we are grateful to all of our contributors for their highly informative, well illustrated, reflective, and practical chapters, and for their patience with the editing process. We would also like to thank our employers and academic institutions – the Edenfield Centre in Greater Manchester Mental Health NHS Foundation Trust and the Centre for Mental Health and Risk at the University of Manchester in England (CL), and Specialist Children's Services in Greater Glasgow and Clyde and Glasgow Caledonian University in Scotland (LJ) – for allowing us the time to edit and also to contribute to this book. We would also like to thank the British Psychological Society for being the impetus for this work and Willan Publishers and now Routledge for agreeing to publish it. We would like too to thank our families for their patience and support in the face of our neglect of them in the last wee while.

Caroline Logan and Lorraine Johnstone
January 2012

Abbreviations

ACF	*Assessment and Classification of Function*
ADHD	attention deficit hyperactivity disorder
AIM	*Assessment, Intervention and Moving on Project*
APA	American Psychiatric Association
ARAI	actuarial risk assessment instruments
ASIST	*Applied Suicide Intervention Skills Training*
ASPD	antisocial personality disorder
AUC	area under the curve
BDI	*Beck Depression Inventory*
BHS	*Beck Hopelessness Scale*
BPD	borderline personality disorder
BSS	*Beck Scale for Suicide Ideation*
CANTAB	*Cambridge Automated Neuropsychological Test Battery*
CAPP	*Comprehensive Assessment of Psychopathic Personality*
CBCL	*Child Behavior Checklist*
CCTV	closed circuit television
CDI	Child Development Institute, Toronto
CFSEI-2	*Culture-Free Self Esteem Inventory-2nd Edition*
CI	confidence interval
COPINE	Combating Paedophile Information Networks in Europe
CPA	care programme approach
CPN	community psychiatric nurse
CU traits	callous-unemotional traits
DCMH	Department of Community Mental Health
DH (also DoH)	Department of Health
DID	dissociative identity disorder
DISCO	*Diagnostic Interview for Social and Communication Disorder*
DLPFC	dorsolateral prefrontal cortex
DMS	Defence Medical Services
DSM-IV	*Diagnostic and Statistical Manual of Mental Disorders 4th Edition*
DSM-5	*Diagnostic and Statistical Manual of Mental Disorders 5th Edition*

DSPD	Dangerous and Severe Personality Disorder (Programme)
EARL-20B	*Early Assessment Risk Lists for Boys*
EARL-21G	*Early Assessment Risk Lists for Girls*
ERASOR	*Estimate of Risk of Adolescent Sexual Offence Recidivism*
ESR	*Estimate of Suicide Risk*
FAM	*Female Additional Manual* (to the HCR-20)
FAM:RV	*Female Additional Manual: Research Version*
FAS	*Fire Assessment Scale*
FEEST	*Facial Expressions of Emotion Stimuli and Tests*
FIRS	*Fire Interest Rating Scale*
Four Ps framework	predisposing, precipitating, perpetuating and protective factors relating to risk of harm
FPR	false positive rate
FSAS	*Fire Setting Assessment Schedule*
GAS	*Goal Attainment Scales*
GGUH	Girls Growing Up Healthy
GLM	good lives model
GPCSL	general personality and social learning theoretical perspectives on crime
GPS	global positioning system
HCR-20	*Historical-Clinical-Risk Management-20* risk assessment guide
HCR:V3	*Historical-Clinical-Risk Management-20 3rd Edition*
HPA	hypothalamic-pituitary-adrenal
ICC	intraclass correlations
ICD-10	*International Classification of Diseases 10th Edition*
ICD-11	*International Classification of Diseases 11th Edition*
ID	intellectual disabilities
IES	integrated emotions systems
IORNS	*Inventory of Offender Risk, Needs and Strengths*
IPDE	*International Personality Disorder Examination*
IVE	Eysenck *Impulsivity-Venturesomeness-Empathy Scale*
J-SOAP II	*Juvenile Sex Offender Assessment Protocol 2nd Edition*
LIT	Leaders-In-Training
LS	*Level of Service*
LSI-R	*Level of Service Inventory-Revised* risk assessment guide
MAPPA	multi-agency public protection arrangements
MATRICS	Measurement and Treatment Research to Improve Cognition in Schizophrenia
MCCB	MATRICS *Consensus Cognitive Battery*
MDO	mentally disordered offender
MDT	multidisciplinary team
MoD	Ministry of Defence
MST	multisystemic therapy
NAPO	National Association of Probation Officers

NAS	*Novaco Anger Scale*
NCCMH	National Collaborating Centre for Mental Health
NCISH	National Confidential Inquiry into Suicide and Homicide
NEO-PI-R	*Neuroticism-Extroversion-Openness Personality Inventory-Revised*
NFRA	*Northgate Firesetter Risk Assessment*
NICE	National Institute for Clinical Excellence
OFC	orbitofrontal cortex
PANSS	*Positive and Negative Syndrome Scale*
PAS-ADD	*Psychiatric Assessment Schedules for Adults with Developmental Disabilities*
PCL-R	*Psychopathy Checklist-Revised*
PDF	probability density function
PEACE	planning and preparation, engagement and explanation, account clarification and challenge, closure, and evaluation
PFC	prefrontal cortex
PFSI	*Pathological Fire-Setters Interview*
PI	prediction interval
PI	*Provocation Inventory*
PPG	penile plethysmography
PRISM	*Promoting Risk Interventions by Situational Management*
PTSD	post-traumatic stress disorder
RAF	Royal Air Force
RCT	randomized controlled trial
RESPONSE	respect, empathy, supportiveness, positiveness, openness, non-judgemental attitude, straightforward talk, and equals talking 'across' to each other
RM2000	*Risk Matrix 2000* risk assessment guide
RMN	registered mental nurse
RN:MH	registered nurse for the mentally handicapped
RNR	Risk-Need-Responsivity
ROC	receiver operator characteristic
RSVP	*Risk for Sexual Violence Protocol* risk assessment guide
SADPERSONS	(male) sex, (older) age, depression, previous attempt, ethanol abuse, rational thinking loss, social supports lacking, organized plan, no spouse, sickness scale for assessing suicide risk
SAM	*Stalking Assessment Manual* risk assessment guide
SAMI	*Suicide Assessment Manual for Inmates*
SAPROF	*Structured Assessment of Protective Factors* for violence risk
SARA	*Spousal Assault Risk Assessment* guide
SAS	Special Air Service
SAVRY	*Structured Assessment of Violence Risk in Youth*
SBRE	*Suicidal Behaviours Risk Evaluation*
SCID-I	*Structured Clinical Interview for DSM-IV Axis I Disorders*

SCID-II	*Structured Clinical Interview for DSM-IV Axis II Disorders*
SIS	*Suicide Intent Scale*
SLO	Service Liaison Officers
SNAP®	Stop Now And Plan
SNAP® GC	SNAP® Girls Connection
SNAP® ORP	SNAP® Under 12 Outreach Project
SOLS	NHS Lothian Sex Offender Liaison Service
SORAG	*Sexual Violence Risk Appraisal Guide*
SPJ	structured professional judgement approach to clinical risk assessment and management
SPS	Scottish Prison Service
S-RAMM	*Suicide Risk Assessment and Management Manual*
SSAFA	Soldiers, Sailors and Airmen's Association
SSPI	*Screening Scale for Paedophilic Interests*
SSS	*Sexual Sadism Scale*
START	*Short-Term Assessment of Risk and Treatability*
STAXI	*State-Trait Anger Expression Inventory*
STORM	*Skills-based Training on Risk Management*
SUMD	*Scale to Assess Unawareness of Mental Disorder*
SVR-20	*Sexual Violence Risk-20* risk assessment guide
TBS order	ter beschikkingstelling, a judicial measure used in the Netherlands imposing mandatory inpatient psychiatric treatment
TCO	threat-control override symptoms of schizophrenia
TOM	theory of mind
TRiM	Trauma Risk Management
VIPA	Veterans In Prison Association
VLPFC	ventrolateral prefrontal cortex
VMPFC	ventromedial prefrontal cortex
VRAG	*Violence Risk Appraisal Guide*
WAIS	*Wechsler Adult Intelligence Scales*
WAIS-III	*Wechsler Adult Intelligence Scales 3rd Edition*
WARS	*Ward Anger Rating Scale*
YOA	Young Offenders Act
ZAS	*Zung Anxiety Scale*

Part I

The need for change

1 Violence risk assessment

From prediction to understanding – or from what? To why?

David J. Cooke and Christine Michie

'Everything in the future is uncertain, as is most of the past; even the present contains a lot of uncertainty . . .'

Dennis Lindley (2006, p. 7)

Risk management: the management of uncertainty

Perhaps Lindley's statement should be on the desk of all forensic practitioners. Risk by definition is about uncertainty (Gigerenzer, 2004). It follows, therefore, that risk management is about the management of uncertainty. Uncertainty about violence engenders anxiety in professionals and the public alike. Fortunately, the last two decades have seen dramatic strides in the technology available to assist uncertainty reduction – the technology of risk management. In retrospect, three eras of risk assessment can be discerned: the era of unstructured professional judgement, the actuarial era, and the era of risk management through structured professional judgement – this final era, we will argue, is transmuting into a fourth era, the era of risk formulation. It is important to recognize the achievements made so far (Otto and Douglas, 2010), but we must also be conscious of the limitations, and indeed the dangers, of some of the approaches that have gained acceptance within criminal justice systems. Lindley's quotation suggests that forensic practitioners should approach the task of risk assessment with transparency, circumspection and humbleness.

Violence risk assessment is at the centre of forensic practice and this is increasingly so as society becomes more risk averse. The focus of this chapter is the *individual* risky offender; the focus is on the provision of useful, valid, ethically sound information, which is probative and not prejudicial, information that can lead to principled and informed decisions. We emphasize this focus on the individual: the individual offender is the primary concern of the forensic practitioner when informing the decision-maker.

Nearly thirty years ago, John Monahan argued that violence risk assessment could only be improved if specific risk factors for violence could be identified. This stimulated a prodigious number of group studies and the field is much better informed about what risk factors need to be considered. We know 'what?' If we are to progress, it is now time to move to the question 'why?': why are people violent, what drives them to violence, what disinhibits or destabilizes them so the likelihood of violence is increased? This focus on 'why?' entails a shift of perspective, from a focus on groups to a greater focus on the individual – from a focus on statistics to a focus on psychological processes. In this chapter, we consider two broad issues which emphasize why such progress is now required.

First, we provide a detailed account of the misuse of so-called actuarial models. In our view, the field has become overconfident about the ability of actuarial procedures to make reliable predictions about whether individuals will be violent (cf. Craig and Beech, 2009; Hanson and Howard, 2010). This misplaced confidence is underpinned by the failure to appreciate the problems of making predictions – with any certainty – for individuals based on aggregate statistics, and importantly, a misunderstanding of the logic and purpose of true actuarial approaches.

Second, we argue that the field of risk assessment can only progress by shifting away from the actuarial paradigm. In our view, for the field to progress, it is necessary to generate both a taxonomy of risk processes and systematic guidance for risk formulation. The development of criteria to validate individual risk formulations is an important – indeed pressing – challenge for the field.

The promise and the peril of the actuarial approach

'The Guide is definite. Reality is frequently inaccurate.'

Douglas Adams

The unstructured clinical approaches of former years have attracted great opprobrium because of their lack of an evidence base, their idiosyncratic nature, and their lack of transparency, replicability and utility (Quinsey, Harris, Rice and Cormier, 1998). As a reaction, attempts were made to impose structure on the decision-making of clinicians through the use of so-called actuarial risk assessment instruments (ARAI) (e.g., Hanson and Thornton, 1999; Quinsey, et al., 1998). These procedures have proved popular amongst practitioners and administators alike. The adoption of ARAI techniques has become widespread: 'In North America and the United Kingdom, actuarial risk assessment has permeated the entire criminal justice system' (Craig and Beech, 2009; p. 197). Khiroya, Weaver and Maden (2009) demonstrated that the Risk Matrix 2000 (RM2000) and *Static-99* were the most commonly used sex-offender assessments in English medium secure forensic units.

While some commentators have contended that the superiority of actuarial scales is a given (Craig and Beech, 2009), other commentators have been less sanguine (Hart, et al., 2003). Empirical evidence suggests that actuarial approaches perform as well as structured professional judgement approaches (SPJ) in terms of predictive validity (e.g., Hanson and Morton-Bouron, 2009; Singh, Grann and Fazel, 2011; Yang, Wong and Coid, 2010a). However, as we demonstrate below, where the actuarial approaches merely claim to estimate the likelihood of an offence, the SPJ approach provides so much more in terms of formulation.

Importantly, SPJ approaches can lead to interventions that are both effective and proportionate.

It is perhaps telling that the proponents of actuarial approaches have derided clinicians' understanding of research methods and statistics (Harris, 2003). But, as we will see, the statistical underpinning of the actuarial approach is, in reality, very shaky. Despite this, proponents have argued for the wholesale adoption of actuarial methods:

> What we are advising is not the addition of actuarial methods to existing practice, but rather the complete replacement of existing practice with actuarial methods . . . actuarial methods are too good and clinical judgment too poor to risk contaminating the former with the latter.
>
> (Quinsey, et al., 1998, p. 171)

In our view, this is a dangerous and scientifically untenable position (Allport, 1940; Harcourt, 2006). We will now explain why this is so.

The basis of the actuarial approach to violence risk assessment

The actuarial paradigm appears simple. A group of offenders, usually prisoners, is assessed – generally characteristics that are easy to measure (and not necessarily clearly criminogenic) are recorded, for example, age, marital status, history of offending, type of victims, and so on. Sometimes the cohort of prisoners is followed up and new criminal convictions are identified from criminal records. More generally, the cohort is followed back, that is, the files of prisoners who have been released and whose convictions status has been monitored, are reviewed. Statistical methods may be used to estimate the characteristics associated with the observed likelihood of reconviction for the group of offenders. Typically, the development sample (the group on which the statistical model was developed) will be divided into risk groups – high, medium or low – then the proportion of each group who reoffended is provided. This information about a group is then used to make a prediction about a new individual, the person who is the focus of the risk assessment decision. Generally, the decision-maker is provided with information about this new individual's likelihood of reoffending using a process of analogy; that is, 'This man resembles offenders who are likely to recidivate, therefore, he *is* likely to recidivate' (Hart, 2003, p. 385). Craig and Beech (2009) recommended the following method of communication:

> Actuarial risk assessment of Mr X using Risk Matrix/Sexual indicates that his score falls within the 'medium' risk category, such a score is associated with a 13% likelihood over five years, 16% over 10 years, and 19% over 15 years, of being reconvicted for a sexual offence (for known and convicted sexual offenders) in a group of sexual offenders with the same score.
>
> (Craig and Beech, 2009, p. 205)

This is a form of inductive logic where it is argued that because Mr X belongs to a group, then the best point estimate of his risk of reoffending is the average for the group. While this may be technically correct, it is fundamentally misleading because of the huge degree of uncertainty associated with this estimate. And of course, argument by analogue falls down further when the offender being assessed is different from the standardization sample; for example, when first offenders are compared with prisoners, or when internet offenders are compared with contact offenders.

While we understand this desire for certainty, we agree with Gigerenzer that certainty in prognostications is an illusion (Gigerenzer, 2002). Unfortunately, this illusion of certainty is bolstered because the actuarial methods wear the clothes of science – samples are collected, data are analysed, arcane statistics are generated, but the product is inherently misleading. Let us consider that contention in more detail.

A signal case

'There is no such uncertainty as a sure thing.'

Robert Burns

Our interest in the uncertainty associated with actuarial tests was triggered when the first author was contacted by a Scottish sheriff (a judge) who was concerned about conflicting expert opinions about an offender. One opinion was based on a frequently used actuarial tool – the RM2000 (Thornton, 2003) – and it was deemed that the offender was at 'high' risk of reoffending. The second opinion, based on a structured clinical judgement approach – the *Sexual Violence Risk-20* (SVR-20, Boer, Wilson, Gauthier and Hart, 1997) – concluded the offender was 'low' risk. The sheriff was concerned; he had to pass a sentence. The first author's initial reaction was one of disquiet when he realized that the actuarial judgment of 'high' risk was founded on only three pieces of information: the offender was 18 years of age, he had not lived in an intimate relationship with someone for two years or more, and he had not met his victim face-to-face before (he and the victim had been in regular contact by phone for five weeks prior to the offence). The offender was convicted of a statutory offence of having sexual intercourse with a minor (see Cooke, 2010a for a fuller account). This case triggered a process of analysis that led to the publication of Hart, Michie and Cooke (2007), a paper which some have regarded as 'controversial' (e.g., Craig and Beech, 2009, p. 203). Below we consider and clarify some of the issues raised in response to previous papers on this issue (Cooke and Michie, 2010; Hart, Michie and Cooke, 2007). We believe that the quantification of uncertainty is key, and that uncertainty is ignored at our peril.

Quantifying uncertainty

'Statistics means never having to say you're certain.'

Anon

Authors and advocates of ARAIs explicitly state that their purpose is prediction; that is, the statement that a specified event will occur in the future. For example, 'RM2000/S is a prediction tool for sexual violence' (RM2000 Scoring Guide February 2007, p. 3), and 'Static-2002 predicts sexual, violent and any recidivism as well as other actuarial risk tools . . .' (Static-2002, Unpublished Manual, p. 1). How certain or uncertain are these predictions? Statistical methods allow the quantification of uncertainty; indeed, a core function of statistical methods is the estimation and quantification of uncertainty. By definition, all estimates are subject to error: the precision of a parameter estimate (e.g., mean rate of sexual recidivism of a group) is specified by a confidence interval (CI), that is, the range of values within which an unknown population parameter is likely to fall. The interval's width provides a measure of the precision – or certainty – associated with the estimate of the population parameter and is determined, in part, by the sample size used to estimate the population parameter.

When we are considering predictions for an individual, there are two stages where uncertainty can be manifest. In the first stage, the parameters (mean, slope and variance) of the regression model specifying the association between the independent variable (e.g., RM2000 scores) and the dependent variable (e.g., likelihood of reconviction) are estimated. Each of these parameters has uncertainty associated with it; this uncertainty can be expressed by a CI around the regression line with data from the group upon which the ARAI was developed being used to assess the degree of uncertainty. In the second stage – the critical stage in this context – a new case for which a decision is to be made is identified, a score is calculated and the likelihood that he will be reconvicted is estimated. This estimate of the likelihood of reconviction for the individual also has a CI – known more specifically as a prediction interval (PI) – that expresses the precision, or uncertainty, that should be associated with the estimated likelihood or reconviction for the new case. The CI for the group and the prediction interval for the individual are very different, both conceptually and in terms of magnitude; the latter is always much wider than the former. This is not new, it is standard and established statistical theory (e.g., Anderson and Bancroft, 1952; Cohen and Cohen, 1983; Vardeman, 1992).

Concern over the case referred to above led us to consider how to quantify the degree of uncertainty associated with the claim that the offender was 'high' risk, that is, he had a 36 per cent chance of recidivating in a sexual manner during the next 15 years. Despite our best efforts, we could not access the raw data on the RM2000. Access to raw data is normally a requirement for the computation of CIs. It is concerning that access to raw data for legitimate reanalysis appears to be a problem in this field (e.g., Waggoner, Wollert and Cramer, 2008).

Fortunately, CIs can be estimated from categorical data by applying a procedure first developed by Wilson (1927). This method is preferred over other possible methods because it is not strongly influenced by extreme values of sample size or the proportion of recidivists, and it does not yield impossible values, such as negative values (Agresti and Coull, 1998). In Hart, et al. (2007), we used Wilson's method to calculate the 95 per cent CI associated with the proportion of recidivists in each of the risk categories for two ARAIs – the *Violence Risk Appraisal Guide* (VRAG, Quinsey, et al., 1998) and the *Static-99* (Hanson and Thornton, 1999). We noted that neither the VRAG nor the *Static-99* were developed using methods (e.g., logistic regression or event history analysis) that allow the derivation of individual regression or survival scores and their respective CIs. We adopted an ad hoc procedure in order to estimate the prediction interval. We checked the ad hoc approach against logistic regression and event history analysis using our own data sets, on which it is possible to generate predictive equations. Wilson's method, adapted in this ad hoc fashion, yielded very similar estimates to the standard measures. The method appeared robust and, in the absence of raw data, it was the only approach possible. The analysis provoked a reaction.

In a letter (non-peer reviewed) published in the *British Journal of Psychiatry*, Mossman and Selke (2007) criticized our approach. The focus of their criticism did not appear to be our application to the group case but our ad hoc adaptation. In our response to their letter, we pled guilty to some of the charges but claimed duress: the developers of the ARAI did not base their tools on statistical methods that allow the reliable estimates of CIs associated with estimates or likelihood or survival time for individuals. Mossman and Selke (2007) are fundamentally incorrect when they assert that 'The 95% CIs for "individual risk" pile nonsense on top of meaninglessness' (p. 561). We respectfully refer them to statistical literature (e.g., Anderson and Bancroft, 1952; Steel, Torrie and Dickie, 1997; Vardeman, 1992). As we demonstrate below, CIs associated with an estimate, whether it is a number such as the number of papers published since graduating with a PhD, or a probability such as the likelihood of having a heart attack in a given time, can be calculated for an individual (Cohen and Cohen, 1983; Steel, Torrie, and Dickey, 1997). This is well recognized in other disciplines (e.g., Henderson and Keiding, 2005; Rose, 1992). Forensic practitioners neglect this fact at their peril.

On reflection, perhaps for many our ad hoc method was a conceptual leap too far. We have carried out further analysis to illustrate our approach (Table 1.1) and to illustrate that reasonable estimates of uncertainty can be achieved when access to the raw data on which the ARAI is based is not achievable – for whatever reason. In Table 1.1, we present an analysis of data from the Scoring Guide for RM2000.8/ SVC, RM2000/S, 1979 discharge sample using the RM2000, an ARAI used primarily for the prediction of sexual recidivism. We have estimated the 95 per cent CIs associated with the observed proportions of recidivists in each of the four groups using Wilson's method. Initially, we carry out the estimation for the actual n in the categories. For purposes of illustration, we then estimate the 95 per cent CI for increasing small sample sizes (n = 50, 10, 5). In essence, we are considering the following question: if you have a group of 10 offenders, what would be the 95 per cent CI associated with the estimated proportion of recidivists? Not surprisingly – indeed it is a matter of first principles – as sample size goes down, the 95 per cent CI widens. While our use of n = 1 in Hart, et al. (2007) may be seen

Table 1.1 Confidence intervals for θ from Risk Matrix 2000/S for different sample sizes, five-year follow-up period

Category	L	M	H	VH
No. in category (n)	86	167	120	56
Proportion reoffending	.03	.13	.26	.50
95% CI	.00 – .09	.09 – .16	.19 – .34	.37 – .63
Sample size 50	.00 – .12	.06 – .25	.16 – .40	.37 – .63
Sample size 10	.00 – 32	.03 – .44	0.9 – .57	.24 – .76
Sample size 5	.00 – .47	.02 – .56	0.6 – 0.67	.17 – .83
Sample size 1	.00 – .81	.00 – 0.84	.02 – .88	.06 – .94

as a leap too far, clearly it takes a greater leap of faith to assume that if precision decreases with decreasing sample size then somehow, when we come to the individual case, we can prognosticate with confidence. As we noted in our reply to Mossman and Selke (2007), our original conclusion stands. The margins of errors for estimates of likelihood for individual cases are either large or unknown. But as we indicate below, they are calculable given access to raw data and the application of appropriate statistical methods. As we will illustrate, Wilson's method – and our ad hoc extension – is in fact robust when compared with other more modern and mathematically secure methods.

Perhaps we may be accused of labouring the point but critics appear not to appreciate the basic statistical principles underpinning the argument (e.g., Hanson and Howard, 2010). We will try to clarify the argument here using the raw data available on the *Static-99* (http://www.static99.org/pdfdocs/detailedstatic-2002rrecidivismtables.pdf). (We used the data from their largest sample, the one that they describe as the 'non-routine sample' for the purposes of illustration. The conclusions reached from analysis of the other samples are the same).

We have argued elsewhere (Cooke and Michie, 2010; Cooke, Michie and Hart, 2010), the hopefully non-contentious point that logistic regression is the appropriate method for modelling the prediction of a binary outcome (e.g. reconviction). Importantly, there are established formal methods for estimating both CIs and PIs when logistic regression is applied (Steel, et al., 1997): these are defined formally, and in detail, in Cooke and Michie (2010).

We estimated the values of the 95 per cent CI and 95 per cent PI associated with the observed group recidivism rates using *Static*-2002 total scores by applying both Wilson's method and logistic regression (see Table 1.2). Examination of Table 1.2 indicates that the values of the 95 per cent CIs calculated are of a similar order of magnitude using the two methods. However, perhaps of greater significance, the 95 per cent PIs calculated using the two methods are very large; our previous estimates using Wilson's method were clearly conservative and the logistic method indicates that the situation is actually worse than we characterized it as being. It is important to remember that all these estimates are optimized, being derived from the development sample; applying them to a new sample will result in the intervals (CIs and PIs) being even wider.

Table 1.2 Confidence intervals for θ from *Static-2002* non-routine sample, five-year follow-up period

Category	n	Mean score	Proportion reoffending	Wilson method		Logistic method	
				CI	PI	CI at mean	PI at mean
1	188	1.2	0.07	0.04–0.12	0.00–0.82	0.06–0.10	0.00–0.95
2	272	3.6	0.14	0.10–0.18	0.00–0.84	0.11–0.15	0.00–0.97
3	305	5.5	0.18	0.14–0.23	0.01–0.86	0.17–0.22	0.01–0.98
4	226	7.5	0.30	0.24–0.36	0.02–0.90	0.24–0.32	0.00–0.99
5	130	9.7	0.38	0.31–0.47	0.03–0.92	0.32–0.45	0.02–0.99

The Wilson method is based on the data for the category and thus is an average for the category. The logistic method calculates the CI and PI at a specific point (the mean score for the category) while estimating variability from the whole sample.

What does this mean in the individual case, the individual being the focus of decision-making in the trials and other tribunals? When it comes to the consideration of an individual case, as we noted above, the PI – rather than CI – is the only relevant measure of uncertainty. For example, an individual with a *Static*-2002 score of 5.2 (i.e., the mean score) will have an estimated likelihood of reoffending of 18 per cent over the next five years. This may seem concerning but this estimate is very imprecise because the 95 per cent PI is 0–98 per cent; that is, the true value of the likelihood would lie somewhere in this range 95 per cent of the time. For an individual with a score in the 'high' risk group, such as a total *Static*-2002 score of 9, the mean likelihood is estimated as 36 per cent over the next five years but the degree of uncertainty is enormous, with the 95 per cent PI indicating that the likelihood actually lies between 0 per cent and 99 per cent. Therefore, the application of ARAIs to predict risk in the individual case is fundamentally misleading.

The illusion of certainty

'The law of probability, so true in general, so fallacious in particular.'
Edward Gibbons

Numerical statements – for example, there is an 18 per cent likelihood that this individual will reoffend sexually in the next five years – are powerful. It is difficult for the decision-maker to disregard the number and alter their evaluation even if presented with detailed, credible and contradictory information. Judges and other decision-makers are not immune from this – the anchoring bias – a well-established cognitive bias that influences all human judgement (Englich and Mussweiler, 2001). This problem is compounded by the tendency to predict rather than forecast, that is, to provide a single value of the likelihood that someone will offend without any indication of the confidence that should be placed on that single value; an indication such as the range of possible values which that likelihood may take. Is the range narrow or wide? It is possible to illustrate the degree of uncertainty associated with an estimated likelihood of reoffending by plotting the probability density function (PDF). PDFs display the shape of the uncertainty. Elsewhere (Cooke, et al., 2010), we demonstrate that PDFs associated with the risk groups in the Static-2002 are so flat, so wide, and so overlapping that knowledge of group membership tells the assessor nothing about an individual's likelihood of recidivism. The PDFs demonstrate that you cannot say, with any reliability, what risk group an individual belongs to.

The problem of making predictions for *individuals* using statistical models is well recognized in other disciplines; it is not merely a function of the inherent complexity and the inherent unreliability of assessing the psychological characteristics of individuals. Almost three decades ago, Rose (1992), discussing preventative medicine, indicated: 'Unfortunately the ability to estimate the average risk for a group, which may be good, is not matched by any corresponding ability to predict which individuals are going to fall ill soon' (p. 48). Individual cases demonstrate the point vividly. Stephen Hawking wryly observed, 'Thirty years ago, I was diagnosed with motor neurone disease, and given two and a half years to live. I have always wondered how they could be so precise about the half.'

That the significance of uncertainty in violence risk assessment based on ARAIs is not widely understood is of great concern – professional and ethical concern. The illusion of certainty created by the provision of a single figure is likely to have a profound effect on legal decision-making. If a decision-maker is persuaded by such figures, it may lead to a lenient sentence when more control is required, or equally, to a disproportionate sentence when such is not required. The problem, of course, is not merely a problem of statistics, it is also a problem of (il)logic.

Life insurance as a false analogue for violence risk assessment

> 'The most misleading assumptions are the ones you don't even know you are making.'
>
> Douglas Adams

A common defence of ARAI is that they are modelled on the practices of life insurance companies; I (DJC) have been told this by judges as well as the proponents of the methods. The analogue is false. The life insurance actuary achieves a profit by predicting the *proportion* of insured lives that will end within a particular time period: the actuary has no interest in predicting the deaths of *particular* individuals and recognizes the impossibility of doing so. By way of contrast, the decision-maker in court is not concerned with the properties of any statistical group, similar, at least in some regard, to the accused; they are only interested in the accused in front of them. As Faigman (2007) notes, giving evidence about an individual based on nomothetic information is one of the greatest challenges to the psychologist giving evidence in court. This distinction between knowledge about groups and individuals has been long recognized:

> While the individual man is an insoluble puzzle, in the aggregate he becomes a mathematical certainty. You can, for example, never foretell what any one man will do, but you can say with precision what an average number will be up to. Individuals vary, but percentages remain constant.
>
> (Conan Doyle, 1890, p. 107)

Sherlock Holmes clearly understood the logical fallacy of division (Rorer, 1990)! The fallacy of division is essentially the drawing of a conclusion about an *individual* member of a group based on the *collective* properties of that group. For example, it is self-evidently fallacious to argue that if, in general, taller people are heavier than shorter people then Bob who is 5ft 3ins will be lighter than Joe who is 6ft. Equally, it is fallacious to argue that although people who score highly on an actuarial risk scale generally reoffend more than people who do not score highly, Hamish in the 'high risk' group will reoffend more often – or more quickly – than Fergus in the 'low risk' group. Rockhill (2005) made the point clearly from the perspective of an epidemiologist:

> This is not just a matter of not including the right 'effect modifiers' in the analysis. Rather, it is a philosophical matter about averages and the inability to draw conclusive statements about individuals based on summary information about classes or groups of individuals.
>
> (Rockhill, 2005, p. 125).

Screening instruments for violence risk assessment

Some recognize the limitations of actuarial instruments and this has led to attempts to salvage something from the wreckage. There appears to be an appetite amongst some researchers, practitioners and, alarmingly, writers of professional practice standards, to use ARAIs to screen offenders for such a purpose (e.g. http://www.rmascotland.gov.uk/ViewFile.aspx?id=363s). This might sound a sensible and reasoned method for allocating resources but, putting it at its most blunt, why would we use a test that is demonstrably not fit for the purpose of prediction for the purpose of screening? In our view, dangerous policies are being promulgated; we remain surprised that they are not subject to more challenge in the courts.

There are two problems with applying ARAIs as screening procedures in the field of violence risk assessment. First, in practice, screening rarely occurs; the practitioners tasked with the assessment generally have neither the training nor the time to move from the so-called screening test to a more comprehensive evaluation. In practice, the decision-maker is merely provided with the results of the actuarial scale. Within our own jurisdiction – Scotland – the Court of Appeal has supported the use of these tests, not merely as screens but as the full assessment. For example, in the appeal Case of HMA–v–Thomas Russell Currie (Appeal No: HCJAC 67 XC227/08), a ground of appeal was that 'The learned trial judge erred in failing to obtain a full risk assessment' (p. 2). Their Lordships' decision was that

> The Risk Matrix 2000 Assessment Tool is regularly and widely used for the purposes of assessing the risk presented by an offender to the public . . . In our view [the trial judge] was entitled to proceed upon the basis of the outcome of the risk assessment carried out using Risk Matrix 2000.
>
> (HMA–v–Thomas Russell Currie, p. 5)

The second problem, in our view, is that it has not been demonstrated that these instruments are effective screens (Cooke, Michie and Hart, 2010).

For a screen to be effective, the risk factors considered must be *very* strongly associated with the disorder being screened for (Wald, Hackshaw and Frost, 1999; see Cooke and Michie, 2010 and Cooke, et al., 2010 for a fuller discussion). In the medical arena, for example, Wald, et al. (1999) indicated that although serum cholesterol is a known and established risk factor for ischaemic heart disease, the belief that it is a useful screen is unwarranted.

Consider Figure 1.1, from Cooke, et al. (2010); the upper panel displays the distributions of serum cholesterol for those who died from ischaemic heart disease and for those unaffected by heart disease over a ten-year period. The distributions overlap to a considerable degree, demonstrating that serum cholesterol level does not provide a useful screen. This contrasts markedly with the distinct distributions displayed in the lower panel, e.g. maternal serum α fetoprotein; this risk factor is an effective screen for open spina bifida.

How does the performance of ARAIs compare to the examples from medicine? The data for recidivists and non-recidivists are displayed in Figure 1.2. It is immediately apparent that this figure is more reminiscent of the serum cholesterol figure than the maternal serum α fetoprotein figure. Visual inspection demonstrates that Static-2002 scores are ineffective screens. The statistics confirm this. The relative odds of reoffending for the top 20 per cent compared with the bottom 20 per cent is 6.8; the detection rate is 14 per cent for a false positive rate (FPR) of 5 per cent. An FPR of 5 per cent is a convention in medicine, the idea being to limit the alarm experienced by those misidentified. Within criminal justice settings, considerations of policy – for example, protection of the public versus concern for the human rights of an offender – might, in the minds of some, justify higher false positive rates. We plotted DR against FPR – this produces a Receiver Operator Characteristic (ROC) curve, a commonly used process to assess 'accuracy' in violence risk assessment. The Area Under the Curve (AUC) achieved was 0.68; this is comparable with many actuarial scales used in violence risk, the effect size being of 'low accuracy' (Akobeng, 2007).

Therefore, in our view, the notion that ARAIs can be used as screening tools is fundamentally flawed. As Scott (1977) observed, it is not possible to ' . . . draw clear lines between the dangerous and non-dangerous . . .' (p. 140). Attempts to use ARAIs for such a purpose are more likely than not to mislead; the public is poorly served by suboptimal decisions.

There is clearly a need for the development of simple methods to identify those individuals who need to be subject to greatest assessment, methods to triage offenders into the clearly risky, the clearly non-risky, and those about whom

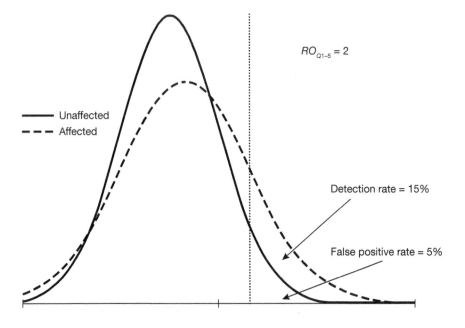

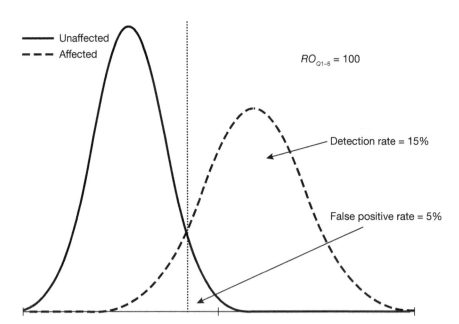

Figure 1.1 Upper panel – serum cholesterol in men who died of ischaemic heart disease and those unaffected; lower panel – serum α fetoprotein and those affected and unaffected by open spina bifida (approximation for illustration after Wald, et al. 1999)

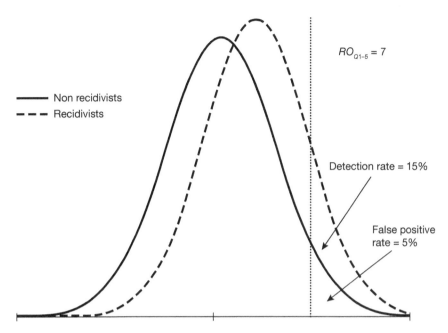

Figure 1.2 Distribution of *Static-2002* scores for recidivists and non-recidivists

uncertainty reigns. However, the development of a screening tool is not straightforward. In order to properly evaluate a screening test, ideally it should be subject to a randomized control trial in order to rule out the many biases that can influence the apparent effectiveness of the screen (Cooke, Michie and Hart, 2010).

The ritual of the ROC

Psychological research is prone to statistical rituals. In *Mindless Statistics*, Gigerenzer (2004) describes what he termed the null ritual; the inappropriate use of null hypothesis testing, a ritual that, because of the sanctions of researchers, editors, teachers and the writers of textbooks, always has to be performed. According to Gigerenzer, the statistical ritual largely eliminates statistical thinking in the social sciences but they assist identification with, and cohesion within, the social group, in this case, other believers in actuarial risk tools – 'Suppression of conflicts and contradicting information is in the very nature of this social ritual' (Gigerenzer, 2004, p. 592). Gigerenzer argues that rituals require cognitive illusions: 'Their function is to make the final product, a significant result, appear highly informative, and thereby justify the rituals' (p. 594).

We see clear parallels in the use of the AUC under the ROC as a simplified summary of a complex situation – it obscures rather than enlightens. We consider that there is evidence of wishful thinking in terms of predictive power. As a summary statistic, the AUC can only describe one facet of the performance of the

ROC, and of course, only performance within the derivation sample, a performance that is optimized (Cook, 2007). While mathematically it is the case, as Rice and Harris (1995) indicated, that the AUC is independent of base rate, this is rarely true in the real world. Brenner and Gefeller (1997) demonstrated that substantial variations in sensitivity and specificity (and thereby AUCs) occur across different populations. This can be explained by the fact that most tests are not inherently diagnostic and the categorization of individuals is influenced both by the distribution of the underlying trait relative to the diagnostic cutoff as well of the level of measurement error that is present.

When it comes to interpreting the magnitude of the AUC as an effect size, different interpretations abound. Akobeng (2007), cited, for example, by Hanson and Howard (2010), described values between 0.5 and 0.7 as 'low accuracy', while those between 0.7 – 0.9 have 'moderate accuracy' and those above 0.9 have 'high' accuracy. In their substantial meta-analytic comparison of nine distinct risk assessment procedures, Yang, Wong and Coid (2010) reported:

> It can be seen that after taking into account the data structure, the country of study, participant's sex, mean age of participants, follow-up time to the outcome, and type of study, the predictive efficacy of the risk instruments all fall between a range of 0.56 and 0.71 in terms of AUC value, with the majority falling within a narrow range 0.65–0.69.
>
> (Yang, Wong and Coid, 2010, p. 753)

In other words, they were of 'low accuracy'. Looking specifically at sex-offender instruments, Hanson, Helmus and Thornton (2010) reported data on the *Static-99* and the *Static-2002*; the majority of the AUC values cited were below 0.7, that is, 'low accuracy'. Barnett, Wakeling and Howard (2010), describing results from a study considering the predictive validity of the RM 2000 in a very large sample, reported an AUC of 0.68 (prediction of sexual violence), which they characterized as being 'moderately accurate', and an AUC of 0.73 (prediction of sexual and/or non-sexual violence), which they characterized as being a 'large' effect. We consider such claims could mislead.

In their magisterial paper, Gigerenzer, Gaissmaier, Kurz-Milcke, Schwartz and Woloshin (2008) identified what they referred to as 'statistical illiteracy' amongst a large number of citizens, including doctors, patients, journalists and politicians – psychologists and other risk assessors are not immune. At its core, statistical illiteracy refers to the inability to understand the meaning of numbers and, critically, the inferences to be drawn from these numbers. Gigerenzer and colleagues demonstrate that in the context of health statistics, the problem is common and it may be exacerbated by non-transparent methods for presenting information – alarmingly, it can also be the consequence of deliberate efforts to obfuscate matters in order to manipulate or persuade decision-makers. Conflicts of interest can result in information being presented in non-transparent ways: such interests could range from the financial (Poythress and Petrila, 2010) through to the championing of a particular ideology by organizations endeavouring to be cost efficient.

As a cure for statistical illiteracy, Gigerenzer, et al. (2008) recommend that data should be presented using transparent indices; they note that:

> Transparent forms include absolute risks, natural frequencies, mortality rates, and, in general, statements about frequencies or depictions of frequencies in pictures. Non-transparent forms include relative risks, conditional probabilities such as sensitivities and specificities, survival rates, and statements about single events that do not specify a reference class.
>
> (Gigerenzer, et al., 2008, p. 77)

We could add to the list of non-transparent forms the oft-preferred measure in the violence-prediction literature, the AUC from ROC analysis. Indeed, the AUC might be considered to be particularly opaque as it is derived from a plot of two non-transparent measures, i.e., sensitivity against 1-specificity.

Relative risks and odds ratios can obscure the true position. For example, a 50 per cent relative risk reduction in offending might be from 20 to 10 offenders in 100 – a sizable effect – or a much less impressive reduction from 2 to 1 offenders in 100. Gigerenzer (2002) argued that representing risk in terms of natural frequencies can reduce innumeracy. Let us apply his cure to our example above.

Let us examine the question, *how well can the Static-2002 identify those who are likely to offend?* The AUC for this sample is 0.68. This would be described by Akobeng (2007) as low accuracy, by others as moderately accurate (Barnett, et al., 2010). To answer the above question, we use natural frequency diagrams displaying data from the *Static-2002* (http://www.static99.org/pdfdocs/detailedstatic-2002 rrecidivismtables.pdf), a sample that contains 1,121 cases. Following Gigerenzer (2002, p. 81 et seq.), in order to present the data transparently, they are first standardized to 1,000 offenders (see Figure 1.3). It will be observed that of 1,000 offenders, 682 are in the 'low risk' group (Categories 1/2/3) while 318 are in the 'high risk' group (Category 4/5).[1] In the 'low risk' group, there are 93 who have offended in the follow-up period. In the 'high risk' group, there are 105 who have offended in the follow-up period. By implementing the *Static-2002*, it might be

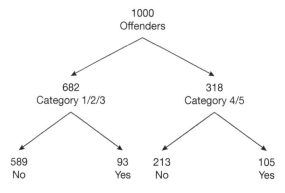

Figure 1.3 Decision tree of *Static-2002* data presented as natural frequencies

concluded that a relative risk reduction of 53 per cent can be achieved (i.e. 105/105+93). This may sound impressive. However, the efficacies of interventions tend to be overestimated when relative risk reduction, rather than absolute risk reduction, is reported (Gigerenzer, et al., 2008). Absolute risk is a more transparent measure when single-event probabilities (i.e., what is the likelihood that this individual will reoffend) are being considered (Gigerenzer, et al., 2008). In the case of the *Static-2002*, the absolute risk reduction is 10.5 per cent (i.e., 105/1000). Another way of looking at this problem is to conclude that out of 100 offenders deemed to be 'high risk', 33 will go on to offend (i.e., 105*100/318), while of those deemed to be 'low risk', 14 will go on to reoffend. Is this good? That question is not amenable to statistical argument; it is a matter of public policy balancing the rights of victims and the rights of offenders, balancing the costs and benefits of effective and ineffective practice.

In sum, we consider that the adoption of the actuarial paradigm in research and practice is a paradigm error; the approach cannot answer the question being posed; that is, How risky is the individual in front of us? Wittgenstein famously remarked that in psychology 'the existence of the experimental method makes us think we have the means of solving the problems which trouble us; though problem and method pass one another by' (Wittgenstein, 1958, p. 232). Other approaches may be required.

From What? To Why?

'The quest for certainty blocks the search for meaning.'

Erich Fromm

If we cannot predict violent outcomes with any certainty, does this mean we should abandon the enterprise of risk assessment? In short, no. Our critique of the precision of ARAIs has lead to the charge that we are promoting the abandonment of evidence-based risk assessment (Harris, Rice, and Quinsey, 2008). This is just plain wrong. The authors confuse 'evidence-based' with 'statistically based'; they confuse problems of structure with problems of process. If we take an analogue beloved of proponents of the actuarial approach (e.g. Hanson and Howard, 2010) – the tossing of coins – this distinction may become clearer. If we want to answer the question 'Did more coins than expected fall as tails?', this can be answered through the application of the binomial distribution. If, however, we want to answer the question 'Why did a particular toss result in a tails?', we would have to consider mechanics. This question cannot be answered by reference to a statistical model. Similarly, with risk assessment, we need to consider psychological theory.

To move from assessment to intervention – and onto effective change – it is necessary to understand process; it is necessary to move from answering the 'What?' question to answering the 'Why?' questions. Why, for example, might a high score on the PCL-R, or a substance misuse problem, or an inability to sustain intimate relationships, lead to an increased risk of violence? Information from an actuarial test, for example, knowing that someone is 18 years old, or has previous convictions, does not lead – in any obvious fashion – to an understanding, or on to effective interventions. Individuals are inherently complex.

Take something as apparently simple as the robust and moderate association between substance misuse and violence (Webster, et al., 1997). Not one but a range of distinct processes may underpin this apparently simple association; there are many answers to the 'Why?' question. Substance misuse may be relevant to future risk because the chemical effect disinhibits aggressive impulses, because it impairs evaluation of relevant social cues (e.g., danger or frustration), it may facilitate the justification of aggressive behaviour ('I need some heroin so I will rob to get money'), it may increase interpersonal conflict and the loss of important supports, it may impair consideration of long-term consequences, the need for illicit drugs may expose the user to violent environments and peers, substance abuse may interact with psychotic symptoms to potentiate violence. For any one individual, substance abuse may be relevant through any one or, indeed, for several reasons. Additionally, there may be synergism with other risk factors, for example, psychotic symptoms or the presence of antisocial peers. This is true for substance abuse, but it is also true of the other risk factors commonly considered by SPJ approaches (e.g., psychopathy, Cooke 2010b). The only way to deal with this complexity is to think psychologically and not statistically, and to think about the process, not the structure.

Thinking about risk processes

One approach might be to consider the underlying risk processes (Cooke and Wozniak, 2010). Risk processes can be regarded as the theoretical constructs that operate in the individual case; they can be thought of as embodying the broad 'Why?' questions. They are the processes by which risk factors result in violence. Three categories are discernable: *drivers* (e.g., a persistent belief in the malevolent intent of others), *disinhibitors* (e.g., the chemical effect of alcohol) and *destabilizers* (e.g., the loss of a key support in a social network). Risk factors, or more probably, elements of risk factors, may be construed as markers of these underlying risk processes. The intellectual challenge is to deconstruct each risk factor to determine which elements are relevant to future violence; relevant in the sense that they may drive, destabilize or disinhibit an individual, increasing his likelihood of future violence. Understanding risk processes – individually and together – can increase the appreciation of, not only the likelihood of future violence, but its likely topography, and perhaps of greatest importance, how to manage the risk.

Figure 1.4 illustrates several HCR-20 risk factors that are considered as being important in a hypothetical case. Risk factors (or elements of risk factors) may be considered to be markers of underlying risk processes in the same way that observable variables are regarded as markers of latent variables in certain forms of factor analysis. To understand the risk processes, we have to engage in what might be described as 'conceptual factor analysis' guided by their understanding – based both on research and clinical knowledge – of the processes that underpin violence.

In this simplified example, we are positing only two underlying risk processes: 'acting without forethought' and 'attachment problems'. We identified that

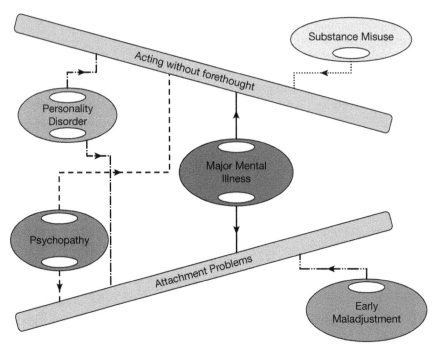

Figure 1.4 Risk processes underpinning risk factors

substance misuse, personality disorder, psychopathy, major mental illness and early maladjustment are present; these risk factors are inherently multi-dimensional. If we consider a putative risk process, 'acting without forethought', on a rational basis it can be seen that dimensions of each of four risk factors – but not all aspects of the risk factors – may contribute to 'acting without forethought'. The chemical disinhibiting effect of some forms of substance misuse (e.g. alcohol) may contribute, the impulsivity inherent in some forms of personality disorder, major mental illness and in psychopathy could also contribute. But other aspects of the latter three risk factors may contribute to another risk process, for example 'attachment problems'. The identification of these risk processes allows those engaging in risk management to manage the complex of risk factors – and their mutual interplays – in such a way that the key risk processes can be identified. It is only when risk processes are identified that they can be managed.

Towards a fourth era of risk assessment: the era of risk formulation

We argued at the outset that there have been three eras of risk assessment – unstructured clinical judgement, actuarial risk assessment and risk manage-ment – but we believe that a fourth era is now discernable: the era of risk formulation. Risk management approaches have evolved out of all recognition.

At their inception, early forms of SPJ gave little, if any, guidance about how to move from the assessment of risk factors to an understanding of the risk posed by an individual; indeed, simplistic summary risk ratings – low, moderate or high – were the primary output of the process (Kropp, Hart, Webster and Eaves, 1994). Rather more guidance was provided in the HCR-20 manual (Webster, Douglas, Eaves and Hart, 1997), but it was not until the publication of the *Risk for Sexual Violence Protocol* (RSVP, Hart, et al., 2003) that a structured process – scenario planning – was adopted to assist the assessor to build a formulation of the nature of the risk posed by an individual.

Building on the venerable tradition of clinical formulation, the last two years have seen signal developments in that risk formulation. Different, yet complementary, methods are evolving and being tested (e.g., Hart, et al., 2003; Hart and Logan, 2011; Logan and Johnstone, 2010). Hart and Logan (2011) explore the various contributions made by four different models and approaches within the forensic arena, from the offence paralleling work of Clark and colleagues (Clark, Fisher and McDougal, 1993) (see Daffern, Jones and Shine, 2010), through the Good Lives Model (Ward, 2003) and the Risk-Needs-Responsivity model (Andrews, Bonta and Hoge, 1990), to the SPJ approach (Hart, et al., 2003). A major challenge is the development of clear – and readily applicable – criteria for assessing the validity of particular formulations about individuals (Cooke, 2010b). In our view, much can be learned from approaches to systematic case studies, whether the target is an individual client or an institution (Cooke, 2010b; Cooke and Wozniak, 2010; Cooke and Johnstone, this volume). The validity of the formulation of a case study starts with the design stage (e.g., employ a theory-driven approach, document the approach adopted with a predetermined protocol) through the evidence-collection phase (e.g., seek multiple sources of evidence, establish the chain of evidence), to, finally, the formulation stage (e.g., pattern matching, explanation building, consideration of rival explanations, and the application of logic models). Validation criteria for risk formulations are the next challenge (Hart, Sturmey, Logan and McMurran, 2011).

Coda: on the misapplication of statistics in forensic practice

'There is a simple solution to every human problem, neat, plausible and wrong.'

Henry Menken

The central thesis of this chapter is that the application of statistically based ARAIs in decisions about individual offenders is fundamentally an error. Statistical evidence can seriously mislead decision-makers. The English case of Sally Clark is a vivid and heart-rending illustration of this point. Sally Clark was a solicitor, and two of her babies died. She was convicted of murder primarily on the basis of 'Meadow's Law'. 'It was stated by Sir Roy [Meadow] at Sally Clark's trial that there were "one in 73 million"; a figure which would suggest that such deaths were beyond coincidence' (Hill, 2004, p. 320) (see Hill, 2004 for a detailed analysis of the statistical arguments). Only after a second appeal was the clearly fallacious reasoning underpinning Meadow's Law accepted by the appeal court; Sally Clark was released but died not long after at the tragically young age of 42.

As a psychologist with a long-standing interest in statistics (DJC) and a professional statistician (CM), we have sympathy with the position statement issued by the Royal Statistical Society in response to the Sally Clark Case:

> Although many scientists have some familiarity with statistical methods, statistics remains a specialised area. The Society urges the Courts to ensure that statistical evidence is presented only by appropriately qualified statistical experts, as would be the case for any other form of expert evidence.
>
> (Royal Statistical Society, 2010)

Clearly, forensic practitioners should remain within their realm of expertise, but perhaps even more importantly we believe that it behoves public bodies that set standards of practice to ensure that they obtain appropriate statistical advice and do not depend upon scientists and practitioners – e.g., psychologists and psychiatrists – who are not qualified statistical experts. The case of Sally Clark is not unique; it should give all forensic practitioners pause for thought.

References

Adams, Douglas, *Hitchhiker's Guide to the Galaxy*, BBC radio.

Agresti, A. and Coull, B. A. (1998) 'Approximate is better than "exact" for interval estimation of binomial proportions', *American Statistician, 52*: 119–26.

Akobeng, A. K. (2007) 'Understanding diagnostic tests 3: Receiver operating characteristic curves', *Acta Paediatrica, 96*: 644–47.

Allport, G. (1940) 'The psychologist's frame of reference', *Psychological Bulletin, 37*: 1–28.

Anderson, R. L. and Bancroft, T. A. (1952) *Statistical theory in reseach*. New York: McGraw-Hill Book Company.

Andrews, D. A., Bonta, J. and Hoge, R. D. (1990) 'Classification for effective rehabilitation: Rediscovering psychology', *Criminal Justice and Behaviour, 17*: 19–52.

Barnett, G. D., Wakeling, H. C. and Howard, P. D. (2010) 'An examination of the predictive validity of the Risk Matrix 2000 in England and Wales', *Sexual Abuse: A Journal of Research and Treatment, 22*(4): 443–70.

Boer, D. P., Wilson, R. J., Gauthier, C. M. and Hart, S. D. (1997) 'Assessing risk of sexual violence: Guidelines for clinical practice', in C. D. Webster and M. A. Jackson (eds) *Impulsivity: Theory, assessment and treatment*, (pp. 326–42), New York: Guilford Press.

Brenner, H. and Gefeller, O. (1997) 'Variations of sensitivity, specificity, likelihood ratios and predicitve values with disease prevalence', *Stastistics in Medicine, 16*: 981–91.

Clark, D. A., Fisher, M. J. and McDougal, C. (1993). 'A new methodology for assessing the level of risk in incarcerated offenders', *British Journal of Criminology, 33*: 436–48.

Cohen, J. and Cohen, P. (1983) *Applied multiple regression/correlation analysis for the behavioural sciences* (2nd edition), London: Lawrence Erlbaum Associates.

Cook, N. (2007) 'Use and misuse of the Receiver Operating Characteristic curve in risk prediction', *Circulation, 115*: 928–35.

Cooke, D. J. (2010a) 'More prejudicial than probative', *The Journal of the Law Society of Scotland, 55*: 20–23.

— (2010b) 'Personality disorder and violence: Understand violence risk', *Journal of Personality Disorders, 24*: 539–50.

Cooke, D. J. and Michie, C. (2010) 'Limitations of diagnostic precision and predictive utility in the individual case: A challenge for forensic practice', *Law and Human Behavior, 34*: 259–74.

Cooke, D. J., Michie, C. and Hart, S. D. Screening for sex offender risk: A Dangerous clinical practice. Manuscript under preparation.

Cooke, D. J. and Wozniak, E. (2010) 'PRISM applied to a critical incident review: A case study of the Glendairy prison riot', *International Journal of Forensic Mental Health Services, 9*: 159–72.

Craig, L. and Beech, A. R. (2009) 'Best practice in conducting actuarial risk assessments with adult sexual offenders', *Journal of Sexual Aggression, 15*: 193–211.

Daffern, M., Jones, L. and Shine, J. (eds) (2010) *Offence Paralleling Behaviour: A case formulation approach to offender assessment and intervention*, Chichester: John Wiley and Sons.

Doyle, A. C. (1890) *The sign of the four* (1994 ed.), Oxford: World's Classics.

Englich, B. and Mussweiler, T. (2001) 'Sentencing Under Uncertainty: Anchoring effects in the courtroom', *Journal of Applied Social Psychology, 31*, 1535–51.

Faigman, D. L. (2007) 'The limits of science in the courtroom', in E. Borgida and S. T. Fiske (eds) *Beyond common sense: Psychological science in the courtroom*, Oxford: Blackwell.

Gigerenzer, G. (2004) *Reckoning with risk: Learning to live with uncertainty*, London: Penguin.

Gigerenzer, G., Gaissmaier, W., Kurz-Milcke, E., Schwartz, L. M. and Woloshin, S. (2008) 'Helping doctors and patients make sense of health statistics', *Psychological Science in the Public Interest, 8*: 53–96.

Hanson, R. K. and Howard, P. D. (2010) 'Individual confidence intervals do not inform decision makers about the accuracy of risk assessment evaluations', *Law and Human Behavior, 34*: 275–81.

Hanson, R. K. and Morton-Bouron, K. E. (2009) 'The accuracy of recidivism risk asessments for sexual offenders: A meta-analysis of 118 prediction studies', *Psychological Assessment, 21*: 1–21.

Hanson, R. K. and Thornton, D. M. (1999) *Static-99: Improving actuarial risk assessments for sex offenders*, Ottawa: Solicitor General Canada.

Hanson, R. K., Helmus, L. and Thomton, D. (2010) 'Predicting recidivism amongst sexual offenders: A multi-site study of Static-2002', *Law and Human Behavior, 34*, 198–211.

Harcourt, B. E. (2006) *Against prediction; Profiling, policing, and punishing in an actuarial age*, Chicago: The University of Chicago Press.

Harris, G. T. (2003) 'Men in his category have a 50% likelihood, but which half is he in? Comments on Berlin, Galbraith, Geary, and McClone'. *Sexual Abuse: A Journal of Research and Treatment, 15(4)*: 389–92.

Harris, G. T., Rice, M. E. and Quinsey, V. (2008) 'Shall evidence-based risk assessment be abandoned?' Letter, *British Journal of Psychiatry, 192*: 154.

Hart, S. D., Kropp, P. R., Laws, R., Klaver, J., Logan, C. and Watt, K. A. (2003) *The Risk of Sexual Violence Protocol (RSVP)*, Burnaby: Mental Health, Law, and Policy Institute, Simon Fraser University.

Hart, S. D. and Logan, C. (2011), 'Formulation of violence risk using evidence-based assessments: The structured professional judgment approach', in P. Sturmey and M. McMurran (eds) *Forensic Case Formulation*, Chichester: John Wiley and Sons.

Hart, S. D. (2003) 'Actuarial risk assessment: Commentary on Berlin et al.', *Sexual Abuse: A Journal of Research and Treatment, 15*: 383–88.

Hart, S. D., Michie, C. and Cooke, D. J. (2007) 'Precision of actuarial risk assessment instruments: Evaluating the "margins of error" of group versus individual predictions of violence', *British Journal of Psychiatry, Supplement, 49,* Vol 190: 60–65.

Hart, S. D., Surmey, P., Logan, C. and McMurran, M. M. (2011) 'Forensic case formulation', *International Journal of Forensic Mental Health, 10*: 118–26.

Hawking, S. BBC interview, 18 February 1996.

Henderson, R. and Keiding, N. (2005) 'Individual survival time prediction using statistical models', *Journal of Medical Ethics, 31*: 703–6.

Hill, R. (2004) 'Multiple sudden infant deaths: Coincidence or beyond coincidence', *Peadiatrics and Perinatal Epidemiology, 18*: 320–26.

Khiroya, R., Weaver, T. and Maden, A. (2009) 'Use and perceived utility of structured violence risk assessments in English medium secure forensic units', *The Psychiatrist, 33*: 129–32.

Knowles, E. (ed.) (2009) *Oxford Dictionary of Quotations*, Oxford: Oxford University Press.

Kropp, P. R., Hart, S. D., Webster, C. D. and Eaves, D. (1994) *Manual for the Spousal Assault Risk Assessment Guide, 1st edition*, Vancouver: The British Columbia Institute for Family Violence.

Lindley, D. V. (2006) *Understanding Uncertainty*, Hoboken: John Wiley & Son.

Logan, C. and Johnstone, L. (2010) 'Personality disorder and violence: Making the link through risk formulation', *Journal of Personality Disorders, 24*, 610–33.

Mossman, D. and Sellke, T. (2007) 'Avoiding errors about "margins of error"', Letter, *British Journal of Psychiatry, 191*: 561.

Otto, R. K. and Douglas, K. S. (2010) *Handbook of violence risk assessment*, New York: Routledge.

Poythress, N. and Petrila, J. P. (2010) 'PCL-R psychopathy: Threats to sue, peer review, and potential implications for science and law. A commentary', *International Journal of Forensic Mental Health, 9*, 3–10.

Quinsey, V. L., Harris, G. T., Rice, M. E. and Cormier, C. A. (1998) *Violent offenders: Appraising and managing risk, 1st edition*, Washington DC: American Psychological Association.

Rice, M. E. and Harris, G. T. (1995) 'Violent recidivism: Assessing predictive validity', *Journal of Consulting and Clinical Psychology, 63*: 737–48.

Rockhill, B. (2005) 'Theorizing about causes at the individual level while estimating effects at the population level: Implications for prevention', *Epidemiology, 16(1)*, 124–9.

Rorer, L. (1990) 'Personality assessment: A conceptual survey' in L. A. Pervin (ed.) *Handbook of personality: Theory and research*, pp. 693–720, New York: Guilford.

Rose, G. (1992) *The strategy of preventative medicine*, Oxford: Oxford Medical Publications.

Royal Statistical Society (2010) 'Royal Statistical Society concerning the issues raised in Sally Clark case'.

Scott, P. D. (1977) 'Assessing dangerousness in criminals', *British Journal of Psychiatry, 131*: 127–42.

Singh, J. P., Grann, M. and Fazel, S. A (2011) 'Comparative study of risk assessment tools: A systematic review and metaregression analysis of 68 studies involving 25,980 participants', *Clinical Psychology Review, 31*: 499–513.

Steel, R. G. D., Torrie, J. H. and Dickey, D. A. (1997) *Principles and procedures of statistics: A biometrical approach*, McGraw Hill.

Thornton, D. M. (2003) *Scoring guide for the Risk Matrix 2000.4.* Unpublished Work.

Vardeman, S. B. (1992) 'What about other intervals?', *The American Statistician, 46*: 193–97.

Waggoner, J., Wollert, R. and Cramer, E. (2008) 'A respecification of Hanson's updated *Static-99* experience table that controls for the effect of age on sexual recidivism among young offenders', *Law, Probability and Risk, 7*: 305–12.

Wald, N. J., Hackshaw, A. K. and Frost, C. D. (1999) 'When can a risk factor be used as a worthwhile screening test?', *British Medical Journal, 319*: 1562–65.

Ward, T. (2003) 'Good lives and the rehabilitation of offenders: Promises and problems', *Aggression and Violent Behavior, 7*: 513–28.

Webster, C. D., Douglas, K., Eaves, D. and Hart, S. D. (1997) *HCR-20 Assessing risk for violence* (2nd ed.), Vancouver: Simon Fraser University.

Wilson, E. B. (1927) 'Probable inference, the law of succession and statistical inference', *Journal of the American Statistical Association, 22*: 209–12.

Wittgenstein, L. (1958) *Philosophical investigations*, Oxford: Blackwell.

Yang, M., Wong, S. and Coid, J. (2010) 'The efficacy of violence prediction: A meta-analytic comparison of nine risk assessment tools', *Psychological Bulletin, 136*: 740–67.

— (2010b) 'The efficacy of violence prediction: A meta-analytic comparison of nine risk assessment tools', *Psychological Bulletin, 136*: 740–67.

Part II
Key areas of practice

2 Violence risk assessment and management

Putting structured professional judgment into practice

Kevin S. Douglas, Adam J. E. Blanchard and Melissa C. Hendry

Forecasting and managing a person's risk for violence is called for in many mental health and criminal justice contexts around the world. In the 1960s and 1970s, legal developments in North America pushed risk assessment – historically also referred to as violence prediction or dangerousness – into the spotlight. And it was not a favourable light in which to be. Scholars derided mental health professionals' abilities to make accurate statements about which patients or offenders were more or less likely to be violent in the future (Cocozza and Steadman, 1976; Ennis and Litwack, 1974). Yet, legal cases (*Barefoot v. Estelle*, 1983; *Re Moore and the Queen*, 1984; *Tarasoff v. Regents of the University of California*, 1976) and statutory enactments such as Sexually Violent Predator civil commitment laws (USA) and Dangerous and Long-Term Offender legislation (Canada) have cemented the role of violence risk assessments in legal contexts. All jurisdictions in the US, Canada and the UK contained 'dangerousness' provisions within civil commitment laws by the 1980s (Wilson and Douglas, 2009).

Whether in countries with long-established risk-relevant law or policy, or in countries in which the legal buzz is more recent, such as Japan (see Yoshikawa and Taylor, 2003), scholarly comment and empirical evaluation of risk assessment is thriving. For instance, a recent count of empirical investigations of one of the most commonly used risk assessment instruments – the Historical-Clinical-Risk Management-20 (HCR-20; Webster, Douglas, Eaves and Hart, 1997) indicated that as of September 2010 it had been translated into 18 languages, and had been the subject of 150 disseminations across 17 countries (see Douglas, Blanchard, Guy, Reeves and Weir, 2010). Studies of contemporary risk assessment instruments reveal that they are statistically associated, with at least moderate effect sizes, with future violence (see, for example, the meta-analysis by Yang, Wong and Coid, 2010). This is decidedly good news for clinicians across the globe who are faced with the daunting task of managing the risk for violence that their patients and offenders might pose. Yet this rich research corpus only goes so far when a clinician is seated in the evaluation room with her patient, or is writing a report to the court about the offender on his caseload who has applied for parole. Of what relevance are the hundreds of studies to the evaluation of *this patient*, and the decisions that must be made about her?

Much of the empirical literature does not address the many tasks and decisions that must be made within the process of a risk assessment. Assuming that we have fairly solid evidence for the association between Risk Measure A, B, or C and future violence, how should we use such instruments at the individual level? This chapter will focus on an approach to violence risk assessment and management called structured professional judgment (SPJ). In our view, it is the best suited of available models to guide clinical practice, as we describe below. In what follows, we will (a) overview the SPJ approach, (b) review research in its support, and then (c) discuss practical considerations in terms of how to use it to assess and manage risk. Topics covered in the latter section of the chapter include (a) determining the individual manifestation and relevance of risk factors, (b) information integration and risk formulation, (c) communicating one's findings, and (d) bridging from risk assessment to risk management.

Structured professional judgment: development and description

A major advancement in the past two decades has been the development and increasing use of the *structured professional judgment* (SPJ) model of violence risk assessment. This approach to risk assessment and management – and how it differs from both actuarial prediction and unstructured clinical judgment – has been described in detail elsewhere (see chapters within Otto and Douglas, 2010), and hence we discuss it only briefly. The SPJ approach was developed in an effort to maintain the strengths of both actuarial and clinical approaches while minimizing their weaknesses (Heilbrun, et al., 2009).

Actuarial approaches rely on the algorithmic combination of risk factors to yield numeric probability estimates of future violence, typically derived from single samples. By contrast, the unstructured clinical approach to decision-making has no rules pertaining to the selection or combination of risk factors – such tasks are entirely at the discretion of the decision-maker. Main strengths of the clinical approach include its focus on individual characteristics and its usefulness with intervention and management strategies (Douglas and Kropp, 2002; Melton, Petrila, Poythress and Slobogin, 2007; Nikolova, Strub and Douglas, 2009). Weaknesses of the unstructured clinical approach include the potential reliance on irrelevant risk factors or disregard of important risk factors, the possibility of inconsistencies across different evaluators and within the same evaluator across assessments, and a lack of transparency (Dawes, Faust and Meehl, 1989; Grove and Meehl, 1996; Hart, 1998; Lavoie and Douglas, 2008). Strengths of the actuarial approach include a strong emphasis on empirical support, operational definition of risk factors, specific coding instructions, and transparency (Dawes, et al., 1989; Hart, 1998; Melton, et al., 2007). Weaknesses of the actuarial approach include a possible lack of generalizability across samples and settings, the potential for omitting relevant risk factors, an overreliance on static (unchangeable) risk factors, a limited bearing on risk management and intervention, the inappropriate weighting of risk factors, and the inclusion of probability estimates regarding the likelihood of future violence for an individual case which have no guarantee of being accurate (Dawes, 1979; Douglas and Reeves, 2010; Hart, 1998; Hart, Michie and Cooke, 2007; Litwack, 2001; Melton, et al., 2007; Otto, 2000).

Structure is imposed in the SPJ approach by (a) the inclusion of a fixed number (20 to 30) of operationally defined risk factors that must be considered in every case, (b) explicit coding rules for each risk factor on a three-point scale (absent, possibly/partially present, definitely present), and (c) explicit instructions for the determination of final decisions about risk (Douglas, Ogloff and Hart, 2003; Douglas and Reeves, 2010; Heilbrun, et al., 2009). This structured approach has also allowed the SPJ model to maintain transparency in the decision-making process. At the same time, the SPJ model incorporates the individualized nature of the clinical approach and links between risk assessment and management strategies. By allowing professionals to use their professional judgment in the final decision-making process and requiring assessors to determine the individual, or idiographic, relevance and manifestations of risk factors, the SPJ model is both structured and individualized.

The SPJ model sets out guidelines that reflect current empirical, theoretical, and clinical knowledge about violence. The guidelines and procedures set out the necessary qualifications for assessors, the relevant information that should be considered, the manner in which information should be ascertained, effective communication strategies, and methods for implementing intervention strategies (Douglas and Kropp, 2002).

Although the SPJ process is very structured, professional judgment is required mainly at three stages. The first involves making a determination regarding the importance of a present risk factor for understanding a given individual's proneness to future violence. That is, after rating the presence of a risk factor, evaluators must determine how that risk factor manifests for a given individual and the relative degree of importance, or relevance, of the risk factor for understanding the individual's risk (Douglas and Reeves, 2010; Hart, et al., 2003; Heilbrun, et al., 2009). The second stage where judgment is necessary is in arriving at a final risk judgment of low, moderate, or high risk, based on the number and relevance of risk factors present and the associated intensity of risk management required to stem risk. The third primary stage at which judgment is required is risk formulation. We will return to these topics later in the chapter in some detail.

Research on structured professional judgment

Although the SPJ approach is intended to guide practice at the individual level, it is important to evaluate it empirically to provide evidence that it works as intended. Typically, this has involved evaluating whether risk factors can be rated reliably across raters, whether risk factors are associated with future violence, and whether judgments (of low, moderate, or high risk) based upon risk factors also are associated with future violence. We will focus on the validity of the SPJ approach, although on average interrater reliability of risk-factor ratings and summary risk ratings have been shown to be acceptable (see chapters within Otto and Douglas, 2010, for reviews).

In our discussion of SPJ's validity, we make use of the research term 'predictive validity' to refer simply to the statistical association in research studies between risk factors or judgments at Time A, and violence at Time B. The SPJ approach is intended to inform the management of risk and prevention of future violence. However, to do so, it is imperative that its constituent elements (risk factors and risk judgments) can be shown to be associated with future violence, so that decisions based upon them are empirically supported. We consider this a vital aspect to the SPJ approach as a whole. Clinicians should know that if they are asked to use a certain approach such as SPJ, the approach goes beyond mere 'good ideas' and has been demonstrated to possess empirical support.

There has been a wealth of research on the SPJ approach to risk assessment, and risk assessment more broadly (see chapters within Otto and Douglas, 2010). In a recent meta-analytic investigation of 113 studies examining the predictive validity of the SPJ model, Guy (2008) found that SPJ instruments in general had good predictive validity with respect to antisocial behaviour. Overall, using total scores (sums of risk factors) of SPJ instruments, Guy found an area under the curve (AUC) ranging from .60 (sexual violence) to .74 (violence). AUC is commonly used as an effect size of predictive validity, where 0 refers to a perfect negative prediction, .5 refers to chance prediction, and 1.0 refers to a perfect positive prediction. Interestingly, though not surprisingly, it was found that effect sizes for SPJ measures were highest for the type of outcome they were designed to predict. For instance, the predictive validity of the HCR-20 was best for violence (as opposed to sexual violence and general recidivism). Further, the definitions of outcomes used by the researchers affected the predictive validity of SPJ measures in that the closer the definition used by researchers was to the actual definition of outcomes as outlined in the measures' manuals, the larger the effect sizes were.

In clinical practice, summary risk ratings (i.e., low, moderate, or high risk) are typically more useful in communicating a client's risk for violence as well as ways of managing this risk than are counts of risk factors. Accordingly, there is an increasing body of literature investigating the predictive validity of these final SPJ judgments. Although this has not been examined as frequently as numerical scores, research demonstrates that there is support for the predictive validity of summary risk judgments with respect to violence (see e.g., Douglas and Reeves, 2010; Heilbrun, et al., 2009, and chapters within Otto and Douglas, 2010, for reviews). Of 12 published studies we could locate, summary risk ratings were associated with future violence in 10 (Catchpole and Gretton, 2003; de Vogel and de Ruiter, 2005, 2006; de Vogel, de Ruiter, van Beek and Mead, 2004; Douglas, Ogloff and Hart, 2003; Douglas, et al., 2005; Enebrink, Långström and Gumpert, 2006; Kropp and Hart, 2000; Pederson, et al., 2010), and not in two (Sjöstedt and Långström, 2002; Viljoen, et al., 2008). Further, a number of these published studies have tested whether final summary risk ratings add incrementally to the prediction of violence, over and above the numerical (or actuarial) use of that instrument, and have demonstrated incremental validity (de Vogel and de Ruiter,

2006; Douglas, et al., 2003; Douglas, et al., 2005; Enebrink, et al., 2006; Kropp and Hart, 2000; Pederson, et al., 2010). Similarly, summary risk ratings have been shown to be as or more strongly related to violence relative to actuarial instruments such as the *Violence Risk Appraisal Guide* (VRAG), the *Sex Offender Risk Appraisal Guide* (SORAG), and the *Static-99* (for reviews, see Guy, 2008; Heilbrun, et al., 2009), as well as relative to the *Psychopathy Checklist-Revised* (PCL-R; Douglas, et al., 2003, 2005; de Vogel and de Ruiter, 2005).

Taken together, these findings point to the conclusion that summary risk ratings of SPJ violence risk assessment instruments have associations with future violence equal or superior to actuarial tools, the numerical use of SPJ instruments (which we do not recommend, but which has been evaluated for research purposes) and the PCL-R. These findings provide strong evidence for clinicians that using their judgment in this structured manner has validity. We will now turn to a discussion of using SPJ in practice.

Using structured professional judgment in practice

In this section, we provide recommendations for conducting a thorough risk assessment and informing risk management, organized according to the following topics: (a) determining the individual manifestation and relevance of risk factors; (b) information integration and risk formulation; (c) communicating one's findings; and (d) bridging to risk management. Table 2.1 presents an overview of these goals of risk assessment and management.

Table 2.1 Overview of the goals of risk assessment and management

1. Determining the individual manifestation and relevance of risk factors
   a. Determine the *presence* of risk factors
   b. Describe the *nature* of risk factors (risk vs. protective factors; static vs. dynamic)
   c. Explicate the *individual manifestation* of risk factors (onset; course; severity; nature of change; acuteness of change; periodicity; recent change; current status; future concerns)
   d. Explain the *idiographic relevance* of risk factors to violence
      i. Causal for this person?
      ii. Use anamnestic assessment and functional analysis
      iii. Role of the risk factor (motivating; disinhibiting; impeding; disorganizing; focusing)
2. Information integration and risk formulation
   a. *Theoretically informed formulation* (social learning; criminological theory; Good Lives Model; tense situations; psychotic action)
   b. *Pragmatically grounded formulation*
      i. Four Ps
      ii. Hierarchy of relevant risk factors
      iii. Risk factor clusters
      iv. Risk factors as portals (warning signs; signature threats; early recognition)

(continued)

Table 2.1 (continued)

3. Communicating one's findings
   a. *Summary risk ratings* (low, moderate, high)
      i. Level of risk and intensity of risk management
4. Bridging to risk management
   a. *General risk management formats* (monitoring; supervision; victim safety planning; treatment)
   b. *Quantity and quality* (nature) of risk management efforts
      i. Risk-Need-Responsivity (RNR)
   c. *Linking to the 'what works' treatment literature*
   d. *Extending formulation into the future* (scenario planning)

Determining the individual manifestation and relevance of risk factors

Any SPJ approach lists and defines risk factors that must be considered in every assessment. It is relatively straightforward to determine whether given risk factors are present, according to the rating guidelines of the instrument(s) at play. In addition to *presence*, however, in order to understand the meaning of risk factors for a given person, evaluators need also to consider the *nature, individual manifestation* and *idiographic relevance* of such factors (Douglas and Reeves, 2010). We discuss each.

Nature

Many scholars have commented on the importance of classifying risk factors as static, or relatively time-invariant, versus dynamic, or time-variant (for a review, see Douglas and Skeem, 2005). Most generally, time-variant risk factors, also called dynamic risk factors or criminogenic needs (Andrews and Bonta, 2006, 2010), can change. Time-invariant factors, also called static factors, cannot change. Most scholars agree that it is essential to identify time-variant risk factors because they represent the best candidates for intervention (Andrews, 2012; Douglas and Skeem, 2005).

Examples of static factors include age at first criminal behaviour and (for adults) history of child abuse. Examples of dynamic factors include psychosis, substance use, and violent ideation. Some dynamic factors (e.g., antisocial attitudes) may take longer to change than others (e.g., negative mood). For this reason, some commentators have further divided dynamic risk factors into *stable* versus *acute* based on their rate of change (Hanson and Harris, 2000). Although there is little research on this distinction in terms of change intervals, it is a useful distinction nonetheless.

By design, all SPJ risk assessment instruments include dynamic factors, and identify them as such. Some other approaches to risk assessment, such as the Level of Service (LS) approach, do as well (see Andrews, et al., 2010; Hoge, 2010, for summaries). However, instruments may not address whether such factors are stable or acute, and how such factors might change. As such, it is important for evaluators to turn their minds to these issues. We would encourage evaluators to consider not just whether a risk factor might change, and how quickly, but the nature of this change as well, a topic we explain in the next section on manifestation. Finally, it is important to point out that a *causal* dynamic risk factor is one that (a) precedes the outcome of interest and (b) when changed, leads to changes in the outcome (Kraemer, et al., 1997).

In addition to the potential changeability of factors, evaluators might benefit from considering whether a factor is a *risk* factor or a *protective* factor. Risk factors, obviously, elevate the probability of future violence. There is no consensus in the literature about whether factors that *decrease* the risk of an outcome should be called strengths, assets, protective factors, or resiliency factors (Perkins and Borden, 2003), or whether such factors exert influence only in the presence of adversity/risk. Further, scholars have proposed several models to explain the interplay between risk and strength factors (main effects model; interaction model). This topic has only recently started to gain traction in the risk assessment field, and scholars will need to wrestle with conceptual issues such as whether strength or protective factors are distinct from risk factors or represent the opposite pole thereof, and whether such factors are only relevant in the face of elevated risk. However, the general concept appears to have promise. (See de Vries Robbé and de Vogel, this volume, for further discussion.)

For instance, some SPJ instruments incorporate positive aspects of individuals that might decrease risk for a range of adverse outcomes. The *Short-Term Assessment of Risk and Treatability* (START; Webster, Martin, Brink, Nicholls and Middleton, 2004) requires each of its factors to be coded *both* as a potential vulnerability and as a potential strength. For instance, a person might show certain problems with substance use, such as continued occasional use of marijuana (moderate vulnerability), but have substantially decreased intake, have stopped using alcohol, and have signed up for community substance-use programs (moderate strength). Research has shown that, in general, vulnerability ratings are associated positively with adverse outcomes, whereas strength ratings are associated negatively with adverse outcomes (e.g., Desmarais, Wilson, Nicholls and Brink, 2010).

The *Structured Assessment of Violence Risk in Youth* (SAVRY; Borum, Bartel and Forth, 2006) has a separate subscale entitled 'Protective Factors', consisting of such factors as prosocial involvement, strong attachment and bonds, and resilient personality traits. Research studies demonstrate that this subscale is inversely related to violence amongst youth (Borum, Lodewijks, Bartel and Forth, 2010). A relatively recent instrument called the *Structured Assessment of Protective Factors*, or SAPROF (de Vogel, de Ruiter, Bourman and de Vries Robbé, 2009) is devoted entirely to protective factors. Its authors concede that they do not adopt any particular theoretical model of protective factors, but that all of its items should be associated with reduced violence. Studies on the SAPROF indicate that it does indeed correlate inversely with violence (de Vogel, et al., 2009).

Individual manifestation

Having identified the presence of violence-relevant factors and their nature, evaluators should next describe what they 'look like' for the case at hand – their *individual manifestation* (Douglas and Reeves, 2010). The rationale for this principle is easily illustrated by contrasting two hypothetical persons with psychosis, one of whom has primarily negative symptoms that are chronic, and the other who is experiencing a rapid first break consisting of acute positive symptoms such as hallucinations and delusions. Despite sharing a common risk factor – psychosis – these individuals differ from one another in meaningful ways.

We recommend that evaluators describe the individual manifestation of risk and protective factors according to the following categories: *onset* (when did the factor first appear?); *course* (how has it progressed over time?); *severity* (mild, extreme?); *nature of change* (increasing, decreasing?); *acuteness of change* (sharp, gradual?); *periodicity* (repeating?); *recent change* (worsening, ameliorating?); *current status* (what does it look like now?); *future concerns* (without intervention, what is the factor's likely course?).

A few words about the nature of change: simply put, it is complex and hard to measure. Factors might increase or decrease, but they can do so differently. Change can be linear (steadily increase or decrease), quadratic (accelerate in increase or decrease), cubic (accelerate then decelerate in increase or decrease), or higher order. As illustrated elegantly by Odgers, et al. (2009), risk factors may fluctuate over time (increase and decrease many times, sometimes unevenly and with different 'wavelengths'). Our basic point is that while it is essential to try to come to terms with how factors change for a given person, it can also be a challenge to do so. To simplify the process, we would recommend that evaluators establish a priori evaluation windows (i.e., change over a set period of time, such as the past six months), re-evaluation schedules (i.e., when re-evaluation should recur), and re-evaluation triggers (i.e., if functioning worsens; prior to any loosening of restrictions or discharge) (see Douglas and Reeves, 2010, Douglas, Hart, Webster and Belfrage, 2011, for a more thorough discussion).

Idiographic relevance

In addition to identifying what risk factors are present, their nature (e.g., are they dynamic?), and how they manifest for a given person (e.g., have they been worsening?), it is vital to add one further step – examine and understand their *idiographic relevance*. That is, in order to identify primary intervention targets, it is important to know what risk factors are most relevant to the violence of the individual person, and which are less so. Simply because a factor has been identified at the nomothetic level as an important risk factor, generally (e.g., substance-use problems), and that it is present in the current case, does not perforce mean that it is terribly important for the individual at hand. What we really are talking about here is whether a risk factor is *causal at the individual level*. Risk factors can be considered to be relevant if they have led to violence in the past (or will do so in the future), or if they interfere with risk management efforts (Douglas and Reeves, 2010; Hart, et al., 2003). Additionally, a risk factor is defined to be relevant to an individual's risk for violent behaviour if it: (a) was a material contribution to past violence; (b) is likely to influence the person's decision to act in a violent manner in the future; (c) is likely to impair the individual's capacity to employ non-violent problem-solving techniques or to engage in non-violent or non-confrontational interpersonal relations; or (d) is necessary to manage this factor in order to mitigate risk (Douglas, et al., 2011). This aspect of an SPJ approach further differentiates it from most actuarial approaches, and increases its suitability for use in treatment planning. Let us describe this concept further.

One reason thought to account for the predictive validity of SPJ instruments is that the model requires the assessor to consider the individual relevance of each risk factor above and beyond the mere presence of the risk factor (Douglas and Reeves, 2010). In the SPJ model, evaluators must consider and rate the presence of a pre-specified set of operationally defined, nomothetically derived risk factors in all cases they encounter. Each of these risk factors has been chosen due to an established relationship with violence in the scientific, theoretical or clinical literature. These risk factors are written essentially as 'templates', or how the risk factor might look in general.

However, for years professionals in the field have been aware that 'factors that are relevant to the risk assessment of one person may not be relevant to the risk assessment of another' (Monahan, et al., 2001, p. 11). Monahan and colleagues (2001) concluded that the multifaceted nature of violence and human behaviour make it understandably difficult, even impossible, to identify variables that are risk factors for every individual. In the SPJ model, subsequent to considering the presence of these nomothetically derived risk factors, assessors must incorporate the idiographic manifestations and idiographic relevance of each risk factor in order to arrive at their final decision. Assessors also consider the presence and relevance of risk factors in determining the case-specific, idiographic, management strategies. The SPJ model thus offers a bridge across the idiographic–nomothetic distinction.

The tension between the nomothetic and idiographic levels of evaluation has been recognized in social and medical science for decades. The basis of the idiographic–nomothetic distinction rests on the statement that 'every man is in certain respects (a) like all other men, (b) like some other men, (c) like no other man' (Kluckhohn and Murray, 1953, p. 53). Essentially, at the most general level there exist universal truths that hold for all people, while at the most specific level there exist individualizing features that are true of only one person (Grice, 2004). Knowledge of parameters and variables that relate to human nature in general (nomothetic knowledge) is fundamental to any assessment. However, knowledge concerning the individual differences and manifestations of variables (idiographic knowledge) is equally important (Stagner, 1979). Idiographic analysis, due to its focus on the unique and individual determinants of behaviour, allows for greater accuracy in understanding and predicting an individual compared to nomothetic techniques (Allport, 1937; Bem and Allen, 1974; Franck, 1982; Paunonen and Jackson, 1986; Runyan, 1983). A thorough understanding of the case particulars is always required to make a prediction, for 'even if all the laws of psychology were known, one could make a prediction about the behavior of a man only if in addition to the laws, the special nature of the particular situation were known'

(Lewin, 1936, p. 11). (See Cooke and Johnstone this volume for additional details). However, when the ultimate goal is idiographic understanding and assessment, it is an erroneous belief that nomothetic data are irrelevant and should not be considered (Grove and Meehl, 1996). The uniqueness of a particular individual is not grounds for the outright rejection of nomothetically derived statistical relations.

As such, a comprehensive assessment of an individual person must be based on nomothetically derived relationships and concepts, but to this must be added an appreciation for the idiographic manifestations and relevance within this individual. Due to the multifaceted and conditional nature of certain behaviours, an assessment tailored to incorporate idiographic manifestations and relevance will allow for more precise identification of functional relations between variables, more useful clinical judgments, more accurate case conceptualizations, and more appropriate intervention strategies (Haynes, Mumma and Pinson, 2009). SPJ tools provide a comprehensive assessment that incorporates both nomothetic and idiographic aspects.

How are we to know whether a risk factor is idiographically relevant or causal? First, the determination of such requires an *anamnestic* assessment of past violence. Second, evaluators need to consider what role a risk factor might play in future violence. Third, a conceptual framework for considering possible roles that risk factors might play in leading to violence can be helpful.

First, evaluators should construct a detailed description of an individual's past violent acts. Anamnestic assessment involves careful examination of past violent events for the purpose of determining their behavioural and situational precipitants (Melton, Petrila, Poythress and Slobogin, 1997, 2007; Otto, 2000). To this we might add affective and interpersonal. The purpose is to understand the factors that led to past violence. There is little research that evaluates anamnestic assessment, although it has high face validity and clinical utility.

Another useful means by which to understand the potential causal relevance of risk factors is to conduct a *functional analysis* of violence. Functional analysis of violence shares with anamnestic assessment the goal of understanding the precipitants of violence. However, it has been set to metric in a line of research conducted in the UK and Australia by Michael Daffern, Kevin Howells, and colleagues (e.g., Daffern and Howells, 2009; Daffern, Howells and Ogloff, 2006). The primary purpose of this approach is to identify the function – or purpose – that violence serves for individuals. Daffern and Howells (2009), using a measure called the *Assessment and Classification of Function* (ACF; Daffern, et al., 2006), determined that violence is often multifunctional. Common functions included the expression of anger, obtaining tangibles, avoiding demands, and reducing tension. In this manner, it can be considered a form of empirically evaluated anamnestic assessment.

Second, armed with knowledge of which risk factors have been most important in leading to violence in the past, evaluators need to consider the role that those risk factors, and others, might play *in future violence*. As Hart (2008) has pointed out, one of the shortcomings of a purely anamnestic approach is that it might lead evaluators to conclude that history is destined to repeat itself. Though it might very well do so, there can certainly be different concerns in the future about which evaluators need to be concerned. Generally, evaluators should consider, based in part on their assessment of the course, current status, and concerns about the future status of the risk factor (see previous section on individual manifestation), whether the risk factor is likely to be important to manage in the future, or if it might interfere with management or intervention efforts. In a criminal justice context, Andrews and colleagues (Andrews and Bonta, 2006, 2010; Andrews, et al., 2010) refer to the latter as 'specific responsivity' factors, a topic we will return to later in the chapter.

Third, in deciding upon the potential individual causal relevance of risk factors, it can be helpful to use a general framework of potential roles that risk factors can play. We provide one example here, though doubtless there are others. As described by Hart (2008, see also Cooke and Michie, this volume), risk factors may be relevant to an individual's violence because they are *motivators, disinhibitors,* or *impeders.* If a risk factor plays a *motivating* role, violence achieves a rewarding or reinforcing role (i.e., armed robbery may alleviate financial problems stemming from unemployment). A *disinhibitor* loosens normal constraints on behaviour (e.g., impulsivity, anger, intoxication). *Impeders* interfere with the potential effectiveness of risk-reduction efforts. A good example is treatment noncompliance. Douglas, Guy and Hart (2009), in the context of psychosis as a risk factor for violence, further discussed the *focusing* or *organizing* role that psychosis might play in violence (i.e., persecutory delusions that focus one's attention on perceived threats and organize defensive action deemed necessary to protect oneself), on the one hand, and the potential *disorganizing* role that it might play on the other (i.e., formal thought disorder that interferes with interpersonal interactions and problem-solving).

Although the determination of idiographic relevance is considered an important aspect of the SPJ approach to assessment and management, its importance has only been reflected formally in recent years through inclusion within SPJ instrument manuals. For instance, the *Risk for Sexual Violence Protocol* (RSVP; Hart, et al., 2003) requires evaluators to rate not only the presence of 22 risk factors for sexual violence, but also their relevance. The upcoming revision of the HCR-20 – called HCR:V3 (Douglas et al., 2011) – will do the same.

There is still little research on relevance as opposed to presence ratings of risk factors. However, the research looks promising. In a recent chapter on the SVR-20 and RSVP by Hart and Boer (2010), the relevance ratings on the RSVP were associated with violence, and could be rated with high levels of interrater reliability. In a retrospective analysis of a draft version of the HCR:V3, Blanchard (2010) found that idiographic relevance ratings (sums for the H, C, R, and Total scores) consistently outperformed presence ratings, and typically achieved large effect sizes. More research on this topic is sorely needed.

Up to this point, we have walked through the anatomy of an assessment in terms of identifying what risk factors are most important in terms of understanding an individual's risk for violence. By establishing the presence, nature, manifestation, and idiographic relevance of risk factors, determined through careful evaluation that incorporates an anamnestic and/or functional approach, the evaluator will have readied herself for the next step – integration and formulation.

Information integration and risk formulation

Determining individual manifestation and relevance, described in the previous section, is a foundational component of risk assessment and management. However, on its own, it is incomplete. Most SPJ risk assessment measures contain 20–30 risk factors. Simply describing each on its own, as if it were unrelated to all others, does not reflect the reality that risk factors, whether considered at the nomothetic or idiographic level, are related to one another. At the nomothetic level, this will be represented by inter-item correlations, or perhaps by scores on principal components or cluster solutions. However, risk factors need to be integrated at the individual level. Ideally, we need to tell a story about an individual that integrates the many pieces of information available to us. We need to derive an *individual theory of risk*, to help us make sense of risk, and therefore how best to intervene and manage such risk. Formulation has its foundation in the general psychotherapy literature. It is intended to facilitate clinicians' conceptualization of the roots of a person's problems with an eye toward intervention.

There is no single theory of violence, and hence no single approach to formulation or conceptualization. It is inherently idiosyncratic, that is, tailored to the individual and intended to explain the behaviour of *just that one individual*. Nonetheless, we recommend structure, and provide some direction for clinicians and criminal justice professionals. We also point out that, just as anamnestic or functional analysis can be used to identify the relevance of risk factors, they can be used to facilitate formulation. Indeed, the two tasks are quite closely aligned.

Lewis and Doyle (2009), in providing an excellent snapshot of the current state of affairs when it comes to formulation in the forensic risk assessment field, described it as follows: 'risk formulation may be regarded as a form of analysis that can assist practitioners to explain the origins, development, and maintenance of risk behaviour, while providing a crucial link between assessment and management in clinical practice' (p. 290). As they pointed out, formulation provides an important bridge between assessment and management, and we will return to it in our section on risk management.

Hart and Logan (2011) have provided an excellent and thorough analysis of the purpose and status of formulation in forensic mental health. As they point out, the process of formulation should be regarded as a core competency in forensic mental health, as it is in broader fields such as medicine and psychology. Hart and Logan discussed essential features of the nature of formulation. In their view, formulation should possess the following characteristics: (a) *inferential* (formulation explains the reasons for or causes of behaviour); (b) *action-oriented* (formulation directs the risk reduction actions of clinicians or criminal justice professionals); (c) *theory-driven* (formulation seeks guidance from an overarching, principled knowledge structure); (d) *individualized* (formulation necessarily seeks to explain the behaviour of a single person); (e) *narrative* (formulation is a qualitative process that produces a temporal story with important 'anchors'); (f) *diachronic* (formulation addresses multiple time periods – past, present, and future); (g) *testable* (formulation should be evaluable); and (h) *ampliative* (formulation creates new information or knowledge about the individual, rather than merely summarizing known facts). We refer readers to Hart and Logan for an extended discussion of these principles, as well as criteria for evaluating the quality of formulations.

In our view, there are two general categories of formulation that can be used within risk assessment: (a) *theoretically informed*, and (b) *pragmatically grounded*. Although Hart and Logan (2011) consider theory a primary feature of formulation, we have observed that there are organizational principles and processes that can help clinicians sort through the vast amount of case information available to them to distil core patterns that are not theories per se. Hence, we discuss these as well. Note that our two approaches are not mutually exclusive. Regardless of approach, in all cases formulation *must* account for the risk factors that were deemed to be relevant in preceding steps. These relevant risk factors are the 'raw data' that are to be synthesized through formulation.

Theoretically informed formulation

As Lewis and Doyle (2009) allude to, clinicians with a cognitive-behavioural theoretical orientation will likely formulate according to reinforcement contingencies (rewards and punishments) and the connection between cognition (particularly distorted cognitions), emotion, and behaviour. Psychodynamic clinicians will organize their formulations around concepts including defence mechanisms and unconscious motivations. Neither is inherently right or wrong, although some theories have more empirical support regarding the role they play in the development and maintenance of violence. For instance, at this very general theoretical level, we would recommend a formulation that draws from social learning and related theories. As Andrews and Bonta (2010) have explained, the *general personality and social learning theoretical perspectives on crime* (GPCSL) has a great amount of empirical support when it comes to explaining crime. Although we lack space to delve into this theory, formulation and treatment essentially involves careful explication of reinforcement contingencies that may have led to the risk factors (i.e., antisocial peers, antisocial attitudes) that maintain antisocial behaviour, and the application of treatments that aim to alter those reinforcement contingencies. One could also turn to criminological theory (e.g., strain theory; social bonding or control theory; social disorganization theory) to derive hypotheses about a person's antisocial behaviour.

At a more specific level, there are several conceptual models of violence that can provide hypotheses to be tested at the individual level. Hiday (1995; 1997), for instance, discussed how, for persons who have a serious mental illness, active symptoms can lead to 'tense situations' through the interaction of the symptoms (their bizarre nature; their effect on the ability to reason and to remain composed) and how some persons might receive them (with fear, anger, or defensiveness). In Baxter's (1997) view, such interactions can lead to disorganized or impulsive violence. Junginger (1996), again in the context of psychosis, has argued that psychosis is more likely to lead to violence when the content and themes of the psychotic symptoms are violence-laden, or consistent with violence. He termed this phenomenon 'psychotic action.' Ward (2002; see also Ward and Laws, 2010) described a 'Good Lives Model' (GLM) to help explain sexual violence and how it may be reduced through treatment. In Ward's view, violence is a means to obtain valued goals. The GLM seeks to promote substitution of destructive means to obtain goals with prosocial means. Ward and Laws (2010), for instance, described a dozen potential prosocial means to help offenders obtain their goals while desisting from violence, and to lead 'good lives.'

Pragmatically grounded formulation

Whereas theoretically informed formulation draws on overarching, substantive ideas to help generate hypotheses about the reasons for violence in any given case, pragmatically grounded formulation provides organizational structure and checklists to facilitate information integration without reference to a specific theory per se. As described by Lewis and Doyle (2009), Weerasekera's (1996) 'Four P' formulation model 'orients the clinician to consider predisposing factors (i.e., longer-term pre-existing vulnerabilities), precipitating factors (more recent triggering events or issues), perpetuating factors (that are maintaining the problem), and protective factors (resources that may mitigate or reduce the impact of the problem)' (p. 287). The clinician would then identify the factors at each of the four stages that fill the respective function. Note that theory may be drawn upon here to facilitate this process. So too may functional analysis.

In our experience, we have found that it is useful to distil relevant risk factors in the following manner in terms of formulation: (a) constructing a hierarchy of relevant risk factors; (b) risk-factor clusters and interactions; and (c) risk factors that serve as portals to a risk process, as described below. In terms of *hierarchy*, in most cases, several risk factors stand out as more important than others. We recommend that evaluators, in addition to considering the relevance of risk factors, also delineate any risk factors that are especially salient. Although all SPJ instruments use unit-weighting to score risk factors, evaluators must then determine which risk factors are most 'troublesome' in terms of violence risk. These will vary across cases, of course, and hence this is a subjective, idiosyncratic judgment. In most cases, there are only a few such risk factors, and these often act as 'portals' or stimulants of other risk factors, in that the exacerbation of a single risk factor can lead to the worsening of other risk factors (discussed in more detail below).

We have also observed benefit from constructing *risk factor clusters* in individual cases. Again, such clusters are inherently idiographic, although evaluators may be guided by theory, as reviewed above. Risk clusters describe the natural covariation amongst risk factors, but at the individual level. As we mentioned earlier, risk factors are rarely uncorrelated with other risk factors, either at the nomothetic or individual level. Reducing the number of 'areas of concern' through identifying risk factors that covary within the individual greatly simplifies implications for risk management, and facilitates the integration of risk information.

We provide an example, drawing on one particular SPJ instrument – the HCR-20. Suppose a patient or offender under evaluation experienced severe abuse as a child at the hands of his father, after his mother abandoned the family when he was six. This abuse and family disintegration created a dismissive attachment style, taught the patient that violence is an effective means by which to solve problems, and instilled a great distrust in authority figures. Ostensibly, such a patient might have several HCR-20 risk factors as a result: H8 (early maladjustment); H9 (personality disorder); H3 (relationship instability); H10 (prior supervision failure); C5 (unresponsive to treatment); R3 (lack of personal support); R4 (noncompliance with remediation attempts). The severe abuse and maternal abandonment fulfills early maladjustment (H8), contributed to the development of a personality disorder (H9, say, borderline personality disorder), created distrust of authority and hence past parole violations (H10), current poor effort in treatment (C5), and concerns about future supervision (R4). It also led to chaotic romantic relationships (H3), and few meaningful connections with friends and family (R4). These risk factors are meaningfully connected with one another *for this person*. They may not be for another person. They cohere through a common antecedent. We have found through practical experience and having engaged in discourse with countless clinicians that for most people, it is possible to identify two to four such clusters of risk factors that cohere in any given case. Typically, such clusters have a common antecedent. (Of note, a similar observation has been observed in terms of situational risk assessment).

Often, such clusters can be 'activated' by *portal* or *gateway* risk factors. How often have the readers of this chapter thought 'she'll be fine, unless . . .?' What follows the 'unless . . .' is often one or two risk factors, that, if they 'act up', could lead to the exacerbation of numerous other risk factors. For instance, a patient's risk might be considered manageable in the community unless she becomes noncompliant with treatment – a single risk factor. If she does, however, then she will experience extreme stress (R5), stop trusting her supervisors (C5, R4), become delusional (C3), be emotionally and behaviourally volatile (C4), not understand how she can deal with her plight (C1), and be unwelcome at her halfway house (R1). Again, through experience and discourse with numerous clinicians, we have found that such a scenario is not uncommon.

This idea of these 'gateway' risk factors is similar to the concept of 'signature risk signs' as embodied in the START. As Webster, et al. (2006) describe them, signature risk signs are 'a specific set of beliefs, symptoms, behaviors, or concerns, which . . . may over time come to be recognized as an early but reliable, unique, and invariant "signature" signal of impending relapse and elevation in risk to self or others' (p. 757). Similarly, Bjørkly (2003) described 'recurrent warning signs as specific individual precursors of violence' (p. 813). In an interesting application of this method, Fluttert, van Meijel, Webster, Nijman, Bartels and Grypdonck (2008) described an 'Early Recognition Method' in which patients and nurses act together to identify the patient's signature threats or warning signs, and then develop risk management strategies to mitigate risk early in the process, before violence occurs. Notably, this model also draws on theory to formulate or conceptualize such warning signs. This method has shown some potential to reduce subsequent violence (Fluttert, van Meijel, Nijman, Bjørkly and Grypdonck, 2010).

Regrettably, as Lewis and Doyle (2009) pointed out, it is this aspect of risk assessment and management that likely has received the least amount of empirical evaluation. Yet clinicians and criminal justice professionals must engage in it. What we *do* know is that when the SPJ model has been evaluated in terms of how it is intended to be used in practice, the results are quite positive, as reviewed earlier in our section on the empirical evaluation of the SPJ model.

Communicating one's findings

Once risk factors have been rated for presence, manifestation, and relevance, and distilled into a coherent formulation, the evaluator must then communicate her findings. Although the precise nature and scope of such communication may differ according to the purpose of the evaluation and who is receiving it (e.g., courts, parole boards, mental health professionals), we recommend that evaluators again use a structured format and then adapt it to their specific context.

We recommend that evaluators use a categorical, non-numeric communication structure that includes case-specific information that provides a rationale for the decision, description of the relevant risk factors, a summary of the formulation, and recommended management strategies. Research has demonstrated that mental health professionals tend to prefer this mode of communication (Heilbrun, et al., 2000; 2004).

All SPJ instruments recommend starting with a basic statement of whether, in an evaluator's judgment, a person should be considered low, moderate, or high risk. As reviewed earlier, this categorical *summary risk rating* is at least as accurate as the numeric (actuarial) use of SPJ instruments and actuarial instruments, if not more so. It also avoids the danger of offering numeric estimates that may very well not be applicable in a given case. The meaning of 'low', 'moderate', and 'high' is intended to capture both the evaluator's concern about the likelihood of future violence, as well as the attendant degree or intensity of management efforts that are required to mitigate risk in the case at hand. These judgments should be informed, but not fixed, by the number of relevant risk factors present in a case. In general, the more risk factors that are present, the higher the risk. However, there may be some cases in which a small number of risk factors are present, although the logical decision should be high risk (say, persecutory delusions coupled with a genuine homicidal threat). Again, all SPJ instruments provide similar definitions of these terms.

In addition to stating a risk category, the evaluator should state *why* this is the case, or provide justification for the decision of low, moderate, or high risk. In fact, the summary risk rating should logically flow from the description of the relevant risk factors, the number of relevant factors, the formulation that integrates them, and the decision about the nature and degree of risk management strategies necessary to mitigate risk. The evaluator should include summary statements (say, in a report, or in oral testimony) about these features of the assessment that provide rationale for his decision about risk level. He should also provide the general definition of the risk category as outlined in SPJ instrument manuals and related sources. Referencing the empirical literature that supports the use of this approach is also recommended.

A brief example – taken from Douglas and Reeves (2010) – will help illustrate communication of risk through the use of the non-numeric categorical summary risk rating system. The following excerpt is taken from Douglas and Reeves (2010), and is the conclusion of a hypothetical written report that used the HCR-20. Note that this excerpt pertains only to the summary risk ratings. Illustration of formulation was provided above, and in Douglas and Reeves (2010).

> Given both the presence of a large number of risk factors, and their relevance to Mr Case's risk for violence, in my judgment Mr Case is a high risk for violence. Furthermore, although history is not destined to repeat itself, consideration of H1 (previous violence) indicates the type of violence that might be of concern if Mr Case were to act violently. That is, in my judgment Mr Case is at high risk for violence that could cause serious injuries to others.
>
> A judgment of high risk means that (a) there is a high likelihood that, if released soon with the current discharge plans, Mr Case will act violently within the next six months; (b) Mr Case should be considered high priority for the delivery of supervision and management resources; and (c) Mr Case requires a high level or intensity of supervision and management in order to mitigate risk. While it is not possible to produce a meaningful numeric estimate of risk, there are numerous risk factors that have not been controlled, and for which there are no future risk management plans in place. I would recommend further efforts to engage Mr Case in drug and alcohol treatment, and to increase his compliance with supervision and treatment efforts, perhaps through establishing a set of contingencies for compliance and non-compliance. It is also important to monitor his psychotic symptoms closely. It may also be worthwhile to foster Mr Case's recent employment success and to assist him in finding employment and stable housing. If Mr Case were to be released, I would recommend frequent (bi-weekly) monitoring and re-evaluation of his risk factors.
>
> Douglas and Reeves (2010, p. 180)

Notice that this brief statement identifies and defines risk level, and specifies both the *intensity* (e.g., how much?) and *nature* (what type?) of risk management strategies. It also recommends a *re-evaluation schedule* (how frequently?) Risk communication should direct action. That is, it should specify what can be done to reduce risk. It should do so by stating what specific risk management strategies should be considered, and the intensity of management efforts that will be required to ameliorate risk level. Recipients of the communication should know what to do if the evaluee comes under their care. As such, it should act as a recipe for and bridge to *risk management*, a topic we consider next.

Bridging to risk management

The ultimate purpose of risk assessment should be to prevent future violence (Hart, 1998). As such, the SPJ approach to risk assessment includes as an integral component the specification of risk management strategies. Indeed, the primary purpose of identifying relevant risk factors and formulating risk is to prepare oneself to enact optimal risk-reduction efforts. In this section, we discuss (a) *general risk management formats* that practitioners or systems can draw upon; (b) *quantity and quality (nature) of risk management efforts*; (c) *linking to the 'what works' treatment literature*; and (d) *extending formulation into the future.*

General risk management formats

There are four basic risk management formats from which decision-makers or agencies can draw (for more extended discussions, see Hart, 2008; Hart, Douglas and Webster, 2001): (a) *monitoring or surveillance*; (b) *supervision or control*; (c) *victim safety planning*; and (d) *treatment*. The purpose of monitoring is essentially to observe the client (e.g., through regular meetings with a case manager or parole officer), in order to determine whether risk changes over time, the necessary frequency of observation, and whether risk management strategies (such as treatment) are having their intended impact.

Supervision or control, on the other hand, involves restricting the liberty of a patient or offender so that it is more difficult for them to act violently. Imprisonment and hospitalization are examples of institutional control. Parole, probation, and conditional releases are examples of community supervision. The former is clearly more restrictive than the latter, although there are degrees of strictness in both institutional and community supervision.

Victim safety planning is typically most relevant when there is an identifiable potential victim (i.e., a spouse) or class of victims (i.e., fellow residents in a supervised housing setting). The essential feature of this management format is to alter the behaviour of the potential victim(s) and their environment so as to reduce their risk of being the recipient of violence by the patient or offender. Finally, treatment addresses aspects of offenders or patients that are associated with violence, such as anger, substance use, antisocial attitudes, or symptoms of psychosis.

Quantity and quality (nature) of risk management efforts

First, the quantity or intensity of risk management efforts must be commensurate with the identified risk level. That is, high-risk people should receive more management efforts than moderate-risk people, who in turn should receive more management efforts than low-risk people. In some cases, this will involve strict curtailing of liberties through supervision or control (i.e., involuntary hospitalization; imprisonment). Although not all options are available to all decision-makers, typically most are in some format. For instance, probation or parole officers can increase or decrease the amount (frequency) of supervision, or can initiate apprehension procedures by law enforcement to deliver their supervisees to imprisonment. Other professionals (psychiatrists, and, in some jurisdictions, psychologists, nurses and social workers) can involuntarily hospitalize patients. Even private practitioners can initiate such proceedings with the assistance of law enforcement. In other situations, as dictated by case specifics, the quantity of management may mean more frequent treatment sessions, or treatment sessions that address a higher number of relevant risk factors.

This basic principle – called the *Risk Principle* (Andrews and Bonta, 2006, 2010) – is absolutely crucial and foundational to effective risk management and the reduction of crime and violence. It is supported by many studies and its effect is summarized quantitatively in various meta-analyses (see Andrews and Bonta, 2010; Andrews, 2012, for reviews). Simply put, there is little reason to believe that deviating from this principle will do anything other than *elevate* risk.

The Risk Principle is one of three main principles that, together, form the Risk-Need-Responsivity (RNR) approach to risk reduction (Andrews and Bonta, 2006, 2010). As with the Risk Principle, the RNR model generally is very well supported empirically (see Andrews et al., 2010, and Andrews, in press, for recent comprehensive reviews). For instance, the more of the RNR principles addressed by correctional intervention studies, the greater the reduction in recidivism (Dowden and Andrews, 2004). Although there have been fewer studies with mentally disordered samples, patterns of findings with such samples are comparable to those based on non-disordered offender samples (Douglas, et al., 2009).

Its second principle, the *Need Principle*, is relevant to the *quality* or *nature* of intervention efforts, and is highly commensurate with the SPJ approach of linking assessment findings to intervention and management efforts. The Need Principle states that management efforts (usually treatment) must focus on *criminogenic needs*, or dynamic (changeable) risk factors, as defined earlier. This is simply logical – one must address the individual causes of violence in order to influence it. This is also why it is so important to identify relevant risk factors and derive a coherent formulation before deciding on the most appropriate management and treatment strategies. Again, this principle is strongly supported across numerous studies. There is a strong linear association between the number of criminogenic needs targeted by a correctional treatment program, and its effectiveness in reducing crime and violence (Andrews and Bonta, 2010). Similarly, the more *non*-criminogenic needs included in a treatment program, the *less* it will reduce recidivism.

The third main principle of the RNR model – *Responsivity* – states that treatment programs should be delivered to offenders in a manner to which they are most responsive. That is, they should align with the learning styles of those who receive them. In correctional and forensic populations, typically this means that programs should be relatively concrete, and follow cognitive-behavioural and social learning principles. These types of interventions typically are identified by meta-analysts as forming the basis of the 'what works' treatment literature, which we review next.

Linking to the 'what works' treatment literature

In addition to identifying the important dynamic risk factors to target in intervention, and the intensity of management plans more generally, clinicians must then choose interventions that work for the nature of the criminogenic needs present in a given case. As this implies, there must be some sort of individualized tailoring of management and intervention strategies to the needs of the particular case in order to maximize the number of relevant criminogenic needs that are targeted, and to minimize the number of non-criminogenic needs that are targeted. To do otherwise will decrease the effectiveness of treatment and may not reduce risk at all.

Fundamentally, in order for treatments to 'work', or reduce risk, they must subscribe to RNR principles – management 'dose' must be titrated according to risk level; the ratio of criminogenic to non-criminogenic needs must be optimized; the format of program delivery must be maximally responsive to learning styles of its participants, as well as any specific responsivity factors unique to individual participants. If these principles are not met, there is little reason to believe that intervention efforts will be successful.

Space precludes a review of effective treatment programs for the reduction of violence and crime (for fuller accounts, see Andrews and Bonta, 2010; Douglas, Nicholls and Brink, 2009). As referred to earlier, the strongest evidence is for programs that use cognitive-behavioural or social-learning approaches. These general orientations can incorporate important dynamic risk factors, such as antisocial attitudes, substance-use problems, anger, or treatment non-compliance. They include emphasis on learning principles such as reinforcement, modeling, and shaping to reward non-violent behaviour and problem-solving (see Douglas, et al., 2009). We should also emphasize that use of psychotropic treatment for major mental illness as a sole risk management strategy is unlikely to be effective in reducing violence, as other violence risk factors that are present must also be targeted (Douglas, et al., 2009).

Extending formulation into the future

Formulation typically focuses on understanding what has happened in the past, though for the purpose of managing risk in the future. Part of bridging from assessment to management is to speculate about what sorts of adverse outcomes might happen in the future. This includes linking relevant dynamic risk factors and risk level with the nature and quantity of future management strategies. However, this process does not explicitly address the nature of the future violent event whose risk must be managed.

Hart, et al. (2003; see also Hart, 2008) proposed that the process of *scenario planning* can facilitate the process of anticipating the type, nature and context of the future violence whose risk must be managed. This is important because it may have implications for the sorts of management efforts that are employed. For example, if we mainly are concerned that a person might lash out reactively during a stressful moment in a crowded place (say, on a city bus), there is little we can do to help potential victims avoid this. However, if we mainly are concerned that a person will kill his ex-intimate partner whom he is stalking, then victim safety strategies are very much necessary.

Scenario planning helps to extend our understanding of a person's past violence – captured through formulation – to an understanding of a person's possible future violence. As Hart and Logan (2011) describe,

> each scenario is a story about violence the person might commit. It is not a prediction about what will happen; rather, it is a general forecast or speculation about what could happen, in light of the evaluator's general knowledge and experience and the specifics of the case at hand.
>
> Hart and Logan (2011, p. 37).

The point is to construct a reasonable number of possible future scenarios that are plausible based on what is known about the case, and then to ensure that risk management strategies are equipped to deal with and prevent these.

As Hart et al. (2003; Hart, 2008) stressed, a person's future violence will not necessarily be a carbon copy of her past violence, although this is one plausible future scenario that clinicians or criminal justice professionals must plan for. As Hart (2008) describes, in addition to planning for a 'repeat scenario', decision-makers can plan for other plausible scenarios, such as an 'optimistic scenario' (the person may engage in less serious violence compared to previous violence), a 'doom scenario' (the person engages in more serious violence), or a 'twist scenario' (the person engages in a different type of violence). Evaluators should plan for such scenarios by asking themselves and their clients what might lead to the various scenarios, whether there are any warning signs or signature threats that signal that a scenario will soon unfold, and what might be done to prevent the various scenarios. Scenario planning in the violence risk field has not yet been empirically evaluated. However, it has very strong face validity and clinical usefulness. As Hart (2008) points out, it also has a long history in other fields that require planning for adverse events in the face of uncertainty (e.g., military; health care).

Conclusion

The field of violence risk assessment has been witness to an extraordinary amount of research and commentary over the past decade or two. Similarly, research on treatment for the purposes of reducing crime and violence offers more now than it ever has. Though assessing and managing risk remains a complex and challenging task, a good deal of guidance is available. One of the more challenging aspects of assessment and management is bridging the nomothetic and idiographic. The vast majority of published work on risk assessment and management focuses on the nomothetic level. Yet clinicians, legal players and criminal justice professionals must make good decisions about individuals.

As such, this chapter was intended to offer guidance at the idiographic level for clinicians who are faced with the task of assessing and managing risk posed by others. Going beyond merely rating the presence of risk factors in a given case, evaluators must consider their individual manifestation and relevance, and integrate them through formulation. This information then needs to be meaningfully communicated to others, and inform risk management plans that are individually tailored, yet based on well-established principles (RNR) and knowledge about treatment. It is our hope that by following some of the recommendations set forth in this chapter, some of the difficulties of working to reduce the violent behaviour of others might be ameliorated.

References

Allport, G. W. (1937) *Personality: A psychological interpretation*, New York: Holt.

Andrews, D. A. (in press) 'The Risk-Need-Responsivity (RNR) model of correctional assessment and treatment', in J. Dvoskin, J. S., Skeem, R. Novaco and K. S. Douglas (eds) *Using social science to reduce crime*, New York, NY: Oxford University Press.

Andrews, D. A. and Bonta, J. (2006) *The psychology of criminal conduct* (4th ed.), Newark, NJ: LexisNexis/Matthew Bender.

— (2010) *The psychology of criminal conduct* (5th ed.), Newark, NJ: LexisNexis/Matthew Bender.

Andrews, D. A., Bonta, J. and Wormith, J. S. (2010) 'The Level of Service (LS) assessment of adults and older adolescents', in R. Otto and K. S. Douglas (eds) *Handbook of violence risk assessment* (pp. 199–225), New York, NY: Routledge/Taylor and Francis.

Barefoot v. Estelle, 463 U.S. 880 (1983).

Baxter, R. (1997) 'Violence in schizophrenia and the syndrome of disorganisation', *Criminal Behaviour and Mental Health, 7*: 131–39.

Bem, D. J. and Allen, A. (1974) 'On predicting some of the people some of the time: The search for cross-situational consistencies in behavior', *Psychological Review, 81*: 506–20.

Bjørkly, S. (2003) 'A brief commentary and a preliminary literature search concerning the role of warning signs in the treatment and prevention of intimate partner violence', *Perceptual and Motor Skills, 96*: 812–16.

Blanchard, A. J. E. (2010) *The Historical-Clinical-Risk Management – Version 3: The inclusion of idiographic relevance ratings in violence risk assessment.* Unpublished Honour's Thesis, Simon Fraser University, Burnaby, BC, Canada.

Borum, R., Bartel, P. and Forth, A. (2006) *Manual for the Structured Assessment for Violence Risk in Youth (SAVRY)*, Odessa, FL: Psychological Assessment Resources.

Borum, R., Lodewijks, H., Bartel, P. and Forth, A. (2010) 'Structured Assessment for Violence Risk in Youth (SAVRY)', in R. K. Otto and K. S. Douglas (eds) *Handbook of violence risk assessment* (pp. 63–79), New York: Routledge/Taylor and Francis Group.

Catchpole, R. E. H. and Gretton, H. M. (2003) 'The predictive validity of risk assessment with violent young offenders: A 1-year examination of criminal outcome', *Criminal Justice and Behavior, 30*: 688–708.

Cocozza, J. J. and Steadman, H. J. (1976) 'The failure of psychiatric predictions of dangerousness: Clear and convincing evidence', *Rutgers Law Review, 29*: 1084–101.

Daffern, M. and Howells, K. (2009) 'The function of aggression in personality disordered patients', *Journal of Interpersonal Violence, 24*: 586–600.

Daffern, M., Howells, K., and Ogloff, J. R. P. (2006) 'What's the point? Towards a methodology for assessing the function of psychiatric inpatient aggression', *Behaviour Research and Therapy, 45*: 101–11.

Dawes, R. M. (1979) 'The robust beauty of improper linear models in decision making', *American Psychologist, 34*: 571–82.

Dawes, R. M., Faust, D. and Meehl, P. E. (1989) 'Clinical versus actuarial judgment', *Science, 243*: 1668–74.

de Vogel, V. and de Ruiter, C. (2005) 'The HCR-20 in personality disordered female offenders: A comparison with a matched sample of males', *Clinical Psychology and Psychotherapy, 12*: 226–40.

— (2006) 'Structured professional judgment of violence risk in forensic clinical practice: A prospective study into the predictive validity of the Dutch HCR-20', *Psychology, Crime and Law, 12*: 321–36.

de Vogel, V., de Ruiter, C., Bouman, Y. and de Vries, M. (2009) *SAPROF. Guidelines for the assessment of protective factors for violence risk*, English Version, Utrecht, The Netherlands: Forum Educatief.

de Vogel, V., de Ruiter, C., van Beek, D. and Mead, G. (2004) 'Predictive validity of the SVR-20 and Static-99 in a Dutch sample of treated sex offenders', *Law and Human Behavior, 28*: 235–51.

Desmarais, S. L., Wilson, C. M., Nicholls, T. L. and Brink, J. (2010, February) *Reliability and Validity of the Short-Term Assessment of Risk and Treatability in Predicting Inpatient Aggression*, paper presented at the annual meeting of the American Psychology-Law Society, Vancouver, BC, Canada.

Douglas, K. S. (2008) 'HCR-20 for violence risk assessment', in B. L. Cutler (ed.) *Encyclopedia of psychology and law* (pp. 353–54), Thousand Oaks, CA: Sage publications.

Douglas, K. S., Blanchard, A., Guy, L. S., Reeves, K. and Weir, J. (2002–10) *HCR-20 violence risk assessment scheme: Overview and annotated bibliography* [Online]. Available: http://kdouglas.wordpress.com.

Douglas, K. S., Guy, L. S. and Hart, S. D. (2009) 'Psychosis as a risk factor for violence to others: A meta-analysis', *Psychological Bulletin, 135*: 679–706.

Douglas, K. S., Hart, S. D., Webster, C. D. and Belfrage, H. (2011) *Historical-Clinical-Risk Management: Assessing Risk for Violence* Version 3, Draft 2.0, Burnaby, British Columbia, Canada: Mental Health, Law, and Policy Institute, Simon Fraser University.

Douglas, K. S. and Kropp, P. R. (2002) 'A prevention-based paradigm for violence risk assessment: Clinical and research applications', *Criminal Justice and Behavior, 29*: 617–58.

Douglas, K. S., Nicholls, T. L. and Brink, J. (2009) 'Reducing the risk of violence among persons with mental illness: A critical analysis of treatment approaches', in P. M. Kleespies (ed.) *Behavioral emergencies: An evidence-based resource for evaluating and managing risk of suicide, violence, and victimization* (pp. 351–76), Washington, DC: American Psychological Association.

Douglas, K. S., Ogloff, J. R. P. and Hart, S. D. (2003) 'Evaluation of a model of violence risk assessment among forensic psychiatric patients', *Psychiatric Services, 54*: 1372–79.

Douglas, K. S. and Reeves, K. (2010) 'The HCR-20 violence risk assessment scheme: Overview and review of the research', in R.K. Otto and K.S. Douglas (eds) *Handbook of violence risk assessment* (pp. 147–85), New York: Routledge/Taylor and Francis Group.

Douglas, K. S. and Skeem, J. L. (2005) 'Violence risk assessment: Getting specific about being dynamic', *Psychology, Public Policy, and Law, 11*: 347–83.

Douglas, K. S., Yeomans, M. and Boer, D. P. (2005) 'Comparative validity analysis of multiple measures of violence risk in a sample of criminal offenders', *Criminal Justice and Behavior, 32*: 479–510.

Dowden, C. and Andrews, D. A. (2004) 'The importance of staff practices in delivering effective correctional treatment: A meta-analysis of core correctional practices', *International Journal of Offender Therapy and Comparative Criminology, 48*: 203–14.

Enebrink, P., Långström, N. and Gumpert, C. H. (2006) 'Predicting aggressive and disruptive behavior in referred 6- to 12-year-old boys: predictive validation of the EARL-20B risk/needs checklist', *Assessment, 13*: 356–67.

Enebrink, P., Långström, N., Hultén, A. and Gumpert, C. H. (2006) 'Swedish validation of the EARL-20B: A decision-aid for use with children presenting with conduct-disordered behaviour', *Nordic Journal of Psychiatry, 60*: 446–68.

Ennis, B. J., and Litwack, T. R. (1974). Psychiatry and the presumption of expertise: Flipping coins in the courtroom. *California Law Review, 62*: 693–752.

Fluttert, F. A. J., van Meijel, B., Nijman, H., Bjørkly, S. and Grypdonck, M. (2010) 'Preventing aggressive incidents and seclusions in forensic care by means of the "Early Recognition Method"', *Journal of Clinical Nursing, 19*: 1529–37.

Fluttert, F. A. J., van Meijel, B., Webster, C. D., Nijman, H., Bartels, A. and Grypdonck, M. (2008) 'Risk management by early recognition of warning signs in forensic psychiatric patients', *Archives of Psychiatric Nursing 22*: 208–16.

Franck, I. (1982) 'Psychology as science: Resolving the idiographic-nomothetic controversy', *Journal for the Theory of Social Behaviour, 12*: 1–20.

Grice, J. W. (2004) 'Bridging the idiographic-nomothetic divide in ratings of self and others on the big five', *Journal of Personality, 72*: 203–41.

Grove, W. M. and Meehl, P. E. (1996) 'Comparative efficiency of informal (subjective, impressionistic) and formal (mechanical, algorithmic) prediction procedures: The clinical-statistical controversy', *Psychology, Public Policy, and Law, 2*: 293–323.

Guy, L. S. (2008) *Performance indicators of the structured professional judgement approach for assessing risk for violence to others: A meta-analytic survey.* Unpublished dissertation, Simon Fraser University, Burnaby, British Columbia, Canada.

Hanson, R. K. and Harris, A. J. R. (2000) 'Where should we intervene? Dynamic predictors of sexual offence recidivism', *Criminal Justice and Behavior, 27*: 6–35.

Hart, S. D. (1998) 'The role of psychopathy in assessing risk for violence: Conceptual and methodological issues', *Legal and Criminological Psychology, 3*: 121–37.

— (2008) 'Preventing violence: The role of risk assessment and management', in A. C. Baldry and F. W. Winkel (eds) *Intimate partner violence prevention and intervention* (pp. 7–18), Nova Science Publishers, Inc.

Hart, S. D. and Boer, D. P. (2010) 'Structured professional judgment guidelines for sexual violence risk assessment: The Sexual Violence Risk-20 (SVR-20) and Risk for Sexual Violence Protocol (RSVP)' in R. Otto and K. S. Douglas (eds) *Handbook of violence risk assessment* (pp. 269–94), New York, NY: Routledge/Taylor and Francis.

Hart, S. D., Douglas, K. S. and Webster, C. D. (2001) 'Risk management using the HCR-20: A general overview focusing on historical factors', in K. S. Douglas, C. D. Webster,

S. D. Hart, D. Eaves and J. R. P. Ogloff (eds) *HCR-20 violence risk management companion guide* (pp. 27–40), Burnaby, British Columbia: Mental Health, Law, and Policy Institute, Simon Fraser University.

Hart, S. D., Kropp, P. R., Laws, D. R., Klaver, J., Logan, C. and Watt, K. A. (2003) *The Risk for Sexual Violence Protocol (RSVP): Structured professional guidelines for assessing risk of sexual violence*, Burnaby, British Columbia: Mental Health, Law, and Policy Institute, Simon Fraser University.

Hart, S. D. and Logan, C. (2011) 'Formulation of violence risk using evidence-based assessments: The structured professional judgment approach', in P. Sturmey and M. McMurran (eds) *Forensic case formulation*, Chichester: John Wiley and Sons.

Hart, S. D., Michie, C. and Cooke, D. (2007) 'The precision of actuarial risk assessment instruments: Evaluating the "margins of error" of group versus individual predictions of violence', *British Journal of Psychiatry, 190*: s60–s65.

Haynes, S. N., Mumma, G.H. and Pinson, C. (2009) 'Idiographic assessment: Conceptual and psychometric foundations of individualized behavioral assessment', *Clinical Psychology Review, 29*: 179–91.

Heilbrun, K., Douglas, K. S. and Yasuhara, K. (2009) 'Violence risk assessment: Core controversies', in J. L. Skeem, K. S. Douglas and S. O. Lilienfeld (eds) *Psychological science in the courtroom: Consensus and controversy* (pp. 333–57), New York: Guilford Publications.

Heilbrun, K., O'Neill, M. L., Stevens, T. N., Strohman, L. K., Bowman, Q. and Lo, Y. W. (2004) 'Assessing normative approaches to communicating violence risk: A national survey of psychologists', *Behavioral Sciences and the Law, 22*: 187–96.

Heilbrun, K., O'Neill, M., Strohman, L., Bowman, Q. and Philipson, J. (2000) 'Expert approaches to communicating violence risk', *Law and Human Behavior, 24*: 137–48.

Hiday, V. A. (1995) 'The social context of mental illness and violence', *Journal of Health and Social Behavior, 36*: 122–37.

— (1997) 'Understanding the connection between mental illness and violence', *International Journal of Law and Psychiatry, 20*: 399–417.

Hoge, R. D. (2010) 'Youth Level of Service/Case Management Inventory', in R. Otto and K. S. Douglas (eds) *Handbook of violence risk assessment* (pp. 81–95), New York, NY: Routledge/Taylor and Francis.

Junginger, J. (1996) 'Psychosis and violence: The case for a content analysis of psychotic experience', *Schizophrenia Bulletin, 22*: 91–103.

Kluckhohn, C. and Murray, H. A. (1953) 'Personality formulation: The determinants', in C. Kluckhohn, H. Murray and D. Schneider (eds) *Personality in nature, society and culture* (pp. 53–67), New York: Knopf.

Kraemer, H. C., Kazdin, A. E., Offord, D. R., Kessler, R. C., Jensen, P. S. and Kupfer, D. J. (1997) 'Coming to terms with the terms of risk', *Archives of General Psychiatry, 54*: 337–43.

Kropp, P. R. and Hart, S. D. (2000) 'The Spousal Assault Risk Assessment (SARA) guide: Reliability and validity in adult male offenders', *Law and Human Behavior, 24*: 101–18.

Lavoie, J. A. A. and Douglas, K. S. (2008) 'Risk assessment approaches', in B. L. Cutler (ed.) *Encyclopedia of psychology and law* (pp.698–701), Thousand Oaks, CA: Sage publications.

Lewin, K. (1936) *Principles of topological psychology*, New York: McGraw-Hill.

Lewis, G. and Doyle, M. (2009) 'Risk formulation: What are we doing and why?' *International Journal of Forensic Mental Health, 8*: 286–92.

Litwack, T. R. (2001) 'Actuarial versus clinical assessments of dangerousness', *Psychology, Public Policy, and Law, 7*: 409–43.

Melton, G. B., Petrila, J., Poythress, N. G. and Slobogin, C. (1997) *Psychological evaluations for the courts: A handbook for mental health professionals and lawyers* (2nd ed.), New York: Guilford.

— (2007) *Psychological evaluations for the courts: A handbook for mental health professionals and lawyers* (3rd ed.), New York: Guilford.

Monahan, J., Steadman, H. J., Silver, E., Appelbaum, P. S., Robbins, P. C., Mulvey, E. P., Roth, L. H., Grisso, T. and Banks, S. (2001) *Rethinking risk assessment: The MacArthur Study of mental disorder and violence*, New York: Oxford University Press.

Nikolova, N., Strub, D. S. and Douglas, K. S. (2009) 'Violence risk assessment', in C. Edwards (ed.) *Encyclopedia of forensic sciences*, Hoboken, NJ: Wiley.

Odgers, C. L., Mulvey, E. P., Skeem, J. L., Gardner, W., Lidz, C. W. and Schubert, C. (2009) 'Capturing the ebb and flow of psychiatric symptoms with dynamical systems models', *American Journal of Psychiatry, 166*: 575–82.

Otto, R. K. (2000) 'Assessing and managing violence risk in outpatient settings', *Journal of Clinical Psychology, 56*: 1239–62.

Otto, R. K. and Douglas, K. S. (eds) (2010) *Handbook of violence risk assessment tools*, New York, NY: Routledge.

Paunonen, S. V. and Jackson, D. N. (1986) 'Nomothetic and idiothetic measurement in personality', *Journal of Personality, 54*: 447–59.

Pedersen, L., Rasmussen, K. and Elsass, P. (2010) 'Risk assessment: The value of structured professional judgments', *International Journal of Forensic Mental Health, 9*: 2, 74–81.

Perkins, D. F. and Borden, L. M. (2003) 'Positive behaviors, problem behaviors, and resiliency in adolescence', in R. M. Lerner, et al. (eds) *Handbook of psychology: Developmental psychology*, Vol. 6 (pp. 373–94), Hoboken, NJ, US: John Wiley and Sons Inc.

Re Moore and the Queen, 10 C.C.C. (3d) 306 (1984).

Runyan, W. M. (1983) 'Idiographic goals and methods in the study of lives', *Journal of Personality, 51*: 413–37.

Sjöstedt, G. and Långström, N. (2002) 'Assessment of risk for criminal recidivism among rapists: A comparison of four different measures', *Psychology, Crime and Law, 8*: 25–40.

Stagner, R. (1979) 'Wundt and applied psychology', *American Psychologist, 34*: 638–39.

Tarasoff v. Regents of the University of California, 551 P2d. 334 (1976).

Viljoen, J. L., Scalora, M., Cuadra, L., Bader, S., Chávez, V., Ullman, D. and Lawrence, L. (2008) 'Assessing risk for violence in adolescents who have sexually offended: A comparison of the J-SOAP-II, J-SORRAT-II, and SAVRY', *Criminal Justice and Behavior, 35*: 5–23.

Ward, T. (2002) 'The management of risk and the design of good lives', *Australian Psychologist, 37*: 172–79.

Ward, T. and Laws, D. R. (2010) 'Desistence from sex offending: Motivating change, enriching practice', *International Journal of Forensic Mental Health, 9*: 11–23.

Webster, C. D., Douglas, K. S., Eaves, D. and Hart, S. D. (1997) *HCR-20: Assessing risk for violence*, Version 2, Burnaby, BC: Simon Fraser University.

Webster, C. D., Martin, M. L., Brink, J., Nicholls, T. L. and Middleton, C. (2004) *Manual for the Short-Term Assessment of Risk and Treatability (START)*, Version 1.0 (consultation ed.), St. Joseph's Healthcare Hamilton: Ontario, Canada–Forensic Psychiatric Services Commission: Port Coquitlam, British Columbia, Canada.

Webster, C. D., Nicholls, T. L., Martin, M. L., Desmarais, S. L. and Brink, J. (2006) 'Short-Term Assessment of Risk and Treatability (START): The case for a new structured professional judgment scheme', *Behavioral Sciences and the Law, 24*: 747–66.

Weerasekera, P. (1996) *Multi-perspective case formulation: A step towards treatment integration*, Malabar, FL: Krieger.

Wilson, C. and Douglas, K. S. (2009) 'Assessment of dangerousness', in C. Edwards (ed.) *Encyclopedia of forensic sciences*, Hoboken, NJ: Wiley.

Yang, M., Wong, S. C. P. and Coid, J. (2010) 'The efficacy of violence prediction: A meta-analytic comparison of nine risk assessment tools', *Psychological Bulletin, 136*: 740–67.

Yoshikawa, K. and Taylor, P. J. (2003) 'Editorial: New forensic mental health law in Japan', *Criminal Behaviour and Mental Health, 13*: 225–28.

3 Working with complex cases

Mental disorder and violence

Lorraine Johnstone

Introduction

At its simplest level, violence refers to a wilful or reckless act perpetrated by one person that is likely to result in harm – physical or psychological – to another individual. This can involve 'actual, attempted or threatened harm' (Webster, Eaves, Douglas and Hart, 1997, p.24). However, an analysis of violence reveals that it is far from simple. Violence varies across type, nature of association between victim and perpetrator, severity, motivation, frequency, imminence and likelihood. Violence is a complex phenomenon. In contemporary society, violence is a major social ill with far reaching, diverse and often devastating consequences. Violence accounts for a significant cause of injury and premature death across all ages. Violence is a major public health problem (World Health Organization, 2002). Faced with this harsh reality, the practice of violence risk assessment is now embedded in criminal justice and forensic mental health practice. Violence risk assessment refers to 'the process of evaluating individuals to (1) characterize the likelihood that they will commit acts of violence and (2) develop interventions to manage or reduce that likelihood' (Hart, 1998, p. 122).

When it comes to assessing violence risk, it would be reasonable to argue that all cases are complex. That said, few if any practitioners would dispute that the following cases are anything but *the* most challenging:

Andrew, who almost killed his brother in the context of an acute psychosis and who has perpetrated multiple acts of violence, across multiple contexts, towards multiple victims, and who has a primary diagnosis of paranoid schizophrenia and a secondary diagnosis of antisocial personality disorder, all in the context of a history of substance abuse and a raft of criminogenic risk factors;

Albert, a promising university student who killed an acquaintance without any apparent motivation (or provocation), in the context of no known history of violence, a complete absence of criminogenic factors, intoxication, or indeed, any other overt risk factors but who suffers from narcissistic personality disorder; and

Gina, who has an appalling childhood abuse history, chronic post-traumatic stress disorder with dissociative symptoms, a long-standing pattern of drug abuse and who attempted to murder her boyfriend and his brother in a ferocious and sustained attack, an event for which she accepts responsibility but claims no memory.

But why are these cases so complex?

One reason they are so complex is that each of the individuals described above suffers from at least one mental disorder or psychopathology that may – or may not – provide some explanatory function for their violence. The extent to which mental disorder is, or is not, relevant to violence has been the subject of a long-standing and controversial debate. Conceptual and methodological confusions pervade the field and, of those conditions that show a statistical link, little is known about why, how or for whom this association exists (Douglas, et al., 2009; Duggan and Howard, 2009; Hart, Sturmey, Logan and McMurran, 2011). As such, risk assessment protocols not only vary, but are contradictory, in terms of how much weight they assign to mental disorder psychopathology. There are many barriers to achieving a robust and reliable risk assessment in those suffering from a mental disorder whereby the relevance of symptoms and traits are properly understood and explained.

Aims and overview

The purpose of this chapter is to explore the link between mental disorder and violence, with the objective of giving the practitioner a framework for making sense of mental disorder in the context of violence risk assessment. Consideration is given to the following key questions: to what extent is mental disorder linked to violence; what is the nature of the link; and how can assessors ensure an appropriate assessment and understanding of symptoms when conducting violence risk assessments? The chapter begins with a brief review of the main findings from the extant literature examining the link between mental disorder and violence. Next, some of the key challenges to understanding this association are explained. Then, options available for assessing violence risk in mentally disordered offenders are described. In keeping with the theme of this book, the structured professional judgement (SPJ) approach is presented as the most appropriate framework for conducting violence risk assessment. Building on the guidelines articulated by Douglas and colleagues (this volume) and other recent developments (Hart and Logan, 2011; Hart, et al., 2011), readers will learn that formulation is a critical stage in the assessment process when dealing with complex cases. Because no single etiological theory of violence or mental disorder exists, risk formulation provides a viable method of understanding the essential features of a person's symptoms and risk in a manner likely to inform and contribute to effective risk management. A case example is used to illustrate how a pragmatically grounded formulation using the 'four Ps' framework may facilitate an understanding of the relevance of mental disorder to violence risk. The chapter closes with some recommendations for future research and theorizing as well as some key points for practice.

Violence and mental disorder: what is the link?

What is a mental disorder?

A mental disorder refers to a 'clinically significant behavioural or psychological syndrome or pattern that occurs in an individual and that is associated with present distress (e.g., a painful syndrome) or disability (i.e., impairment in one or more important areas of functioning) or with significantly increased risk of suffering death, pain, disability or an important loss of freedom' (American Psychiatric Association, 1994, p.xxi). Two formal nosological systems – the *Diagnostic and Statistical Manual of Mental Disorders 4th Edition* (DSM-IV; American Psychiatric Association [APA], 1994) and the *International Classification of Diseases 10th Edition* (ICD-10; World Health Organization, 1994) – exist to facilitate the reliable assessment and diagnosis of each condition. In each system, a set of criteria and symptoms are specified for achieving a diagnosis.

There are many different types of disorders – for example, anxiety disorders, mood/affective disorders, schizophrenia and other psychoses, substance-use disorders, sexual and gender identity disorders, and personality disorder. Some conditions reflect an acute form of psychological disturbance that marks a significant and observable departure from the person's usual presentation (e.g., mood, anxiety and psychotic disorders), whereas others (e.g., sexual deviation) characterize the person's typical way of being and there are few, if any, outwardly apparent or overt symptoms of dysfunction. Outside the formal psychiatric categories, there are other forms of psychopathology that are generally accepted by practitioners and researchers as meaningful constructs. Psychopathic personality disorder (PPD), as operationalized by Hare in the *Psychopathy Checklist-Revised* (PCL-R; Hare, 1991; 2003) and more recently by Cooke, Hart, Logan and Michie in the *Comprehensive Assessment of Psychopathic Personality* (see http://www.gcu.ac.uk/capp/developers/index.html), is an important example.

Is mental disorder a risk factor for violence?

For mental disorder to have any explanatory function in violence risk assessment, there must be evidence to support its role as a putative risk factor. Establishing causality is difficult: Arboleda-Florez, et al. (1998) explained, 'any attempt to outline specific causal criteria must be tempered by the knowledge that philosophers have been absorbed by this question for centuries' (p. 39). Nevertheless, it is important to pursue this issue. Based on the work of Haynes (1992), Duggan and Howard (2009) have accepted that, for a variable such as mental disorder to be accepted as a causal risk factor, the following conditions must be met:

> (1) covariation between variables, i.e., there needs to be an association between the predictor and outcome variables; (2) temporal precedence, i.e., mental disorder must precede violence; (3) exclusion of an alternative, i.e., no

other explanation (or variable) can account for the association between the mental disorder and violence; and (4) logical connection, i.e., there must be a clear rationale for expecting mental disorder and violence to be linked. The extent to which these conditions have been satisfied in terms of mental disorder is addressed below.

Covaration between mental disorder and violence

On reviewing the extant literature, it is apparent that a number of mental disorders show a statistical association with violence. An overview of the main findings is presented below.

SCHIZOPHRENIA AND PSYCHOSIS

Schizophrenia is a mental illness characterized by a particularly severe and debilitating combination of symptoms, including some or all of the following: hallucinations, delusions, disorganized thoughts, speech and behaviour, social withdrawal, and emotional blunting. McMurran, et al. (2009) noted that while most people with schizophrenia *do not* commit violence, there is an elevated risk of violence – around four to ten times – in this population. Individuals suffering from a comorbid alcohol or substance-use problem and/or personality disorder are most at risk. In a recent meta-analysis designed to explore the link between psychosis (linked to any form of major mental illness) and violence, Douglas, et al. (2009) confirmed this finding. Psychosis was reliably and significantly associated with a 49 per cent to 68 per cent increase in violence risk. In terms of the nature of the violence, individuals suffering from psychosis tended to behave violently towards family members (Arboleda-Florez, et al., 1998; Douglas, et al., 2009). Others have reported that the type of symptomatology is relevant: where command hallucinations and delusions are present, the risk of violence is significantly increased (Fazel, Gulati, Linsell, et al., 2009; Taylor, 1998). Furthermore, O'Reilly, Marshall, Carr and Beckett (2004) summarized the available research and confirmed an association between psychosis and sexual offending.

AFFECTIVE/MOOD DISORDERS

Affective/mood disorders refers to a range of conditions where the person suffers a serious disturbance in their mood. Unipolar depression or major depression involves a significant lowering of mood alongside some or all of the following symptoms: loss of interest and pleasure, lack of energy, appetite and sleep disturbance, cognitive difficulties (e.g., impaired concentration and attention), psychomotor agitation or retardation, feelings of worthlessness, hopelessness, despair and guilt, and thoughts of death and suicide. Bipolar depression is characterized by fluctuating mood. Periods of major depression are accompanied by periods of mania where the clinical presentation is one of elevated or irritable mood co-occurring with symptoms such as: inflated self-esteem or grandiosity, reduced need for sleep, excessive talkativeness, flight of ideas or racing thoughts, distractibility, agitation, and excessive involvement in pleasurable activities. (Psychotic symptoms can be a feature of both unipolar and bipolar disorders.) There is a positive association between mood disorders and violence. Dell and Smith (1983) and Taylor (1986) found affective disorders in a significant proportion (3 to 37 per cent) of people charged with or convicted of murder. In a follow-up study by Hodgins, Lapalmec and Toupin (1999), 33 per cent of patients with a major affective disorder were more likely to have perpetrated a violent offence after two years (although substance use influenced the level of violence risk). Gonzalez-Ortega, Mosquera, Echebura and Gonzales-Pinto (2010) reported that 40 per cent of inpatients suffering from mania engaged in aggressive and violent behaviours. Research has also documented an association with mood disorder and sexual violence (Kafka and Prentky, 1994; Raymond, et al., 1999).

POST-TRAUMATIC STRESS DISORDER (PTSD)

PTSD is an impairment that occurs following exposure to a traumatic event, during which the person directly experiences or observes actual or threatened death or serious injury to either themselves or others. Symptoms can include recurrent and intrusive images and dreams, re-experiencing the traumatic event, intense psychological distress, physiological reactivity, inability to recall aspects of the trauma, diminished interest in activities, feelings of detachment or estrangement from others, restricted range of affect, sense of foreshortened future, sleep problems, irritability and anger, difficulties concentrating, hypervigilance, and active attempts to avoid thinking, talking or being exposed to reminders of the event. There is a link between post-traumatic stress disorder and violence. This has been reported in cases of domestic violence (Parrott, Drobes, Saladin, Coffey and Dansky, 2003; Sippela and Marshall, 2011) and in the violence perpetrated by war veterans (McFall, Fontana, Riskind and Rosenheck, 1999; Lasko, Gurvitis, Kuhne, Orr and Pitman, 1994; see also Marham, this volume).

DISSOCIATIVE DISORDERS

Dissociative disorders are characterized by a 'disruption in the usually integrated functions of consciousness, memory, identity, or perception of the environment' (APA, p. 477). There are four different dissociative disorders: (1) dissociative amnesia, which refers to a condition whereby the person is unable to recall personal details, often involving past trauma or distressing events; (2) dissociative identity disorder (DID), which refers to a phenomenon whereby the person has at least two different and distinct identities; (3) dissociative fugue, which is a condition whereby an individual will suddenly travel away from their home or place of work, have an inability to recall their past, be confused about who they are and may assume a new identity; and (4) depersonalization disorder, which refers to a condition whereby the person experiences chronic feelings of detachment from their own mental processes and/or their body but is, at the same time, able to engage in appropriate reality testing. In a review of the literature, Moskowitz (2004) examined the relationship between dissociation and violence and found research documenting significant levels of dissociative disorders among violent offenders. He estimated that between 6 and 21 per cent of adult violent and sex offenders suffered DID and between 14 and 39 per cent suffered from any dissociative disorder. Moskowitz (2004) also noted high rates of DID and dissociative disorders in adolescents, with figures reportedly being 28.3 per cent and 14.3 per cent respectively. However, Moskowitz cautioned that these figures likely reflected an underestimate of the true prevalence of this disorder among violent offenders, as detection rates among samples were low.

PERSONALITY DISORDERS

A personality disorder refers to an 'enduring pattern of inner experience and behaviour that deviates markedly from the expectations of the individual's culture, is pervasive and inflexible, has an onset in adolescence or early adulthood, is stable over time, and leads to distress or impairment' (APA, p. 629). There are several different forms of personality disorder. The DSM-IV differentiates between clusters A, B and C. Cluster A refers to disorders where the prominent features are odd or eccentric behaviours. Paranoid personality disorder, schizoid personality disorder and schizotypal personality disorder are included in this category. Cluster B refers to those conditions where the prominent features include a dramatic and flamboyant presentation and includes antisocial personality disorder, borderline personality disorder, histrionic personality disorder and narcissistic personality disorder. Cluster C refers to conditions where the main presentation involves anxiety and fearfulness and includes avoidant personality disorder, dependent personality disorder, and obsessive-compulsive personality disorder. The ICD-10 conceptualizes personality disorders in a similar manner. There is a sizeable literature demonstrating a link between personality disorder and violence (see Logan and Johnstone, 2010). Several studies are mentioned below to provide some illustrative examples.

Antisocial personality disorder was observed to increase the odds ratio of homicidal violence tenfold in men and fiftyfold in women, in a study by Eronen, Tiihonen, and Hakola, et al. (1996). Borderline personality disorder has been shown to be related to intimate-partner violence (Critchfield, et al., 2007) and explosive and impulsive violence (Baros and de Pádua Serafim, 2008). Psychopathy is linked (albeit with small to moderate effect sizes) to all forms of serious violence (Hart and Dempster, 1997; Hart and Hare, 1997; Hart, et al., 2003; Porter and Woodworth, 2006; Salekin, Rogers and Sewell, 1996) and narcissistic personality disorder also, though more tenuously (Logan, 2009; Warren and South, 2009). Finally, Jamieson and Taylor (2004), in a 12-year follow-up of 204 patients discharged from high-secure forensic psychiatric facilities, reported that the odds of committing a serious reoffence were seven times higher for those with a personality disorder diagnosis compared to those with a mental illness diagnosis alone.

SUBSTANCE-USE DISORDERS

Substance-use disorder refers to a condition where the person engages in a maladaptive pattern of drug and/or alcohol use that leads to clinically significant impairment or distress. Symptoms include excessive use, tolerance, withdrawal effects, and clinical and social dysfunction in important areas such as social, occupational or recreational activities. Substance-use disorders show a significant association with violence. They are related to sexual violence (Abracen, Looman and Anderson, 2000), homicide (Putkonen, et al., 2004; Violence Reduction Unit, 2006), domestic abuse (Klostermann and Fals-Stewart, 2006), and gang-related violence (Violence Reduction Unit, 2006). Furthermore, the transport and supply of drugs is a feature of organized criminality and violence.

SEXUAL DEVIATION/PARAPHILIAS

Paraphilias are characterized by 'recurrent, intense sexual urges, fantasies, or behaviours that involve unusual objects, activities, or situations and cause clinically significant distress or impairment in social, occupational or other important areas of functioning' (APA, 1994, p.493). By definition, some of the sexual deviations are violent *viz-a-viz* exhibitionism, paedophilia, sexual sadism, and sexual masochism. In these instances, sexual deviation may serve as the main driver for violent behaviour. In those rare but extreme cases involving predatory sexual homicide, sexual sadism is often a prominent feature, with the violent act resulting in sexual gratification (Kirsch and Becker, 2007; Knoll and Hazelwood, 2009; see also Russell and Darjee, this volume).

PERVASIVE DEVELOPMENTAL DISORDERS

Pervasive developmental disorders are characterized by 'severe and pervasive deficits and impairments across multiple areas of development, such as reciprocal social interaction and communication, which occur in the presence of stereotyped behaviour, interests and activities' (DSM-IV, APA, p. 38). Autistic and Asperger's disorder are included in this category. Considering the relationship between pervasive developmental disorder and violence, most of the literature has focused on Asperger's syndrome and autism. The findings are inconclusive. Touhami, Ouriaghli and Manoudi, et al. (2011) and Farmer and Aman (2001) reported an increased likelihood of violence as well as covert and verbal aggression in those with autism, while Bjørkly (2009) found that there was no stable or consistent link between autism and violence.

Conceptual and methodological limitations and implications for practice

Based on the above review, there is evidence to suggest that some forms of mental disorder are associated with violence, and the relationship seems to hold across design, samples (inpatients, outpatients, community samples and prison populations), and methods of measurement (e.g., official statistics, case notes, formal records, self-report). However, there are major limitations with the extant research. First, there is a dearth of studies examining the full range of mental disorders and violence. Investigators have tended to focus on psychosis and schizophrenia (Blaumenthal and Levander, 2000; Douglas, et al., 2009) or cluster B and psychopathic personality disorders. However, as others have noted, absence of evidence is not evidence of absence. There are important implications associated with the dearth of good research: practitioners might adopt an empiricist standpoint. They may simply fail to consider the broad set of psychopathology when conducting an evaluation or, even if a disorder is identified, the knowledge that there is no known statistical link or that the findings are equivocal might result in the clinician dismissing the condition as irrelevant. On both counts, the result could be an unreliable and misleading assessment. Second, it is unclear whether particular symptoms, constellations of symptoms, intensity of symptoms, level of severity, extent of impairment associated with symptoms, pattern of relapse, and so on are more or less relevant to violence. Indeed, we know very little about what actually accounts for the statistical link.

Third, many seriously violent offenders do not fit neatly into any particular typology of violence or maintain absolute fidelity to one type of conduct. Those who perpetrate harmful acts are a heterogeneous group. Despite some apparent assumptions that offenders specialize (Kunelsman, 2001; Schwaner, 1998, 2000), 'exclusives'[1] as they are referred to by Loucks (2002), are in fact rare. For example, men who have convictions for violent offending often have a history of domestic violence (Cadksy and Crawford, 1988; Campbell, Webster, Koziol-McLain, et al., 2003; Hilton, et al., 2001, 2004; Kropp, 2009). Research has also documented an association between spousal assault, sexual assault, and stalking (Home Office, 2004), and sexual offenders often have a history of violent offending (Prentky, Knight and Lee, 1997; Rasmussen, 1999). Also, there are some rare cases where a person's violent conduct is so unusual (or bizarre) that their acts could be considered idiopathic. Examples would include apparently 'motiveless murders' (Burgess, Hartman, Ressler, Douglas and McCormack, 1986), filicide, matricide, patricide, infanticide, lust-murder, and so on. There is very little evidence in the literature to suggest that attempts have been made to fully explore the specificity of effects and the nature of the relationship between mental disorder pathologies, symptoms, and constellations of symptoms, and violence types (although see Green, Schramm, Chiu, McVie and Hay, 2009, who found that Capgras delusions and command hallucinations were associated with homicide, and that threat-control override symptoms and grandiose delusions were associated with assault). Consequently, Elbogen and Johnson (2009) observed that

> ... empirical studies often combine all violent acts into one composite variable owing to limited statistical power to distinguish specific forms of violent acts ... leaving unanswered the question of whether mental illness predicts some kinds of violence but not others (e.g., substance-related violence).
>
> Elbogen and Johnson (2009, p. 153)

CONCLUDING COMMENTS

While covariation among some forms of mental disorder and violence has been reported in the literature, the extent to which mental disorder has status as a putative risk factor cannot be established from these findings. We need to consider the other criteria.

Temporal precedence

In terms of 'temporal precedence', it is very difficult to be precise regarding the date of onset of a mental disorder, or for that matter violence. For example, prodromal phases are common in schizophrenia, and conduct disorder in childhood is a prerequisite for a diagnosis of antisocial personality disorder (ASPD). Furthermore, other disorders are often invisible to even the most expert of clinicians (*viz.* dissociation) and diagnoses made only after an act of violence has brought the person to the attention of the authorities. It is therefore difficult to ascertain, with any degree of certainty, which came first. Furthermore, most human beings have to unlearn aggressive behaviour. Taking a developmental perspective, toddlers are notoriously naughty – biting, kicking and hair pulling are all part of the territory for the 'terrible twos'. Thus, we have a real chicken-and-egg conundrum to disentangle if other mechanisms, such as social learning, poor parenting, and so on, are to be discounted. McMurran, et al. (2009) illustrated this when she explained how a diverse set of phenomena might explain the association between schizophrenia and violence. She drew attention to the fact that variables such as developmental problems, conduct problems and substance abuse often predate the onset of psychoses, and that all of these variables are also known risk factors for violence.

CONCLUDING COMMENTS

Disentangling symptoms of mental disorder (and violent behavioural problems) and then accurately locating the onset of dysfunction remains a difficult task. Temporal precedence is not yet established.

Exclusion of an alternative third variable

When it comes to understanding the relationship between mental disorder and violence, it is virtually impossible to exclude a third variable. Note Rutter's point:

> There is abundant evidence that, with rare exceptions, mental disorders are multifactorial in origin – meaning an interplay among multiple environmental and multiple genetic influences. Moreover, the particular pattern or interplay will vary among individuals.
>
> Rutter (2011, p. 648)

Furthermore, comorbidity in mental disorders is common across all groups – adult, juvenile, male, female, prisoner or patient populations (Blackburn, Logan,

Donnelly and Renwick, 2003; Coid, Kahtan, Gault and Jarman, 1999; Duggan and Howard, 2009; Eaves, Tien and Wilson, 2000). For example, mood disorders are associated with substance use, and heavy alcohol consumption may be associated with depression and mania, as well as aggressive and violent behaviour (Eaves, Tien and Wilson, 2000). Taylor (1998) found that more than half of offenders with personality disorder had more than one diagnosis and around 20 per cent of psychotic offenders had a personality disorder. Furthermore, studies have reported an additive effect of comorbidity. For example, Dean, Walsh and Moran (2006) concluded that personality disorder with mental illness appears more predictive of future violence. Thus, it is very difficult to ascertain primacy to one difficulty or disorder over another.

Notwithstanding the covariation among mental disorders, acute and chronic forms of mental disturbance also correlate with other known risk factors for violence (Monahan and Steadman, 1983). Indeed, the concerns exposed as a result of this fact led to a reasoning that it was these criminogenic risk factors and not mental disorder per se that accounted for the observed association with violence. This would seem an erroneous conclusion. It is neither necessary nor sufficient to have criminogenic risk factors for violent behaviour to occur. Mental state is relevant.

There is also the problem with the tautological nature of the link. Various authors have illustrated the point using antisocial personality disorder as an example. Given that aggressiveness is a diagnostic feature of the condition, it is little surprise that violence is associated with this group (Blaumenthal and Levander, 2000; McMurran, et al., 2009). The same argument applies to other conditions (see Skeem and Cooke, 2010, for an informative discussion on how this relates to psychopathy). This tautology in terms of diagnoses and aetiology is a serious problem. According to Arboleda-Florez, et al. (1998):

> Confounding by definition seriously mars any causal inferences that could be made based on empirical evidence showing a statistical association between mental illness and violence. By embedding etiologic inferences in diagnostic formulations we seriously undermine our ability to conduct risk factor studies.
>
> Arboleda-Florez, et al. (1998, p. 41)

CONCLUDING COMMENTS

Confounding definitions in mental disorder and violence, comorbidity among disorders, and multifarious confounding variables in terms of criminogenic factors, do much to confuse the picture. Third variables are not yet fully excluded.

Logical connection

In terms of 'logical connection', as mentioned above, this requires a definitive statement of how and in what way the variable leads to the outcome – in this case how mental disorder leads to violence. To date, no such definitive statement exists, although some suggestions have been made for some symptoms. For example,

Eaves, Tien and Wilson (2000), on discussing mania, explained that violence could follow on from feelings of irritability or anger when the person, who has grandiose delusions, is challenged, thwarted or feels undermined in some way. Similarly, another well-known example (although debated) of symptom-level explanations is the use of the threat-control override (TCO) symptoms of schizophrenia to explain psychotically driven violence (e.g., Link and Stueve, 1994). TCO symptoms may result in the patient believing that external factors are in control of them and that, within that context, their violence is both logical and rational. To illustrate: a person suffering from a delusional belief that he is the son of God and his father is the devil will have some 'logic' for perpetrating violence towards his father as he will likely believe that his father is his enemy intent on harming him. However, these propositions are fairly blunt and, as indicated above, lack specificity or depth of explanation. Logan and Johnstone (2010) have also offered several hypotheses to explain the link between personality disorder and violence.

CONCLUDING COMMENTS

While there are theoretically consistent explanations of why various symptoms might drive, destabilize or disinhibit a person's violence risk, as it stands at present, the field does not have access to a definitive theory of mental disorder or of violence. The logical connection is a tenuous one.

Overall conclusion

In sum, a range of mental disorders show a statistical link to violence but a full understanding of the nature of the relationship evades us. There is a pressing need to conduct robust and systematic research into all of the mental disorders and violence in an attempt to establish the existence (and strength) of any associations. Studies must control, as far as possible, for the myriad of confounding (and confusing) factors that currently muddy the waters. In addition, research and theory-building is needed to explain the nature and direction of the relationships. Not only will the resolution to these issues take sophisticated and continuous theorizing, hypothesis testing, and research, it will also take time. Of course, that is of little consolation to both patients and clinicians who currently face the challenge of understanding and managing mental disorder and violence risk. How then can assessors ensure an appropriate assessment and understanding of mental disorder when conducting violence risk assessments? This is the subject of the next section.

Assessing and understanding mental disorder in violence risk assessment

There are three main approaches to violence risk assessment: (1) the unstructured clinical judgement approach; (2) the actuarial risk assessment approach; and (3) the structured professional judgement (or SPJ) approach. Suffice it to say, the SPJ approach is accepted as best practice. While there are many papers and chapters dedicated to evidencing this position, less information exists to guide practitioners on the mechanics of the process, and there is a lack of detailed guidance on how to deal with the issue of mental disorder specifically. As such, in the section that follows, key considerations and recommendations are made for the purposes of assisting practitioners to work within the confines and constraints of the extant knowledge base regarding mental disorder. Before describing these stages, and for the sake of completeness, the main limitations undermining the utility of the other methods for assessing and understanding mentally disordered offenders are briefly mentioned. Because the pros and cons of each of these methods has been the topic of much research, discussion and debate (see Otto and Douglas, 2010, also Douglas, et al. and Cooke and Michie, this volume), it is unnecessary to reiterate or rehearse the arguments again in detail.

Unstructured clinical judgement

The unstructured clinical judgement method is used to predict who is most likely to perpetrate acts of harm. This approach refers to a process of risk assessment in which the evaluation is conducted at the discretion of the assessor and relies on their experience and skill. This type of assessment occurs in the absence of any formal structure or system and, as such, is highly variable in approach. While advocates point to the person-centeredness, flexibility, and time-effectiveness of these methods, they have been heavily criticized for their lack of transparency and consistency and for their highly unsatisfactory levels of reliability and validity (Borum 1996; Grove and Meehl 1996). There is consensus among experts – both clinical and legal – that this is a highly inappropriate and indefensible method for reaching an opinion about risk. This approach should not be used when assessing violence risk in mentally disordered offenders.

Actuarial risk assessment

At the other end of the continuum, actuarial risk assessment (e.g., Hanson and Thornton, 1999; Quinsey, Harris, Rice and Cormier, 1998) exists to impose a systematic and consistent structure around risk assessment. This method is highly organized and provides an easy-to-follow process for scoring a set of risk factors derived from theory or research. Actuarial risk assessment is concerned with risk prediction and uses mathematical models for predicting likelihood of recidivism over a given period. Derived from statistical or theoretical frameworks, it has been praised for its face validity, its transparent and conceptually appealing process, as well as its easy-to-use method of assessing risk. Actuarial assessment tools are commonly used. However, they have serious limitations, including an emphasis on static risk factors, a lack of emphasis on risk management, poor generalizability, and the use of a mechanistic process that disengages the practitioner from the client, and eliminates relevant knowledge and expertise in reaching a judgement (Department of Health, 2007; Douglas and Kropp, 2002). Furthermore, they lack specificity in the individual case and fail to provide any predictive validity beyond a group average (Cooke, 2010; Cooke and Michie, this volume; Hart, Cooke and Michie, 2007).

Considering their utility for assessing mentally disordered individuals, many of the more widely used actuarial risk assessment tools do not reflect the extant literature. For example, the *Violence Risk Appraisal Guide* (VRAG; Quinsey, Harris, Rice, et al., 1998), one of the most widely used actuarial tools for violence prediction, argues that schizophrenia is negatively associated with risk and no other acute forms of mental disorder are included in this protocol. Thus, applied to a mentally disordered population and particularly cases with low base-rate psychopathology such as rare forms of mental disorder, an actuarial risk assessment such as the VRAG might yield highly misleading opinions. In sum, actuarial tools provide an unsatisfactory alternative to the unstructured approach and lack utility in assessing violence risk in mentally disordered populations.

Structured professional judgement

The SPJ approach reflects a conceptual shift away from predicting dangerousness to managing risk. It is an evidence-based approach to risk assessment (Hart and Logan, 2011). SPJ retains the strengths of both the clinical and actuarial approaches in that it is grounded in empirical research but, crucially, it allows the clinician to exercise discretion and professional judgement. The reliability and validity of this approach is well established (see Douglas, et al., this volume). The approach requires the assessor to follow a series of stages to ensure a systematic, robust and individualized evaluation of a person's level and nature of risk. Central to the SPJ paradigm is decision theory. According to decision theory, a person ultimately will 'choose' whether or not to perpetrate a violent act after considering the probable outcomes of their behaviour and, at some level, deciding this is the most effective method of achieving their preferred outcome at that point in time. However, in terms of violent conduct, these decisions will be influenced by a multitude of individual, relational, and contextual factors, thus the SPJ demands a comprehensive and detailed analysis at each of these levels. The steps involved are described in the preceding chapter by Douglas and colleagues and elsewhere (see also Hart, et al., 2003) and they include: (1) background history; (2) risk factor ratings of presence *and* relevance; (3) risk formulation and scenario planning; (4) risk management planning; and (5) summary judgements. (The SPJ approach is illustrated in Figure 3.1.) Specific issues concerning the assessment and understanding of mental disorder and violence within the SPJ approach are explained below.

Background history

As with all forms of assessment, a comprehensive history-taking exercise constitutes an essential first step. It is only by conducting a detailed examination of the person's development, family history, educational and occupational history, interpersonal and relationship functioning, substance use, physical and mental health, as well as their forensic and violence histories, that risk factors and risks

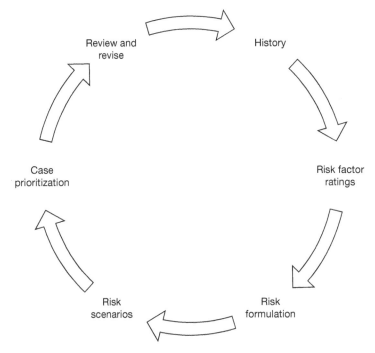

Figure 3.1 The structured professional judgement paradigm

can be identified. In order to reach an opinion about mental disorder and violence, interviews and testing of the offender will be required, as will interviews with families, friends and other collateral informants. There should also take place discussions with professionals who have knowledge of the case (e.g., psychiatrists, social workers, nurses) and a review of records is fundamental, including case-notes, legal documentation, victim statements, court judgements, social, health and educational records. It is critical to gather information from a range of sources to ensure that, if mental-disorder symptoms are present in the case, the nature, onset, course and duration of disorder and difficulties are identified. Assessors should use timelines to facilitate the temporal sequencing of dysfunction – and to disentangle the proverbial chicken from the egg.

Risk factors

In the next stage, assessors are required to consider the extent to which the known risk factors for violence occur in the case being evaluated. Several manualized guidelines exist to facilitate this process and assessors should select one or more to guide their assessment. Protocols exist for assessing interpersonal violence (i.e., the *Historical Clinical Risk-20* or HCR-20, Webster, et al., 1997), sexual violence (the *Sexual Violence Risk-20* or SVR-20; Boer, Hart, Kropp, et al., 1997; the *Risk for Sexual Violence Protocol* or RSVP; Hart, et al., 2003), spousal assault (the

Spousal Assault Risk Assessment or SARA; Kropp and Gibas, 2010), and stalking (the *Stalking Assessment Manual* or SAM; Kropp, et al., 2008). Furthermore, when assessing mental disorder, and in particular acute forms of dysfunction, the *Short Term Assessment of Risk and Treatability* (START; Webster, Martin, Brink, et al., 2004) is an important protocol. It is important to emphasize, however, that these tools do not equate with a risk assessment. Each of these protocols includes only a minimum set of risk factors to be considered. Assessors should select those that match the violence that has occurred in the case under consideration.

Assessing mental disorder

The assessment of mental disorder is an essential part of violence risk assessment. For example, judgements about mental disorder are relevant to many risk factors in the HCR-20 (e.g., H6 'major mental illness', H7 'psychopathy', H9 'personality disorder', C1 'lack of insight', C3 'negative attitudes', C4 'impulsivity', C5 'unresponsive to treatment') and in the RSVP (e.g., item 11 'sexual deviance', item 12 'psychopathic personality disorder', and item 13 'major mental illness').

There are some specific issues with regard to assessing mental disorder. First, assessors must possess the requisite competencies in psycho-diagnosis. Assessors must be able – and legally entitled – to assess both violence and mental disorder. In most jurisdictions, this will fall to psychiatrists and clinical psychologists. Practitioners must have a core training and knowledge base that enables them to recognize and diagnose acute and chronic forms of psychopathology. In some settings, this might be optimally achieved by working in a multi-disciplinary team setting where mental health professionals are able to contribute this information. Where a professional conducting a risk assessment is not a diagnostician, Hart and colleagues have indicated that it is permissible for assessors to (a) assess mental disorder under supervision from a qualified colleague; (b) refer to findings reported by others; (c) rate risk factors provisionally and have these confirmed by a qualified colleague; or (d) omit the items and state this limitation in their overall opinion (Hart, et al., 2003, pp. 21–22).

Second, assessors should utilize standardized protocols. In terms of assessing mental disorder, the SPJ manuals recommend the use of guidelines such as the *International Personality Disorder Examination* (IPDE; Loranger, 1999), the *Psychopathy Checklist Revised* (PCL-R; Hare, 1991, 2003), and the *Structured Clinical Interview for DSM-IV Axis I and Axis II Disorders* (SCID-I and II; First, Spitzer, Gibbon, et al., 1994; 1997). Procedures such as the Wechsler Scales (Wechsler, 2008) would be appropriate for assessing cognitive impairment and protocols such as the *Diagnostic Interview for Social and Communication Disorder* (DISCO; Leekam, Libby, Wing, Gould and Taylor, 2002; Wing, Leekam, Libby, Gould and Larcombe, 2002) for assessing autistic spectrum disorders. Notwithstanding the ongoing debate about the construct, classification and diagnosis of mental disorder per se (Rutter, 2011), structured protocols are recommended to enhance the reliability and consistency in reaching diagnoses and drawing comparisons across groups. (It is important to reiterate here that these protocols also exist to structure – not determine – diagnoses; clinical skill is paramount to the process.) The position is stated as follows by Loranger (1999):

> The IPDE presupposes a thorough familiarity with either the DSM-IV or ICD-10 classification systems of mental disorders, as well as considerable training and experience in making psychiatric diagnoses. As is true of any semi-structured clinical interview, the reliability and validity of the IPDE are inseparable from the qualifications and training of the person using it. It is designed for experienced psychiatrists, clinical psychologists, and those with comparable training who are capable of making independent psychiatric diagnoses without a semi-structured interview.
>
> Loranger (1999, p. 8)

Third, categorical and dimensional models should be used. A further advantage of using standardized protocols is that this proffers the opportunity for the analysis and documenting of both categorical and dimensional models of psychopathology. While categorical models enable comparisons to be drawn from other individuals with the same diagnoses, dimensional models allow the evaluator to summarize symptom-level information, thereby reducing the concerns and complexities associated with comorbidity (Blaumenthal and Levander, 2000). Symptom-level analyses are likely to be far more informative and comprehensive in terms of informing risk assessment and management than simply reaching a view as to whether or not a diagnostic threshold has been achieved. By considering each symptom in turn, the nature, individual expression, and relevance of the trait or symptom to risk and risk management will be more apparent. To illustrate: psychosis for one person might result in a delusional belief system whereby they believe they are the Son of God, whose purpose in life is to spread peace to all – for this person, violence might be unlikely. For another person, who also believes he is the Son of God, his particular delusion might be that his task is to rid the world of sinners and he may thereby plan and plot to perpetrate mass killing. Violence is more of a possibility in the second scenario. In addition, for each disorder and symptom per se, the onset, course, severity, stability and treatability should be examined. It is likely that with such detailed analyses, key information about the possible links to violence, priority for treatment, and likely response to intervention, will be better understood and thereby managed.

Fourth, a comprehensive differential diagnosis is critical. It is vital that those conducting risk assessments are able to engage in the process of differential diagnosis. Many disorders share the same overt symptoms. Thus, it is essential that evaluators are aware of the nuances and aetiological theories for various disorders to ensure an accurate diagnosis. Furthermore, because the bulk of research has concentrated on the relationship between psychosis and personality disorders, there is a possibility that assessors might fail to consider other diagnoses. O'Rourke's chapter (this volume) underscores the need for comprehensive assessments of cognitive functioning. The consequences of misdiagnoses can be catastrophic. Indeed, Maden observed that in homicide inquiries, schizophrenia was often misdiagnosed as antisocial personality disorder (Maden, 2007). Similarly, a person with neurological impairment might also be vulnerable to receiving a personality-disorder diagnosis, especially if they are a poor historian, give inconsistent information and confabulate.

Finally, consideration must be given to low base rate/case-specific psychopathologies. Related to the above, assessors must be able to detect low-base-rate phenomena, and/or other idiosyncratic presentations. As such, 'case-specific' psychopathologies may be included in the risk analysis. Of course, the assessor should acknowledge the caveats and limitations associated with drawing from such literature but nevertheless, this is a preferable method to dismissing an important feature of the person's presentation as irrelevant.

As described by Douglas, et al. (this volume), all risk factors are then rated according to whether they are present and relevant. This is a key stage in making sense of mental disorder. Presence is relatively straightforward to establish and guidelines exist to aid the assessor. In terms of relevance, assessors must consider whether a risk factor is functionally linked to violent outcomes and consider whether it is a driver, destabilizer or disinhibitor (or whether it is irrelevant). An example is given to illustrate this process: If a person who has perpetrated several armed robberies also has a history of child maltreatment for which they show no objective, and deny any subjective, long-term effects, it may be concluded that the risk factor is present but not relevant to their ongoing risk of harm. However, if another person has a long-standing, early onset, alcohol-abuse problem and batters his partner each and every time he is intoxicated (but never when sober), this risk factor is both present and relevant. This would seem a fundamental step in working with mental disorder. By considering relevance in addition to presence, the hypothetical logical connection can be articulated and tested at the idiographic level.

Configurative risk models

When dealing with mental disorder, it is important that assessors use the SPJ paradigm as a configurative (not cumulative) risk model. Leading on from the points made above, practitioners should acknowledge (and educate decision-makers about) the fact that, in some cases, mental disorder might be the only single risk factor that is present in a particular case and that having only one risk factor does not equate with low risk. Configurative models offer far more in terms of explanatory information than a simple totting-up of items. For example, in Albert's case from the vignette at the beginning of this chapter, his narcissistic personality disorder may provide the answer to his violence. Individuals with this pathology are highly vulnerable to experiencing narcissistic rage – a state associated with violence and that can lead to offending in the absence of other criminogenic variables (Logan, 2009; Logan and Johnstone, 2010). Similarly, the onset of a psychotic illness might result in a person perpetrating an extremely violent offence in the absence of any criminogenic or indeed warning signs. By detailing the relevance of any particular symptoms to risk outcomes, the number of risk factors becomes less relevant and an explanatory paradigm can be achieved where criminogenic (or other third) variables are clearly not necessary for violence to occur. This is especially useful when dealing with a low base rate or complex forms of psychopathology.

Risk formulation

Building on the points made above, formulation is considered a critical stage in violence risk assessment. Formulation provides a framework for structuring and organizing the information into a theoretically and conceptually consistent frame-work. Formulation requires the assessor to produce a set of hypotheses that help integrate the available information about static and dynamic aspects of the person's context to explain the onset, development and maintenance of their present-ing problems (in this case mental disorder and violence and any other presenting problems). Formulation is not a new or novel concept in general terms; it is used in each of the main models of psychotherapy – behavioural, cognitive-behavioural, psychodynamic, systemic and integrative approaches (Johnstone and Dallos, 2006). However, it has only relatively recently been proposed as a stage in the violence risk assessment process.

Johnstone and Dallos (2006) and Hart, et al. (2011) have noted that the core elements of formulation are the same regardless of the underpinning model or subject. Formulation is all of the following: (a) a summary of the person's main presenting problems; (b) an inferential explanation for their difficulties, (c) action-oriented in that it assists the practitioner to prioritize the presenting problems and to ensure the correct planning, sequencing, implementation of any treatments or interventions; (d) theory-driven, and thereby developed and articulated in accord-ance with at least one but typically more theoretical models; (e) individualized and entirely concerned with the person being assessed, their specific problems, experi-ences and contexts – it is not about generalities or averages; (f) narrative, in that it provides qualitative descriptors of the person's difficulties – it tells their story; (g) diachronic and thereby relevant across time, and takes account of the past, the present and the person's likely futures; (h) testable and produces hypotheses which can be evaluated; (i) open to revision and reformulation; and (j) it is ampli-ative and results in new information which broadens and deepens our understand-ing of the client.

Douglas, et al. (this volume) differentiate between theoretically informed formulation and pragmatically grounded formulation. The former refers to model-specific analyses; for example, a cognitive-behavioural formulation, which might include explanatory mechanisms that link early experiences to core schema and emotions, cognitions and behaviours, or a psychodynamic formulation, which might organize the information into defence mechanisms or unconscious desires. In contrast, the pragmatically grounded formulation is broader in its scope and leaves the assessor to draw from an eclectic theoretical framework. I would concur with Douglas, et al. (this volume) that this latter approach seems a more appropriate method of encapsulating and explaining violence risk since no definitive theory or model exists to explain either violence or psychopathology. Weerasekera's (1996) 'four Ps' model is a valuable framework.

The four Ps model requires the assessor to organize risk factors according to whether they are *predisposing* (i.e., risk factors in the individual's past that may increase his proclivity or vulnerability to violence); *precipitating* (i.e., events or circumstances that may trigger the behaviour or disinhibit usual behavioural controls); (3) *perpetuating* (i.e., risk factors that cause the risk to remain); or (4) *protective factors* (i.e., aspects of the offender's functioning or circumstances that moderate the risk). This model is accessible to a range of professionals, allows for a biopsychosocial explanation of the person's difficulties, and enables a temporal sequencing of events (and symptoms). Thus, it is likely to facilitate broad-based explanations drawn from a range of theoretical frameworks and, therefore, more explanatory function.

Notwithstanding the sound rationale for including this stage in risk assessment, Hart and colleagues have cautioned that, as yet, formulation has not been shown to have predictive or clinical utility. Furthermore, with the exception of only a few papers, little guidance exists on *how* to achieve risk formulation in practice. Assessors must therefore be transparent about the limitations to their knowledge. While that evidence base accrues, practitioners should consult Hart and Logan (2011), Hart, et al. (2011) and Logan and Johnstone (2010) for relevant guidance. For the purpose of this chapter, I have summarized the principles developed by Hart and colleagues (Hart, et al., 2011). The authors have provided a set of principles for developing formulations and criteria by which they can be adjudged. These include the following: *external coherence* (the formulation is consistent with theory); *factual foundation* (the information used is of an acceptable standard); *internal coherence* (the formulation is consistent and compatible, and not contradictory); *explanatory breadth* (ties together multiple facets or features of the presentation); *diachronic* (knits together information relevant to the past, present and future); *simplicity* (is free from unnecessary information); *reliability* (consistent with the formulations generated by others); *generativity* (produces detailed and testable hypotheses); *accuracy* (the hypotheses are correct); and *acceptability* (the content is accepted by others – professionals and patients alike). In cases where mental disorder is present, assessors should ensure that these criteria are achieved.

Scenario planning

In this step, the evaluator considers all of the available information in order to produce a theoretically and empirically guided speculation about the most plausible scenarios to be managed. Assessors must consider scenarios along the following dimensions: nature, severity, imminence, frequency, and likelihood. This process aims to ensure that the risk being identified as a concern is well defined and well described. Considering mental disorder, as indicated above, a patient's clinical presentation might traverse many diagnostic criteria and their violence might be diverse. Within the SPJ model, assessors should consider the relevance of each disorder and symptom to each potential violent outcome (in other words, for each scenario the relevance of any mental disorder symptomatology should be clear). Whilst only the RSVP and SAM give explicit instructions in the manuals to follow scenario planning, it is applicable in all cases and for all items. (The forthcoming version three of the HCR-20 manual will do so also). Furthermore, because one particular process might function for one form of harm, it is not necessarily the case that it will be the same for all forms of violence. To articulate a scenario, mental disorder symptoms should be considered in relation to the nature, severity, imminence, and likelihood of *all* potential violent outcomes for the person. For those experiencing acute disturbances, scenarios for when well and when unwell should be included.

Risk management recommendations

Assessors are then required to provide a set of risk management recommendations for countering the risk. The RSVP, SAM and the Risk Management Authority, Scotland (2007) have produced guidelines for developing recommendations. It is generally accepted in forensic practice that a risk management plan should cover the following areas: (1) supervision; (2) monitoring; (3) treatment (the provision of (re-)habilitative interventions to improve psychosocial functioning); (4) victim-safety planning; and (5) other (see Douglas et al., this volume, for more details).

Where mental disorder is present, the steps involved in managing the associated risks should be clearly explained. In terms of treatment, formulation should directly guide the prioritization and type of interventions delivered. For example, a person with acute psychosis who has perpetrated a violent offence may have diverse treatment needs but it is important that his or her treatment needs are properly sequenced. For example, even if a cognitive-behavioural intervention for violence seems merited, there is no point in delivering this first if the person is acutely unwell. The priority is to stabilize the person's mental state. This might require medication. However, the building blocks of a psychological therapy formulation will already be in place and the subsequent intervention will be able to focus on the particular schema, symptom, or psychological vulnerability that elevates violence risk potential when the person is ready. Nevertheless, the formulation should ensure a treatment plan for the immediate, medium and long term. In terms of monitoring, it is likely that detailed assessments and risk formulations will provide important information about warning signs or signature risk signs or symptoms. For example, some people's delusions have unique features – signature risk signs – and this should be included in their management plan. This should optimize the effectiveness of the intervention, permit early intervention by highlighting early warning signs, thus ensuring appropriate supports and responses are provided. By achieving this level of analysis and understanding in the risk assessment, and by detailing it in the formulation, the risk management and treatment success is likely to be optimized. Formulation promises clarity in relation to the *what, why and how* of violence risk and, as such, risk management may be optimized.

Summary judgement

In this final stage, the assessor is expected to reach an overall conclusion. Generally, this is given as a broad statement as to whether the individual merits high, medium or low case prioritization and this informs the nature, type and intensity of risk management required.

Case example: Andrew

In an attempt to illustrate the utility of the SPJ in dealing with mental disorder psychopathology and risk, an overview of Andrew's case – presented as a brief vignette at the beginning of this chapter – is presented below.

Index offence

Nine years ago, when Andrew was 27, he was charged with the attempted murder of his brother. Acquitted on the grounds of insanity and diagnosed as suffering from paranoid schizophrenia, he was detained for eight years in a high security hospital. In the last 18 months, his presentation has settled and he is now requesting discharge to the community. A risk assessment report was required to assist tribunal members to reach a decision in this regard.

Relevant findings

Andrew's index offence occurred in the context of a long history of convictions for multiple forms of violence (reactive, instrumental, acquisitive and psychotically driven violence) towards multiple victim-types (he has targeted male, female, stranger and acquaintance victims) and with varying degrees of severity (minor injuries to life-threatening assaults). His prior violence involved weapon use, including knives, to threaten and harm others.

Brief social history

Andrew was raised in a violent household characterized by domestic violence. He also recalled violence in the home between other adults. He said this typically followed on from weekend drinking parties enjoyed by his parents and others. His parents were described as rejecting and neglectful towards him. His mother suffered periods of hospitalization due to psychotic illness. He showed an early onset conduct disorder and he has admitted to delinquent activities. However, records suggest that he stole items such as food and clothes to meet his basic needs. His childhood was spent between home and residential care settings. He started to drink alcohol at around 11 years and his substance-use problems also onset at that time. He did poorly in education and, despite being offered employment training opportunities, he failed to engage. By his early adulthood, Andrew had developed a serious substance-abuse problem and used heroin on a daily basis. He has a history of unstable relationships – also characterized by domestic violence leading to convictions. Prior to the index offence, he had accrued 13 convictions for assault and robbery, 28 convictions for assault and 6 convictions for serious assault. Andrew has minimized the extent of his difficulties and has impressed as having poor insight and as lacking in remorse or regret. He is candid in his views that crime and gambling are a way of life for him and he claimed that, at the time of admission, he owed about £50,000 in gambling debts.

Progress in hospital

During the first several years of his hospital admission, Andrew was very difficult to manage. He has shown a variable degree of compliance (and response) to medication and he has relapsed on several occasions whereby he has become deluded about his brother, believing that his brother was plotting to murder him. Andrew's illness takes a predictable form. Early warning signs include decreased levels of interaction with others, social withdrawal, avoidance of recreational and occupational activities on the ward, physiological arousal, poor self-care, and a reluctance to eat hospital food, preferring to purchase packaged items from the hospital shop. Within a week or two, he begins to ruminate and to show paranoid ideation. He will often begin to ask staff about his brother – whether he has been in touch, if he has 'a pass' for the hospital, if he could be masquerading as a staff nurse. In acute phases, Andrew articulates the belief that the general manager is in fact his brother and he looks out for him on the hospital grounds. His thoughts and speech become disorganized. When in this stage, Andrew has a history of making targeted threats to the general manager. Andrew has told patients and staff to pass on messages to the general manager and he has written long letters to him detailing complex delusional beliefs – and threats to harm him. Thus far, Andrew has experienced a relapse of such a nature on three occasions. However, in the last 18 months, Andrew has been compliant with clozapine therapy and has been viewed as showing an excellent response in terms of his mental state. That said, he continues to refuse all psychological therapies and refuses to acknowledge a prior substance-misuse problem. He remains procriminal in his attitudes, he has lost contact with family and friends such as they are, and he is adamant that he has a number of enemies in the community who, due to past transgressions, would seek revenge. He claims to be able to be able to 'handle' this.

Assessment of mental disorder

A cognitive assessment using the *Wechsler Adult Intelligence Scales* (WAIS) indicated that Andrew was in the normal range of intellectual functioning (Full Scale IQ = 103, 95 per cent Confidence Interval 99 – 107; Verbal IQ = 101, 95 per cent Confidence Interval 96–106, Performance IQ = 106, 95 per cent Confidence Interval, 99–112). In terms of mental disorder, using the IPDE, Andrew met diagnostic criteria for antisocial personality disorder. There is a long-standing pattern of the following criteria: early onset conduct disorder; a failure to conform to social norms; impulsivity and failing to plan ahead; irritability and aggressiveness; and a pattern of consistent irresponsibility and lack of remorse. Andrew also showed traits of narcissistic personality disorder, specifically a sense of entitlement, a tendency towards interpersonal exploitation, a lack of empathy, and arrogant and haughty behaviour. On the PCL-R, Andrew showed definite evidence of proneness to boredom/need for stimulation, conning and manipulative, lack of remorse or guilt, shallow affect, callous/lack of empathy, parasitic lifestyle, promiscuous sexual behaviour, early behaviour problems, lack of realistic, long-term goals, impulsivity, many short-term marital relationships, juvenile delinquency, and revocation of conditional release.

In terms of acute mental illness, using the SCID-I, it was possible to confirm his diagnosis of paranoid schizophrenia with a definite history of paranoid delusions (particularly concerning his brother whom he believed had plotted to kill him), hallucinations (he complained of being able to hear his brother threatening to murder him and of 'bargaining' with him whereby he would suggest that if he killed himself or another person, his brother would 'forgive' him his transgressions). Andrew also described hearing female voices outside his head, which gave a highly critical and demeaning commentary on him (they called him pathetic and weak and swore at him). He also showed a history of disorganized speech and behaviour (including copious letter writing to the general manager of the hospital), and some negative symptoms. Andrew also met diagnostic threshold for a past diagnosis of alcohol and opioid dependence.

Analysis of risk factors using the HCR-20

Andrew shows definite or partial evidence of the following historical risk factors: 'previous violence', 'young age at first violent incident', 'relationship instability', 'employment problems', 'substance use problems', 'major mental illness', 'psychopathy', 'early maladjustment', 'personality disorder' (antisocial), and 'prior supervision failure'. Clinically, he shows a lack of insight, negative attitudes, impulsivity, and is unresponsive to treatment (specifically, psychological, occupational and offending-behaviour programmes). In terms of risk management items, there is a high or moderate probability of the following in a community (and hospital setting): his plans lack feasibility, he will be exposed to destabilizers, he will lack personal support, he will be non-compliant with remediation attempts, and he will experience and struggle to cope with stress. Other case-specific factors include a history of serious gambling.

Risk formulation

Many factors may have predisposed Andrew to having violent behaviour problems. From a social-learning perspective, he would appear to have experienced a difficult and traumatic childhood where the adults in his life – at home and in care – frequently displayed violence. As such, he is likely to have learned that violence was an acceptable and effective method of having his needs met. Furthermore, drawing from personality theory, it is possible that the consequent trauma of witnessing such events might have led to some emotional blunting and numbing, thereby increasing his risk of deficient affective experience (lack of empathy, remorse, regret, and so on). In addition, his early experiences of neglect and abandonment will likely have taught him that he is very much alone in life and that others are not to be trusted or depended upon to meet his needs. This might have led him to have suffered significantly impaired attachments and resulted in him having an inability to form and sustain meaningful and functional emotional relationships with others (in other words, he shows shallow affect) as well as causing him to be undependable and irresponsible. By dint of his early experiences, Andrew has not been able to maximize opportunities to develop prosocial and adaptive living skills. Instead, he used substances and perpetrated antisocial acts as a means of surviving and, over the years, it would appear that these became deeply entrenched habitual methods of living and interacting with others and his environment. It would appear that, as he matured, these premorbid difficulties caused him to develop the range of symptoms associated with personality disorder.

Andrew has a complex presentation and his earlier psychiatric history suggests that he is particularly vulnerable to experiencing psychotic symptoms associated with severe paranoid ideation. When such symptoms are present, he perceives hostile intent in the benign actions of others, he will ruminate on his concerns, and he will withdraw socially and from activities.

In terms of precipitating risk factors for violence, it would appear that Andrew's premorbid personality coupled with substance use (effects of disinhibition) and psychotic illness were critical factors to his index offence, whereby he seems to have decompensated into a psychotic state with paranoid symptoms. He was feeling at risk of harm and viewed violence towards his brother as a logical and justified behaviour and an effective method of self-preservation – in other words, he made a rational choice in the context of irrationality. A range of indicators have been viewed as possible warning signs for a repeat of a similar event in the future. When unwell, Andrew shows high levels of physiological arousal, hostility, anxiety and insomnia. He voices feelings of disgruntlement and he is prone to feeling aggrieved when something does not go his way. He also quickly shows a deterioration in his self-care and he becomes markedly withdrawn.

In terms of other offending, such as instrumental violence, it would appear that substance use and his antisocial personality disorder again are key drivers to this behaviour. However, merely having a desire to achieve a secondary goal (acquisition of money, alcohol, drugs, and so on) has been a sufficient precipitant for a violent offence such as robbery in the past.

Andrew's reactive violence seemed to occur in response to him experiencing a frustrating event or his needs being unmet. He would appear to have made a decision to use violence in order to eliminate the source of frustration, gain control over his environment and satisfy his needs.

The perpetuating risk factors in this case are Andrew's mental illness status, his negative attitudes, his antisocial personality disorder, his ongoing risk of alcohol and substance misuse, his limited insight, lack of opportunities in employment, poor attitude towards treatment, his vulnerability to stress and exposure to destabilizers, and his lack of personal support. He also shows a pervasive mistrust of others and struggles to be open and candid with people who are available to support him. As such, a further consideration is his non-compliance and problems with risk management.

Risk scenarios

The following scenarios would be most relevant if Andrew was residing in a community setting.

Interpersonal and psychotically driven violence

This refers to an incident involving verbal or physical violence directed towards another person that may be reactive or impulsive in nature. A repeat scenario would involve recidivistic offending of a similar nature as he has shown before; the most likely scenario would be a verbal altercation, which could escalate into a physical assault or fight. The most likely victim would be a stranger or an acquaintance, a professional with whom he felt a strong dislike or mistrust, or the police. The physical consequences would most likely be mild to moderate injuries such as bruising. In the present circumstances, while he is in receipt of good risk management, is mentally stable and sober, this would be moderately likely. In the absence of close monitoring and robust risk management, I would consider such an event to be highly likely. An escalation or worst-case scenario refers to a reoffence that involves outcomes that are more serious. In this case, this would involve a more serious physical or fatal attack and would likely be the result of Andrew carrying a weapon such as a knife. His brother and the general manager of the hospital, or any other person he believes is associated with these two people, would be at particular risk. The circumstances detailed above would be similar but perhaps more related to difficulties coping, coupled with acute mental-illness symptoms. Similarly, if he had been using drugs and was intoxicated, this would be more likely. In the absence of close monitoring and robust risk management, this outcome would be moderate to highly likely.

Instrumental violence

This refers to violence perpetrated for a secondary gain, for example, to obtain money or goods. Andrew admits to having perpetrated a number of crimes involving instrumental violence whereby he would rob stores such as off-licence premises. It would appear that he would threaten staff with a knife and would tell them they were at risk of lethal harm. A repeat scenario is therefore possible. If he was residing in the community, lacked financial resources or was using substances or alcohol, there is a significant risk of a repeat scenario. An escalation or worst-case scenario would involve a similar offence but more serious physical harm. This would be more likely if Andrew was intoxicated and/or experiencing poor mental health and/or he was challenged by the person he was attempting to rob.

Other scenarios

Given Andrew's history, he must be considered at risk of perpetrating other forms of harm, including domestic violence in his intimate relationship or familial violence. Harassing others by prolific letter-writing is another potential risk.

Risk management

In order to optimize the likelihood of effective risk management, the following interventions are recommended. In terms of supervision, Andrew suffers from a major mental illness and personality disorder. He is subject to the Mental Health Act and as such will be supervised by mental health and criminal justice agencies. He will require intensive and long-term supervision. In respect of monitoring, while Andrew is under the auspices of mental health and criminal justice care and supervision, he should be closely monitored for relapse in his mental state, associations with antisocial peers, use of drugs and alcohol, contact with past rivals and access to weapons, and how he is meeting his financial needs. He should be subjected to blood tests to measure compliance with medication and he should be subjected to routine and regular mandatory drug testing. Steps should also be put in place to ensure that he does not have access to weapons while incarcerated and, if possible, subsequent to his discharge. His attempts to contact others, most notably his brother and the general manager, should also be monitored.

In respect of treatment, Andrew has many identifiable treatment targets including his mental-illness problems, addictions, poor anger control, inadequate problem-solving and coping skills, negative pro-violence attitude, and his personality disorder pathology. He is, however, not motivated to engage in anything other than psychopharmacological treatment and his compliance with this has varied across time. As such, motivational interviewing and rapport building may be a necessary first step before more intensive or structured treatments are attempted. In terms of victim safety planning, Andrew's brother and the general manager are identifiable potential victims. A victim safety plan should therefore be developed to protect them. In addition, close monitoring for the inclusion of others in Andrew's delusional belief system should be done and a victim safety plan developed for any other identifiable person.

In respect of occupational skills training, Andrew has failed to establish skills or experiences in either education or employment opportunities. This will likely pose a significant barrier for him should he wish and attempt to reintegrate into the community. He should be supported in accessing and benefitting from vocational and skills training. Similarly, Andrew identifies strongly with a criminal subculture. He lacks in skills of daily living and he has little in the way of community ties or prosocial interests. If he is to progress towards an offence-free lifestyle, he will need to learn to identify and engage in more prosocial activities. He should be supported in identifying and developing appropriate interests and behaviours.

Regular reassessment of risk

Andrew's risk status and risk management needs should be regularly reviewed. It is likely that, given the early onset, persistent, chronic and multifaceted difficulties experienced by Andrew, risk management interventions will have to be complex, multifaceted, stringent, and long-term. It would be essential that a mechanism be in place to re-evaluate and realign his risk management should any indicators of relapse in his major mental illness emerge.

Case prioritization

Andrew requires high-intensity risk management.

Summary and recommendations for practice

In this chapter, the link between mental disorder and violence has been examined. An overview of the key findings from the extant literature was presented – covariation between at least some forms (but not all) and violence has been established. Next, consideration was given to what can (and what cannot) be inferred from the nature of this association. Temporal precedence and the exclusion of an alternative variable is difficult to ascertain. There is, however, a logical connection between mental disorder and violence, and through the use of the structured professional judgement paradigm, incorporating the critical risk formulation stage, it might be possible to work within the confines and constraints of the extant literature. However, it is apparent that we are far from achieving a panacea in the field of violence risk assessment; much work remains to be done. In the meantime, it is envisaged that the guidelines and illustrations contained in this chapter will be of assistance to those tasked with assessing and understanding violence risk in complex cases.

Note

1 An offender might be considered 'exclusive' if he or she perpetrates the same type of offence, in the same context, for the same reasons, against the same victim types, in the same manner and with the same outcomes.

References

Abracen, J., Looman, J. and Anderson, D. (2000) 'Alcohol and drug abuse in sexual and non-sexual violent offenders', *Sexual Abuse: A Journal of Research and Treatment*, 12: 263–74.

American Psychiatric Association (1994) *Diagnostic and Statistical Manual of Mental Disorders 4th Edition*, Washington, DC: APA.

Arboleda-Florez, J., Holley, H. and Crisanti, A. (1998) 'Understanding causal paths between mental illness and violence', *Social Psychiatry and Epidemiology*, 33: 38–46.

Baros, D. M. and de Pádua Serafim, A. (2008) 'Association between personality disorder and violent behavior pattern', *Forensic Science International*, 179, 19–22.

Bjørkly, S. (2009) 'Risk and dynamics of violence in Asperger's syndrome: A systematic review of the literature', *Aggression and Violent Behaviour*, 14: 306–12.

Blackburn, R., Logan, C., Donnelly, J. and Renwick, S. (2003) 'Personality disorders, psychopathy and other mental disorders: Co-morbidity among patients at English and Scottish high security hospitals', *Journal of Forensic Psychiatry and Psychology*, 14: 111–37.

Blaumenthal, S. and Levander, T. (2000) *Violence and Mental Disorder: A Critical Aid to the Assessment and Management of Risk*, London: Zito Trust.

Boer, D. P., Hart, S. D., Kropp, P. R. and Webster, C. D. (1997) *Manual for the Sexual Violence Risk – 20: Professional Guidelines for Assessing Risk of Sexual Violence*, Vancouver, British Columbia: British Columbia Institute on Family Violence and Mental Health, Law and Policy Institute, Simon Fraser University.

Borum, R. (1996) 'Improving the clinical practice of violence risk assessment: Technology, guidelines and training', *American Psychologist*, 51: 945–56.

Burgess, A. W., Hartman, C. R., Ressler, R. K., Douglas, J. E. and McCormack, A. (1986) 'Sexual homicide: A motivational model', *Journal of Interpersonal Violence*, 1: 251–72.

Cadksy, O. and Crawford, M. (1988) 'Establishing batterer typologies in a clinical sample of men who assault their female partners', Special issue: Wife battering: A Canadian Perspective, *Canadian Journal of Community Mental Health*, 7: 119–27.

Campbell, J. C., Webster, D., Koziol-McLain, J., Blick, C., Campbell, D., Curry, M. A., Gary, F., Glass, N., McGArlane, J., Sachs, C., Sharps, P., Ulrich, Y., Wilst, S. A., Manganello, J., Xu, X., Schollenberger, J., Frye, V. and Laughon, K. (2003) 'Risk factors for femicide in abusive relationships: Results from a multi-site case control study', *American Journal of Public Health*, 93: 1089–97.

Coid, J., Kahtan, N., Gault, S. and Jarman, B. (1999) 'Patients with personality disorder admitted to secure forensic psychiatry services', *British Journal of Psychiatry*, 175: 528–36.

Cooke, D. J. (2010) 'Acturial risk assessment: More prejudicial than probative', *Scots Law Times*, 10th January.

Cooke, D. J. and Michie, C. (this volume) 'Violence risk assessment: From prediction to understanding – or from what? to why?', in C. Logan and L. Johnstone (eds) *Managing Clinical Risk: A Guide to Effective Practice*, Oxford: Routledge.

Critchfield, K. L., Levy, K. N. and Clarkin, J. F. (2007) 'The Personality Disorders Institute/ Borderline Personality Disorder Research Foundation randomized control trial for borderline personality disorder: Reliability of Axis I and II diagnoses', *Psychiatric Quarterly*, 78: 15–24.

Dean, K., Walsh, E., Moran, P., Tyrer, P., Creed, F., Byford, S., Burns, T., Murray, R. and Fahy, T. (2006) 'Violence in women with psychosis in the community: A prospective study', *British Journal of Psychiatry*, 152: 91–96.

Dell, S. and Smith, A. (1983) 'Changes in the sentencing of diminished responsibility homicides', *British Journal of Psychiatry*, 142: 20–34.

Department of Health (2007) *Best Practice in Managing Risk: Principles and Evidence for Best Practice in the Assessment and Management of Risk to Self and Others in Mental Health Services*, London: Department of Health.

Douglas, K. S., Blanchard, A. J. E. and Hendry, M. C. (this volume) 'Violence risk assessment and management: Putting structured professional judgement into practice', in C. Logan and L. Johnstone (eds) *Managing Clinical Risk: A Guide to Effective Practice*, Oxford: Routledge.

Douglas, K. S., Guy, L. S. and Hart, S. D. (2009) 'Psychosis as a risk factor for violence to others: A meta-analysis', *Psychological Bulletin*, 135: 679–706.

Douglas, K. S. and Kropp, P. R. (2002) 'A prevention based paradigm for violence risk assessment: Clinical and research applications', *Criminal Justice and Behavior*, 29: 617–58.

Duggan, C. and Howard, R. C. (2009) 'The functional link between personality disorder and violence: A critical appraisal', in M. McMurran and R. C. Howard (eds) *Personality, Personality Disorder and Violence*, Chichester: Wiley-Blackwell.

Eaves, D., Tien, G. and Wilson, D. (2000) 'Offenders with major affective disorders', in S. Hodgins and R. Müller-Isberner (eds) *Violence, Crime and Mentally Disordered Offenders: Concepts and Methods for Effective Treatment and Prevention*, Chichester: John Wiley and Sons.

Elbogen, E. B. and Johnson, S. C. (2009) 'The intricate link between violence and mental disorder: Results from the National Epidemiologic Survey on Alcohol and Related Conditions', *Archives of General Psychiatry*, 66: 152–61.

Eronen, M., Hakola, P. and Tiihonen, J. (1996) 'Mental disorders and homicidal behaviour in Finland', *Archives of General Psychiatry*, 53: 497–501.

Eronen, M., Tiihonen, J. and Hakola, P. (1996) 'Schizophrenia and homicidal behavior', *Schizophrenia Bulletin*, 22: 83–89.

Farmer, C. A. and Aman, M. G. (2001) 'Aggressive behaviour in a sample of children with autistic spectrum disorders', *Research in Autism Spectrum Disorders*, 5: 317–23.

Fazel, S., Gulati, G., Linsell, L., Geddes, J. R. and Grann, M. (2009) 'Schizophrenia and violence: Systematic review and meta-analysis', *PloS Medicine*, 6.

Gibbon, M. B., Spitzer, R. L., Williams, J. B. W. and Benjamin, L. S. (1997) *Structured Clinical Interview for DSM-IV Axis II Personality Disorders* (SCID-II), Washington, D. C.: American Psychiatric Press, Inc.

Gonzalez-Ortega, I., Mosquera, F., Echebura, E. and Gonzales-Pinto, A. (2010) 'Insight, psychosis and aggressive behaviour in mania', *European Journal of Psychiatry*, 24: 70–77.

Green, B., Schramm, T. M., Chiu, K., McVie, K. and Hay, S. (2009) 'Violence severity and psychosis', *International Journal of Forensic Mental Health*, 8: 33–40.

Grove, W. M. and Meehl, P. E. (1996) 'Comparative efficiency of informal (subjective impressionistic) and formal (mechanical, algorithmic) prediction procedures: The clinical-statistical controversy', *Psychology, Public Policy and Law*, 2: 293–323.

Hanson, R. K. and Thornton, D. (1999) The Static-99. http://www.static99.org

— (2000) 'Improving risk assessments for sex offenders: A comparison of three actuarial scales', *Law and Human Behaviour*, 24: 119–36.

Hare, R. D. (1991) *Manual for the Hare Psychopathy Checklist Revised*, Toronto: Multi-Health Systems.

— (2003) *Manual for the Hare Psychopathy Checklist Revised, 2nd Edition*, Toronto: Multi-Health Systems.

Hart, S. D. (1998) 'The role of psychopathy in assessing risk for violence: Conceptual and methodological issues', *Legal and Criminological Psychology*, 3: 121–37.

Hart, S. D., Cooke, C. and Michie, C. (2007) 'Precision of actuarial risk assessment instruments: Evaluating the "margins of error" of group v. individual predictions of violence', *British Journal of Psychiatry*, suppl. 49: 60–65.

Hart, S. D. and Dempster, R. J. (1997) 'Impulsivity and psychopathy', in C. D. Webster and M. A. Jackson (eds) *Impulsivity: Theory, Assessment and Treatment*, New York: Guilford.

Hart, S. D. and Hare, R. D. (1997) 'Psychopathy: Assessment and association with criminal conduct', in D. M. Stoff, J. Brieling and J. Maser (eds) *Handbook of Antisocial Behaviour*, New York: Wiley.

Hart, S. D. and Logan, C. (2011) 'Formulation of violence risk using evidence-based assessments: The structured professional judgement approach', in P. Sturmey and M. McMurran (eds) *Forensic Case Formulation*, Chichester: Wiley-Blackwell.

Hart, S. D., Kropp, P. K., Laws, D. R., Klaver, J., Logan, C. and Watt, K. A. (2003) *The Risk for Sexual Violence Protocol: Structured Professional Guidelines for Assessing Risk of*

Sexual Violence, Vancouver, Canada: Mental Health, Law and Policy Institute, Simon Fraser University.

Hart, S. D., Sturmey, P., Logan, C. and McMurran, M. (2011) 'Forensic case formulation', *International Journal of Forensic Mental Health*, 10: 118–26.

Haynes, S. N. (1992) *Models of Causality in Psychopathology*, New York: Macmillan.

Hilton, N. Z., Harris, G. T. and Rice, M. E. (2001) 'Predicting violence by serious wife assaulters', *Journal of Interpersonal Violence*, 16: 408–23.

Hilton, N. Z., Harris, G. T., Rice, M. E., Lang, C. and Cormier, C. A. (2004) 'A brief actuarial assessment for the prediction of wife assault recidivism: The ODARA', *Psychological Assessment*, 16: 267–75.

Hodgins, S., Lapalmec, M. and Toupin, J. (1999) 'Criminal activities and substance use of patients with major affective disorders and schizophrenia: A 2-year follow-up', *Journal of Affective Disorders*, 55: 187–202.

Home Office (2004) *The British Crime Survey*, London: HM Stationery Office.

Jamieson, L. and Taylor, P. J. (2004) 'A reconvictions study of special (high security) hospital patients', *British Journal of Criminology*, 44: 783–802.

Johnstone, L. and Dallos, R. (2006) *Formulation in Psychology and Psychotherapy: Making Sense of People's Problems*, London: Routledge.

Kafka, M. P. and Prentky, R. A. (1994) 'Preliminary observations of DSM-III-R axis I comorbidity in men with paraphilias and paraphilia-related disorders', *Journal of Clinical Psychiatry, 55*: 481–7.

Kirsch, L. and Becker, J. (2007) 'Emotional deficits in psychopathy and sexual sadism: Implications for violent and sadistic behaviour', *Clinical Psychology Review*, 27: 904–22.

Klostermann, K. and Fals-Stewart, W. (2006) 'Intimate partner violence and alcohol use: Exploring the role of drinking in partner violence and its implications for intervention', *Aggression and Violent Behavior*, 11: 587–97.

Knoll, J. and Hazelwood, R. (2009) 'Becoming the victim: Beyond sadism in serial sexual murders', *Aggression and Violence Behaviour*, 14: 106–14.

Kropp, P. R. (2009) 'Intimate partner violence risk assessment', in J. L. Ireland, C. A. Ireland and P. Birch (eds) *Violent and Sexual Offenders: Assessment, Treatment and Management*, Cullompton: Willan Publishing.

Kropp, P. R. and Gibas, A. (2010) 'The Spousal Assault Risk Assessment Guide (SARA)', in R. K. Otto and K. D. Douglas (eds) *Handbook of Violence Risk Assessment*, New York: Routledge.

Kropp, P. R., Hart, S. D. and Lyon, D. R. (2008) *Guidelines for Stalking Assessment and Management (SAM) Manual*, Vancouver, Canada: British Columbia Institute on Family Violence.

Kunelsman, J. C. (2001) *Desistance among Specialized Persistent Felony Offenders: A Policy Analysis of a Criminal Statute in Kentucky*, Dissertation Abstracts International, The Humanities and Social Sciences, 61: 3362-A.

Lasko, N., Gurvitis, T., Kuhne, A., Orr, S. and Pitman, R. (1994) 'Aggression and its correlates in Vietnam veterans with and without chronic posttraumatic stress disorder', *Comprehensive Psychiatry*, 35: 373–91.

Leekam, R. S., Libby, S. J., Wing, L., Gould, J. and Taylor, C. (2002) 'The Diagnostic Interview for Social and Communication Disorders: Algorithms for ICD-10 childhood autism and Wing and Gould autistic spectrum disorders', *Journal of Child Psychology and Psychiatry*, 43: 327–42.

Link, B. G. and Stueve, A. (1994) 'Psychotic symptoms and the violent/illegal behaviour of mental patients compared to community controls', in J. Monahan and H. J. Steadman (eds) *Violence and Mental Disorder: Developments in Risk Assessment*, Chicago: University of Chicago Press.

Logan, C. (2009) 'Narcissism', in M. McMurran and R. Howard (eds) *Personality, Personality Disorder and Violence*, Chichester: Wiley-Blackwell.

Logan, C. and Johnstone, L. (2010) 'Personality disorder and violence: Making the link through risk formulation', *Journal of Personality Disorders*, 24: 610–33.

Loranger, A. W. (1999) *International Personality Disorder Examination, DSM-IV and ICD-10 Interviews*, Lutz, FL: Psychological Assessment Resources, Inc.

Loucks, N. (2002) *Recidivism Amongst Serious Violent and Sexual Offenders*, Edinburgh: Scottish Executive Social Research.

Maden, T. (2007) *Treating Violence: A Guide to Risk Management in Mental Health*, Oxford: Oxford University Press.

Marham, J. (this volume) 'Clinical risk assessment and management with military personnel and veterans: The tip of a camouflaged iceberg', in C. Logan and L. Johnstone (eds) *Managing Clinical Risk: A Guide to Effective Practice*, Oxford: Routledge.

McFall, M., Fontana, A., Riskind, M. and Rosenheck, R. (1999) 'Analysis of violent behavior in Vietnam combat veteran psychiatric inpatients with posttraumatic stress disorder', *Journal of Traumatic Stress*, 12: 501–17.

McMurran, M., Khalifa, N. and Gibbon, S. (eds) (2009) 'Mental disorder and offending', in M. McMurran, N. Khalifa and S. Gibbon, *Forensic Mental Health*, Cullumpton: Willan Publishing.

Monahan, J. and H. J. Steadman (eds) (1983) *Violence and Mental Disorder: Developments in Risk Assessment*, Chicago: University of Chicago Press.

Moskowitz, A. (2004) 'Dissociation and violence: A review of the literature', *Trauma, Violence and Abuse*, 5: 21–46.

O'Reilly, G., Marshall, W. L., Carr, A. and Beckett, R. C. (2004) *The Handbook of Clinical Intervention with Young People who Sexually Abuse*, New York: Brunner-Routledge.

Otto, R. K. and Douglas, K. S. (eds) (2010) *Handbook of Violence Risk Assessment*, New York: Routledge.

Parrott, D., Drobes, D., Saladin, M., Coffey, S. and Dansky, B. (2003) 'Perpetration of partner violence: Effects of cocaine and alcohol dependence and posttraumatic stress disorder', *Addictive Behaviors*, 28: 1587–1602.

Porter, S. and Woodworth, M. (2006) 'Psychopathy and aggression', in C. J. Patrick (ed.) *Handbook of Psychopathy*, New York: Guilford.

Prentky, R. A., Knight, R. A. and Lee, A. F. S. (1997) 'Risk factors associated with recidivism among extrafamilial child molesters', *Journal of Consulting and Clinical Psychology*, 65: 141–49.

Putkonen, A., Kotilainen, I., Joyal, C. C. and Tiihonen, J. (2004) 'Comorbid personality disorders and substance use disorders of mentally ill homicide offenders: A structured clinical study on dual and triple diagnoses', *Schizophrenia Bulletin*, 30: 59–72.

Quinsey, V., Harris, G., Rice, M. and Cormier, C. (1998) *Violent Offenders: Appraising and Managing Risk*, Washington, DC: American Psychological Association.

Rasmussen, L. (1999) 'Factors related to recidivism among juvenile sexual offenders', *Sexual Abuse: A Journal of Research and Treatment*, 11: 69–85.

Raymond, N. C., Coleman, E., Oherlkling, F., Christenson, G. A. and Miner, M. (1999) 'Psychiatric comorbidity in pedophilic sex offenders', *American Journal of Psychiatry*, 156: 786–88.

Risk Management Authority (2007) *Standards and Guidelines for Risk Management of Offenders Subject to an Order of Lifelong Restriction*, www.rmascotland.gov.uk.

Russell, K. and Darjee, R. (this volume) 'Managing the risk posed by personality-disordered sex offenders in the community: A model for providing structured clinical guidance to support criminal justice services' in C. Logan and L. Johnstone (eds) *Managing Clinical Risk: A Guide to Effective Practice*, Abingdon: Routledge.

Rutter, M. (2011) 'Child psychiatric diagnosis and classification: Concepts, findings, challenges and potential', *Journal of Child Psychology and Psychiatry*, 52: 647–60.

Salekin, R. T., Rogers, R. and Sewell, K. W. (1996) 'A review and meta-analysis of the Psychopathy Checklist and Psychopathy Checklist Revised: Predictive validity and dangerousness', *Clinical Psychology: Science and Practice*, 3: 203–15.

Schwaner, S. L. (1998) 'Patterns of violent specialisation: Predictors of recidivism for a cohort of parolees', *American Journal of Criminal Justice*, 28: 371–84.

— (2000) '"Stick 'em up, buddy": Robbery, lifestyle and specialisation within a cohort of parolees', *Journal of Criminal Justice*, 28: 371–84.

Sippela, L. M. and Marshall, A. D. (2011) 'Post-traumatic stress disorder, intimate partner violence perpetration, and the mediating role of shame processing bias', *Journal of Anxiety Disorders*.

Skeem, J. L. and Cooke, D. J. (2010) 'Is criminal behavior a central component of psychopathy: Conceptual directions for resolving the debate', *Psychological Assessment*, 22: 433–45

Spitzer, M.B., Gibbon, R.L. and Williams, J.B.W (1996) *Structured Clinical Interview for DSM-IV Axis I Disorders, Clinician Version* (SCID-CV), Washington, D.C.: American Psychiatric Press, Inc.

Taylor, P. J. (1986) 'Psychiatric disorder in London's life-sentenced offenders', *British Journal of Criminology*, 26: 63–78.

— (1998) 'When symptoms of psychosis drive serious violence', *Social Psychiatry and Psychiatric Epidemiology*, 33: 47–54.

Touhami, M., Ouriaghli, F., Manoudi, F. and Asri, F. (2011) 'Pervasive developmental disorders and violence', *European Psychiatry*, 26, Abstracts of the European Congress of Psychiatry.

Violence Reduction Unit (2006) *Reducing Violence: An Alliance for a Safer Future*, UK: Violence Reduction Unit.

Warren, J. and South, S. (2009) 'Cluster B psychopathology among incarcerated women: Issues of internal consistency and construct validity', *International Journal of Law and Psychiatry*, 32: 10–17.

Webster, C. D., Douglas, K. S., Eaves, D. and Hart, S. D. (1997) *HCR-20: Assessing Risk for Violence* (Version 2), Burnaby, BC: Mental Health Law and Policy Unit, Simon Fraser University.

Webster, C. D., Martin, M-L., Brink, J., Nichols, T. L. and Desmaris, S. L. (2004) *The Short Term Assessment of Risk and Treatability (START)*, BC Mental Health and Addiction Services and St. Joseph's Healthcare, Hamilton.

Wechsler, D. (2008) *Wechsler Adult Intelligence Scale, 4th Edition*, Pearson Assessment.

Weerasekara, P. (1996) *Multi-perspective Case Formulation: A Step Towards Treatment Integration*, Malabar, FL: Krieger.

Wing, L., Leekam, L., Libby, S., Gould, J. and Larcombe, M. (2002) 'The Diagnostic Interview for Social and Communication Disorders: Background, inter-rater reliability and clinical use', *Journal of Child Psychology and Psychiatry*, 43: 307–25.

World Health Organization (1994) *International Classification of Diseases 10th Edition* (ICD-10), Geneva: World Health Organization.

— (2002) *World Report on Violence and Health*, Geneva: World Health Organisation.

4 Managing the risk posed by personality-disordered sex offenders in the community

A model for providing structured clinical guidance to support criminal justice services

Katharine Russell and Rajan Darjee

Introduction

There is a significant literature on assessing and managing risk in sexual offenders. Much has been written about aetiology (Ward, Polaschek and Beech, 2005), risk factors (Hanson and Morton-Bourgon, 2005, 2009), risk assessment instruments (Beech, Craig and Browne, 2009), treatment (Marshall, et al., 2006; Siegert, et al., 2007) and risk management (Siegert, et al., 2007). There are probably more instruments for sex offenders than any other offender group. Most sex offenders in the community in the UK are managed by probation services (or criminal justice social work services in Scotland) and the police. A significant minority are clinically complex with severe personality disorders and paraphilias providing particular challenges. Community forensic mental health services focus on severe mental illness and provide little input for these conditions. Risk assessment instruments used by criminal justice agencies and standard approaches to community management may be insufficient to properly manage these cases. Over the last four years, we have developed a service model for providing clinical input to help criminal justice agencies manage sexual offenders with personality disorders and paraphilias in South East Scotland. We present this model in this chapter to illustrate a practical approach to delivering evidence-based clinical risk management in a multi-agency community context with challenging and complex sexual offenders.

To provide a context for this, in the first part of this chapter we will examine the following issues: the nature and scope of sexual offending; mental health and legal responses to sex offenders both in the UK and abroad; and the process of assessing risk in sex offenders. We will then devote the second part of this chapter to an examination of the particular demands personality-disordered sex offenders present to services and make recommendations for how they may be managed in community settings. We will use the example of the Sex Offender Liaison Service based in Edinburgh, Scotland, to illustrate some key practice points we wish to make about risk assessment and management with this population. The chapter will then set out some observations about the clinical risk assessment and management of other special groups of sex offenders whom we have found to pose particular challenges. We will conclude with a set of good-practice recommendations.

Nature and scope of the problem

Sexual offending covers behaviours from indecent exposure and voyeurism, through sexual assault and rape, to sexually motivated homicide. Sex offenders are feared and vilified more than any other group daily by the media, politicians and the public. In this context, taking an objective, evidence-based approach can be difficult. Understanding the prevalence of sex offending, the characteristics of sex offenders, reoffending rates and the factors associated with sex offending is important so that risk management is proportionate and focused on the right issues.

Prevalence

There are difficulties specifying the prevalence of sexual offending due to low reporting rates, low conviction rates and definitional issues. In the UK, there are 50,000–60,000 sexual offences reported to the police annually, sexual offences account for 1–2 per cent of recorded crime, and for every sexual offence there are two to three non-sexual offences against the person (Page, et al., 2010; Walker, et al., 2009). According to the British Crime Survey, 3 per cent of women and 1 per cent of men were sexually assaulted in a year (Walker, et al., 2009). There were approximately 38,000 sex offenders subject to notification requirements under UK legislation living in the community on 31 March 2010 (Ministry of Justice, 2010a). About 10 per cent of UK male prisoners have committed sexual offences (Ministry of Justice, 2010b).

Recidivism

Recidivism rates of 10 to 20 per cent have been reported for a new sexual offence over 5–10 years (Craig, Browne and Beech, 2008; Hanson and Bussière, 1998). In a meta-analysis of studies of sexual offenders with an average follow-up of 5–6 years (Hanson and Morton-Bourgon, 2004), the rate of sexual recidivism was 13.7 per cent, of non-sexual violent recidivism 14.0 per cent, of violent recidivism (sexual or non-sexual) 25.0 per cent, and of general recidivism 36.9 per cent. Offenders with adult victims have higher rates of violent and general recidivism compared to offenders with child victims. Rates of sexual recidivism are highest in extra-familial child molesters, lowest in intra-familial child molesters and intermediate in adult rapists (Hanson, 2002). Many offenders do not fall neatly into these categories. Offenders with adult and child victims, or with male and female victims, have higher rates of recidivism than 'non-diverse' offenders (Heil and Simmons, 2008). High rates of reoffending have been reported in men who indecently expose (Murphy and Page, 2008). Very low rates of new offences have been reported in sexual offenders after they reach the age of 60 (Hanson, 2001). Unsurprisingly very different rates of 'recidivism' are reported if non-convicted allegations or concerning behaviours are included (Falshaw, et al., 2003). The length of follow-up is important; not all reoffending occurs within five or ten years, about a fifth of reoffending occurs more than ten years after release (Home Office, 2004). Despite adjustments to figures to take account of under-reporting, the majority of sexual offenders do not reoffend, and when they do they are more likely to commit a non-sexual offence. As a group, sexual offenders have lower recidivism rates than almost all other types of offenders (Home Office, 2001).

Typologies and aetiological models

Sex offenders are heterogeneous in motivations, personal characteristics, psycho-sexual functioning, propensity to reoffend, and responsiveness to interventions. Two types of models have sought to bring understanding and organisation: typologies (Knight and Prentky, 1990) and aetiological models (Ward and Beech, 2006).

There are typologies of rapists (Knight and Prentky, 1990), sexual murderers (Proulx, et al., 2007), child molesters (Knight and Prentky, 1990), internet offenders (Beech, et al., 2008), indecent exposers (Morin and Levenson, 2008), and female offenders (Gannon and Cortoni, 2010). For example, studies of rapists seem to point to sadistic, angry, opportunistic and sexual types (Canter and Heritage, 1989; Groth, 1979; Knight and Prentky, 1990; Kocsis, 2010). It is important not to squeeze individuals into typological boxes and many offenders do not fit perfectly into categories. Few typologies have been empirically validated or empirically linked to risk, but using typologies can help when formulating a case.

Similarly, aetiological models can provide a framework for case formulation (Ward, et al., 2005). There are single-factor theories, but given the complexity of sexual offending, we find multifactor aetiological models more useful. Most aetiological models describe the distal and proximal factors and processes that lead to sexual offending. Ward and Beech's (2006) unified theory is a comprehensive bio-psycho-social model that fits with current models of risk (Beech and Ward, 2004). Note that many of the factors that appear in aetiological models of sexual offending mirror those of relevance to personality disorders; for example, genetic vulnerabilities, early attachment experiences, and maladaptive schema.

Mental health and legal responses: a comparison across jurisdictions

Legal responses

Given political and public concerns, most jurisdictions have their own specific laws and sentences. Some apply to sex offenders and some to other 'dangerous' offenders too. Some legal measures require an assessment of risk before imposition, some assume risk for certain types of offenders, and others allow for generic or specific risk management strategies to be put in place.

Indeterminate sentences are used in several jurisdictions for offenders considered to pose an ongoing risk to the public. These are used disproportionately for sex offenders (Darjee and Russell, 2011; McSherry and Keyzer, 2009). Uniquely in Scotland, a structured professional judgement formulation-based assessment is required by statutory guidance before the imposition of such sentences. Other sentences used for sex offenders include extended sentences, determinate sentences and probation orders. Extended sentences in the UK allow for longer than usual, but not indeterminate, statutory supervision following release from prison. In some jurisdictions, post-sentence commitment allows detention in hospital (e.g. sexually violent predator laws in the USA; Miller, Amenta and Conroy, 2005) or prison (e.g. Australia; Mercado and Ogloff, 2007) following a determinate sentence. In England and Wales, mental health legislation is sometimes used to detain personality-disordered offenders in secure hospitals at the end of a prison sentence. Concerns have been raised about such post-hoc measures (McSherry and Keyzer, 2009).

Since 1997 in the UK, convicted sex offenders in the community have been required to notify certain personal details to the police for a determinate or indeterminate period, depending on their sentence. This is known colloquially as signing the 'sex offenders register', although unlike other jurisdictions, such as most US states, there is no publically available register. Notification allows police to put in place monitoring arrangements. Some offenders who had received long sentences were subject to notification requirements indefinitely without review, but this was recently found to breach the European Convention on Human Rights. Now there has to be periodic review of such cases with a test based on risk of sexual harm. In the UK, a range of civil orders is available to restrict individuals considered to pose a risk of sexual harm; for example, sexual offences prevention orders, risk of sexual harm orders, and foreign travel orders. In England and Wales, legislation allows mandatory polygraph testing in the supervision of sex offenders in the community (Grubin, Wilcox and Madsen, 2007).

Electronic tagging and GPS tracking are used to restrict and monitor the movements of sex offenders. There is limited evidence that they reduce reoffending (Button, et al., 2009; Mair, 2005). In some US states, exclusion zones are such that it can be impossible for sex offenders to live near other people, which can lead to individuals becoming isolated and going missing (Council of State Governments, 2010). Community notification in the USA may require individuals to place notices on their property and cars, and allows public access to details of sex offenders in the community via websites and mobile phone apps. In the UK, disclosure to certain individuals (e.g. employers, accommodation providers, schools) may occur if this is merited in an individual case. A scheme to allow parents to seek information from the police regarding individuals they are concerned about (e.g. a new partner who has access to their children) has been extended across Scotland. Blanket notification (like restriction zones) can alienate sexual offenders and perhaps increase risk. Although blanket or limited notification may reassure the public, there is no evidence that it contributes to reducing the risk of sexual violence.

Multi-Agency Public Protection Arrangements (MAPPA) are a statutory framework in the UK to ensure multi-agency cooperation in the management of high-risk sex offenders in the community. Agencies involved include: police, criminal justice social work/probation, prison, housing, health service, other social services, and some voluntary sector agencies. At the core of MAPPA is information sharing and joint risk management. Within MAPPA, cases are allocated to one of three levels, depending on the complexity of risk management. Of those allocated to the highest levels (2 and 3), almost all have significant personality disorders.

Mental health responses

Many sexual offenders have mental disorders considering the range of conditions in ICD-10 and DSM-IV. Most common are personality disorders, paraphilias and substance-related disorders. Severe mental illnesses, mood disorders, anxiety disorders, organic disorders and learning disabilities are less common, but more prevalent than in the general population. (Alden et al., 2007; Fazel et al., 2007).

There is a traditional mental health model used for offenders with severe mental illness and marked learning disability in the UK and other jurisdictions. Sexual offenders with these conditions are usually diverted into forensic mental health services where they are provided with care and treatment. The assumption is that treating the mental illness will reduce the risk. The problem is that research shows most mentally ill sex offenders have the same criminogenic needs as non-mentally ill sex offenders (Drake and Pathé, 2004). The implication is that the same risk assessment, treatment and risk management strategies used for non-mentally ill sexual offenders are relevant to mentally ill offenders. The challenge is to integrate good risk management with mental health treatment.

Sex offenders with personality disorders and paraphilias do not fit this traditional model. But they pose challenges for criminal justice agencies both in prison and the community. The challenge with these offenders is to provide clinical input to enhance understanding of cases, risk assessment and risk management in criminal justice settings, to both support criminal justice agencies and reduce risk. Some jurisdictions have tried a primarily mental health approach to personality-disordered offenders, including sex offenders (e.g. Dangerous and Severe Personality Disorder or DSPD Programme services in secure hospitals in England and Wales, and Sexually Violent Predator commitment in the USA). Such services rely on an approach very close to the traditional mental health model, which whilst appropriate for individuals with severe mental illness does not work well for individuals with personality disorders. There is little to recommend this approach for personality-disordered sexual offenders (Tyrer, et al., 2010; Duggan, 2011). In England and Wales, the future focus is likely to be on management in criminal justice rather than mental health settings (Department of Health, 2011).

Assessing risk in sex offenders: Models and minefields

Sexual violence risk factors fall into three categories: static, stable dynamic and acute dynamic (Table 4.1). These categories can be mapped onto aetiological models (Beech and Ward, 2004), which describe distal developmental factors (such as attachment problems, genetic vulnerability, abuse or rejection) that lead to psychological vulnerabilities or traits (sexual problems, dysfunctional attitudes, emotional and interpersonal difficulties, self-regulation problems), heightening the risk of particular states of mind, leading to offending. Static factors are markers for psychological vulnerabilities and traits. All three categories have factors specifically associated with sexual recidivism and factors associated with recidivism of any type (sexual and non-sexual). Please see Table 4.1 for more information about risk factors for sexual reoffending.

Systematic reviews have summarized static and stable dynamic factors (Hanson and Brussière, 1998; Hanson and Morton-Bourgon, 2004; Mann, et al., 2010). Previously, denial and victim empathy were considered important factors, featuring heavily in assessments conducted by practitioners and in treatment programmes. No research has shown lack of victim empathy is related to future sexual offending (Hanson and Morton-Bourgon, 2004), and denial has largely been found to be the same, albeit with some interesting exceptions (denial has been found to be related

Table 4.1 Static, stable dynamic and acute dynamic risk factors for sexual re-offending

Historic/Static	Stable/Dynamic	Acute

• Sexual violence history
• Non-sexual violence history
• Childhood problems
• Young age
• Employment problems
• Relationship problems
• Substance misuse
• Response to supervision
	• Social influences
	• Intimacy deficits
	  o Capacity for relationship stability
	  o Emotional identification with children
	  o Hostility towards women
	  o General social rejection
	  o Lack of concern for others
	• Pro-offending attitudes
	  o Rape-supportive attitudes
	  o Child-molester-supportive attitudes
	  o Sexual entitlement
	• General self-regulation
	  o Impulsive
	  o Poor problem-solving
	  o Negative emotionality
	• Sexual self-regulation
	  o Sexual preoccupation
	  o Sex as coping
	  o Deviant sexual preference
	• Cooperation with supervision
		Triggers
		• Increase in substance misuse
		• Deteriorating relationships
		• Increased contact with pro-offending peers
		• Problems getting or keeping work
		• Increased access to potential victims
		
		Situation/State
		• Increased sexual preoccupation
		• Mood/mental state
		• Creating opportunities or making plans to offend
		• Using drugs/alcohol to deal with negative emotions
		• Isolation
		• Increasingly chaotic lifestyle

to reoffending in some incest offenders but to be protective in some higher risk offenders; Mann, et al., 2010). Despite research evidence, practitioners, in our experience, are reluctant to ignore these factors. Acute dynamic factors are less easy to research as they act over minutes, hours or a few days.

Two clinical conditions, personality disorder and sexual deviance, are particularly important when assessing risk in sex offenders (Hanson and Morton Bourgon, 2005). Personality disorder, antisocial personality disorder, and particularly psychopathy, are associated with general, violent and sexual reoffending. A close look at stable dynamic factors reveals that many may be underpinned by dysfunctional personality traits and sexual disorders (see Table 4.2).

There is not a consensus on the best way to identify risk factors or to combine them in a systematic and meaningful way (although see Douglas et al., this volume). As with other areas of violence risk assessment, there are arguments as to the relative merits of actuarial and structured professional judgement (SPJ)

Table 4.2 An example of how personality disorder traits and paraphilias may underpin stable dynamic risk factors, using Stable 2007 and DSM-IV personality disorders and paraphilias

Stable Dynamic Factor from Stable 2007	Relevant disorders from DSM-IV
Significant social influences	-
Capacity for relationship stability	Paranoid Schizoid Schizotypal Borderline Antisocial Narcissistic Histrionic Avoidant Dependent Obsessive-compulsive
Emotional identification with children	Schizoid Avoidant Borderline
Hostility toward women	Paranoid Antisocial Narcissistic
General social rejection	Paranoid Schizoid Schizotypal Avoidant
Lack of concern for others	Narcissistic Antisocial Schizoid
Impulsive	Antisocial Borderline

Stable Dynamic Factor from Stable 2007	Relevant disorders from DSM-IV
Poor problem solving	Paranoid Borderline Antisocial Avoidant Dependent Obsessive-compulsive
Negative emotionality	Paranoid Borderline Avoidant
Sex drive/preoccupations	-
Sex as coping	-
Deviant sexual preference	Paraphilias
Cooperation with supervision	Paranoid Schizoid Antisocial Narcissistic Borderline

approaches (see Cooke and Michie, this volume; also Cooke and Michie, 2011; Hart and Boer, 2010; Hart and Logan, 2011; Quinsey, et al., 2006), and evidence that unstructured approaches are poor (Hanson and Morton Bourgon, 2009). It is important that practitioners are trained in any risk assessment instrument or tool they use, have the necessary competence to use the tool, and understand its scope and limitations. They also need to know how to interpret the output of any tool so as to reach appropriate conclusions and plan risk management appropriately. SPJ approaches involving an individualized formulation of risk are particularly useful with complex cases with underlying personality disorders (Hart and Logan, 2011; Logan and Johnstone, 2010).

Risk assessment should lead to proportionate, individualized, defensible risk management. Monitoring and restrictions should be based on the particular issues of concern in a case (e.g. access to children, alcohol/substance misuse). In too many cases, one-size-fits-all generic management plans are used for sex offenders as a group or for types of sex offenders (e.g. child molesters or rapists; 'low', 'medium' or 'high' risk cases) and defensive rather than defensible practice creeps in. This can be avoided by using an evidence-based individualized approach. Scenario planning as part of an SPJ assessment can help achieve this (Hart and Boer, 2010), particularly where cases are complex and/or concerning (Hart and Logan, 2011). It is important to prioritize and put in place the key measures necessary, particularly in complex cases with an overwhelming myriad of risk factors, few if any protective factors, a complex formulation, and future scenarios pointing towards a seriously harmful outcome. A common mistake is to put in place far too many risk management strategies in such cases.

The challenge of assessing and managing sexual offenders with personality and sexual disorders

There are high rates of personality disorders in sexual offenders (Fazel, et al., 2007). Over a third, and perhaps more than half, of sexual offenders have personality disorders (Dunsieth, et al., 2004; Fazel and Danesh, 2002; Fazel, et al., 2007; Raymond, et al., 1999). Personality disorder is particularly prevalent in high-risk cases receiving long or indeterminate prison sentences (Coid, et al., 2007), and amongst difficult to manage offenders in the community (Craissati, et al., 2011). Personality pathology is heterogeneous. High rates of antisocial, narcissistic, paranoid and psychopathic traits have been described in adult rapists (Chantry and Craig, 1994; Craissati, Webb and Keen, 2008; Oliver, et al., 2007; Porter, et al., 2000). There may be higher rates of avoidant, schizoid and obsessional traits in child sexual offenders and internet offenders (Webb, Craissati and Keen, 2007). High rates of borderline personality disorder have also been reported (Turner, Miller and Henderson, 2008). Psychopathy is associated with sexual and non-sexual violent recidivism (Hildebrand, deReiter and deVogel, 2004). Psychopathy is also associated with poor engagement in supervision, dropping out of treatment and poor response to treatment (Lösel, 1998). The accepted wisdom that treatment makes psychopaths more likely to reoffend has been questioned by recent reviews (D'Silva, 2004). Personality disorder more generally can cause difficulties with treatment and management (Craissati, et al., 2011). A number of stable dynamic risk factors (see Table 4.2) are manifestations of dysfunctional personality traits.

Unsurprisingly, paraphilias (also known as disorders of sexual preference) are associated with sexual offending. But not all sex offenders have paraphilias, and most people with paraphilias do not commit sexual offences. The prevalence of paraphilias in sex offenders is put at between 25 per cent and 75 per cent (Dunsieth, et al., 2004; Hanson and Harris, 2000; Raymond, et al., 1999). In child molesters, extra-familial offenders have high rates of paedophilia, but most incest offenders are not paedophilic. Most adult rapists do not have paraphilias and a rare minority are sexually sadistic. There is some controversy as to whether a preference for coercive sex should be recognized as a paraphilia in DSM-5 (Knight, 2010). Some sex offenders have multiple paraphilias (Freund, 1990). Deviant sexual interests, particularly paedophilia, sexual sadism and multiple paraphilias, are associated with sexual recidivism (Becker and Murphy, 1998; Hanson and Bussière, 1998; Kafka, 2003). Rates of paraphilias in sexual murderers are as high as 80 per cent (Hill, et al., 2007; Proulx, et al., 2007). Phallometric assessments of internet child pornography offenders show they have higher rates of paedophilia than contact offenders (Quayle, 2008). Hypersexual arousal (a suggested sexual dysfunction for DSM-5) is associated with reoffending in sexual offenders (Kafka, 2003).

Assessing personality disorders and paraphilias is important in sex offenders who have these conditions. Where cases are unusual, concerning or challenging, this is particularly important. Understanding the role of these conditions in the risk posed by a sexual offender requires evidence-based assessment and a comprehensive case formulation, leading to a management plan which takes personality disorder and/or paraphilia into account.

The NHS Lothian Sex Offender Liaison Service (SOLS)

The Scottish context

In Scotland, forensic mental health services focus on offenders with severe mental illness and learning disabilities. A primary diagnosis of personality disorder does not result in a mental health disposal (Darjee and Crichton, 2004). There is little interest or expertise in personality disorder within forensic mental health services. Offenders with personality disorders are managed within the criminal justice system, in prison and the community, with very limited if any clinical input.

In Scotland, the two agencies most closely involved with sex-offender management in the community are the police and criminal justice social work. The police, through specific offender-management units, monitor all registered sex offenders in the community. Criminal justice social work supervise those on probation or those released from prison on parole. About a third of registered sex offenders in the community are also under criminal justice social work supervision. Criminal justice social work deliver accredited group treatment programmes. In prison, sex offenders are offered sex offender and other treatment programmes, but unlike England and Wales, there is no specific provision for prisoners with personality disorders. Treatment programmes in prison are run by forensic psychologists with the support of prison officers and social workers. Mental health teams in prison are not involved with these programmes and focus instead on identification and treatment of prisoners with mental illness.

National guidance compels criminal justice agencies to use actuarial static (*Risk Matrix 2000*) and dynamic (*Stable and Acute 2007*) instruments. SPJ purists would argue against using such tools at all (Cooke, 2010; see also Cooke and Michie, this volume), but it would be unrealistic to use a comprehensive SPJ approach for all sex offenders. However, actuarial instruments are particularly limited with the complex personality-disordered sexual offenders who are challenging and concerning. In such cases, an SPJ formulation approach is particularly useful when planning risk management (Hart and Logan, 2011), but requires a degree of clinical expertise not widely available to criminal justice practitioners in Scotland.

There has been limited opportunity for joint working between criminal justice and mental health services involved with personality-disordered sex offenders. Most community forensic mental health services do not accept referrals of offenders with primary personality disorder, and focus on individuals with schizophrenia and other mental illnesses. Many forensic services do not take direct referrals from criminal justice agencies in the community, and when they do, it is not uncommon for an assessment of a personality-disordered offender (if undertaken at all) to conclude with the unhelpful (and very insightful!) comment that the person is 'not mentally ill'.

The introduction of MAPPA in 2007 provided an opportunity for greater joint working, as the NHS became a partner agency in the management of sex offenders in the community. Forensic mental health services, as part of the NHS in Scotland, have varied in the extent to which they have used this to develop closer working ties with criminal justice agencies.

SOLS: service development, model and description

Criminal justice agencies were frustrated by the lack of input from mental health services with their more difficult and complex offenders and the focus purely on mental illness. They were also limited when managing difficult personality dis-ordered and paraphilic sexual offenders by not having access to an SPJ formulation approach. Forensic mental health clinicians were resistant to becoming involved with criminal justice's difficult and concerning sex offenders, fearing that they would be left 'holding the baby'. SOLS sought to address these issues by providing clinical input to support criminal justice agencies in the management of challenging sex offenders in the community. It addressed the above problems by providing clinical input in a criminal justice context without turning offenders into 'patients' within the traditional mental health model described above.

The service is different from traditional forensic mental health services in Scotland in a number of ways. It is not psychiatry-led, but jointly led by psychology and psychiatry. The service is small: NHS Lothian fund half a consultant forensic psychiatrist, a full-time consultant clinical psychologist, and full-time adminis-trative support, with some additional input from the trainee psychologists and psychiatrists we supervise. The service has always focused on how to use a limited resource to help with as many cases as possible and that is the reason behind the use of a consultation/liaison model.

We provide varying levels of input to support criminal justice services, from telephone advice through to comprehensive clinical assessments (see Figure 4.1). The service has developed over the last four years, adapting to the demands placed on it. We have very few referral criteria; we are basically interested in discussing anyone who has a history of sexual offending (including allegations) or who is considered to be at risk of sexual offending (even if they do not have a sexual conviction) whom agencies are struggling to understand or manage. We do not use personality disorder as a referral criterion as referrals come from non-clinicians (usually criminal justice social workers or police officers). We are therefore happy to consider anyone who is 'tricky, difficult, challenging, causing concern, causing agencies or staff to fall out, or unusual'. We do not have referral forms but encour-age people to phone or email us with cases that are causing concern. Our close working relationships with criminal justice agencies locally facilitate the referral process and we very rarely receive inappropriate referrals.

All referrals are allocated for a case discussion where we meet the referrer and any other staff involved for one and a half hours. At this meeting we attempt to gain an understanding of the offender and the issues of concern; we review the case information available, we construct a preliminary case formulation, and

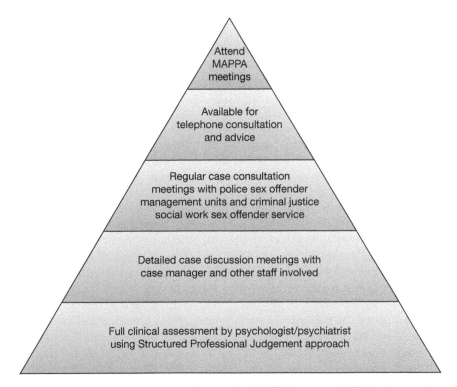

Figure 4.1 Sex Offender Liaison Service, levels of clinical input to criminal justice agencies

provide 'on-the-spot' advice and consultation. We use SPJ tools to help structure consideration of the case. In some cases this is sufficient, although we are always happy to discuss cases again in the future if there are further issues. If the case is too complex or we do not have a good enough understanding of the case from the material available, we will undertake a comprehensive clinical assessment of personality and risk.

A full assessment involves a minimum of two two-hour interviews with two members of SOLS staff, a review of all records from every agency that has been involved with the client (prison, police, social work, mental health, courts), interviews with staff who know the client, and sometimes interviewing partners or family members. Interviews are conducted by two staff of different genders to allow for an assessment of how the individual interacts differentially with males and females. This has been particularly informative in assessing the attitudes, interpersonal functioning and emotional reactions of rapists. Having two staff involved also provides supervision, support, safety, and consensus scoring of instruments.

We use a number of structured instruments: the *Psychopathy Checklist-Revised* (PCL-R; Hare, 2003), the *International Personality Disorder Examination* (IPDE; Loranger, 1999), the *Sexual Sadism Scale* (SSS; Marshall, et al., 2002), the *Screening Scale for Paedophilic Interests* (SSPI; Seto and Lalumière, 2001), the

RSVP and the RM2000. The RM2000 provides a useful nomothetic starting point for considering risk, but does not contribute much to our assessments. In using the RSVP, given recent evidence, we place little weight on the denial/minimization factor and routinely consider the additional factors, in particular, sexual preoccupation and sexualized coping. If warranted, we also use the HCR-20, the *Spousal Assault Risk Assessment Guide* (SARA; Kropp, et al., 1999), the *Stalking Assessment Manual* (SAM; Kropp, Hart and Lyon, 2008) and selected neuropsychological assessments. Our assessments use an SPJ approach, and the key aspects of our assessments are comprehensive case formulation and narrative risk scenarios, leading to pragmatic risk management advice for community criminal justice agencies.

The individuals we assess have significant personality dysfunction, most have personality disorders, and a significant minority have psychopathy (see Table 4.3). So assessing personality disorder comprehensively and in a way that helps inform management is crucial. We favour a dimensional approach to understanding personality disorder and keenly await the introduction of the 5th edition of the *Diagnostic and Statistical Manuals* (DSM-5; Widiger, 2011). In the meantime, we are more interested in what the IPDE and PCL-R tell us about personality dysfunction and dimensions, rather than using them as diagnostic tools with cutoffs. We are less interested in whether a person meets four or five narcissistic criteria than in the implications of their narcissistic traits for understanding interpersonal development, offending and how management should be delivered (Logan and Johnstone, 2010).

Paraphilias need to be assessed appropriately. The use of interviews and self-report measures can be problematic. Penile plethysmography (PPG) is not available

Table 4.3 Characteristics of 82 sexual offenders fully assessed by NHS Lothian Sex Offender Liaison Service (SOLS) between May 2007 and June 2011 (excluding consultation-only cases)

$N =$		No.	%
82	*Referred by:*		
	Criminal justice social work	36	43.9
	Police	20	24.4
	Mental health services	17	20.7
	Court	8	9.8
81	*Offending history:*		
	Internet offending	15	18.5
	Other non-contact (e.g. exhibitionism)	27	33.3
	Contact offending	59	72.8
	Penetrative offending	37	45.7
	Sexual homicide	5	6.2
	Non-sexual violent offending	31	38.3
	Non-sexual non-violent offending	45	55.6
	Sexual offending against child	56	69.1
	Sexual offending against adult	38	46.9
	Sexual offending against male	26	32.1
	Sexual offending against female	60	74.1
	'Seriously harmful' offending	50	61.7

N =		No.	%
71	*Any personality disorder:*		
	Any personality disorder	55	77.5
	Cluster A	20	28.2
	Paranoid	10	14.1
	Schizoid	12	16.9
	Schizotypal	8	11.3
	Cluster B	39	54.9
	Antisocial	29	40.8
	Borderline	10	14.1
	Histrionic	2	2.8
	Narcissistic	17	23.9
	Cluster C	13	18.3
	Avoidant	12	16.9
	Dependent	0	0
	Obsessive-compulsive	4	5.6
69	PCL-R Score 0–19	51	73.9
	Score 20–29	9	13
	Score 30+	9	13

'Seriously harmful' = behaviour which is life threatening and/or traumatic and from which the victim's recovery, whether physical or psychological, can be expected to be difficult or impossible.

in Scotland. Although there are arguments that PPG is unreliable and adds little to the assessment of sex offenders (e.g., Marshall 2006), PPG-assessed sexual deviance is an important risk factor (Hanson and Morton Bourgon, 2005). Alternative methods of assessing paraphilias include viewing time measures (Abel and Wiegal, 2009; Harris, et al., 1996) and behavioural ratings of objective offence behaviours. We use two behavioural rating scales: the *Sexual Sadism Scale* (SSS; Marshall and Hucker, 2006) and the *Screening Scale for Pedophilic Interests* (SSPI; Seto and Lalumiére, 2001). We have not used viewing time measures, but will shortly commence using Affinity 2.5 (Glasgow, 2009) to assess individuals where sexual interest in children is an issue.

In our formulations, we always consider childhood, adolescent and adult development, personality functioning, sexual development and functioning, and offence analysis. This enables us to consider predisposing, precipitating and perpetuating factors of relevance to offending. We also explicitly consider protective factors, including those of relevance to desistance (Laws and Ward, 2011). We use scenarios to give a narrative conclusion to inform risk management recommendations, and never use terms like 'low', 'medium' or 'high risk'. Why not? When cases are referred, the risk assessment tools already used will have provided a score and an attached risk level. The reason for referral is usually that staff feel they do not really understand the offence or how the person is presenting, and therefore struggle to manage risk. By providing a formulation of past offences, scenarios of potential future offending and an understanding of interpersonal dynamics, we provide a unique and practical contribution to managing the case.

A significant part of our risk management recommendations focuses on relationships that criminal justice staff have with the offender. This is based on what we learn about the offender's previous attachments, particularly with parents, but also with friends, partners and victims. The interpersonal dynamics of early attachments, offences, and supervisory relationships often mirror each other (Craissati, et al., 2011). We try to help staff engage positively and productively with offenders, and to avoid getting drawn into unhelpful ways of interacting.

We attempt to make our reports concise and user-friendly. No one wants to read a 30–50-page report, no matter how erudite it is! We make sure we focus on the specific practical issues that are causing concern (see Figure 4.2). Once completed, the report is sent to the referrer, we make it available to the offender, and it is shared with all those involved with the case. We attend risk management meetings to feed back the conclusions of the assessment, and provide ongoing advice and consultation on the cases we have seen.

SOLS: successes and challenges

The service aims to provide clinical input (within an SPJ framework) to support criminal justice agencies (particularly the police and criminal justice social work) to manage personality-disordered sex offenders in the community. Feedback from the agencies we work with indicates that we have managed to achieve that aim and are now seen as an intrinsic part of the multi-agency management of sex offenders in the Lothian and Borders area of Scotland. The aspects of the service that are

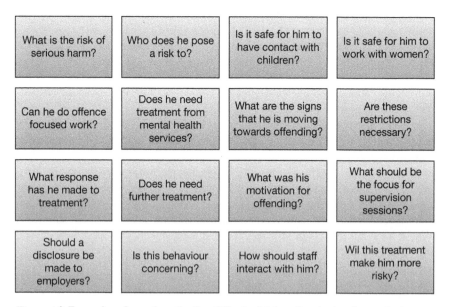

Figure 4.2 Examples of questions the Sex Offender Liaison Service has been asked to consider

responsible for its success are good working relationships with other agencies; providing support and advice which is of direct practical relevance; making sure other agencies understand what we can (and cannot) do, and our understanding of the role of other agencies; fitting the service into criminal justice systems and structures, rather than mental health systems and structures; support from our organization (NHS Lothian) and support from staff at all levels in other MAPPA agencies; the enthusiasm, commitment and expertise of our staff; making links with other clinicians who work with sex offenders internationally for advice and peer support; and being flexible and adapting to use our resources in the most effective way as demands change.

As the service has developed, we have been seeing increasingly disturbed individuals who sometimes engender strong or unusual counter-transference reactions. Recently we have started having regular reflective practice supervision from a psychodynamic psychotherapist. This has helped us to understand our reactions and formulate cases. We now see this as a crucial aspect of supervision within our service. Other aspects of supervision are equally important: we ring-fence regular time to discuss cases and formulations, and informal peer support is always available. This is not work that should be done in isolation.

We see many individuals who have unmet treatment needs, particularly the need for psychological treatment for personality disorders or for sex offender treatment that cannot be provided by criminal justice social work. Sometimes they can access treatment through services that are available locally (e.g. psychotherapy services), but there is a dearth of treatment services for the types of individuals we see. Within the resources and remit of our service, we are not able to provide treatment, although we have started to think about the potential development of treatment approaches.

Another challenge in multi-agency working with sex offenders in the community is the tension between restrictive approaches to management (curfews, tagging, minders, limiting work opportunities, disclosures, and so on) and a more positive approach informed by desistance and good-lives models. Although we occasionally find ourselves recommending very restrictive measures (e.g. where a psychopathic sexual sadist is being released from prison at the end of a determinate sentence), we also find ourselves questioning some of the restrictions that other agencies consider necessary. Sometimes the restrictions imposed make it inevitable that a person will fail (and be recalled to prison) and occasionally restrictions increase risk (e.g. by making the person frustrated and angry). Rather than causing overt conflict this tension usually leads to healthy debate and a more considered approach by the agencies involved. The most important thing is that those involved in imposing restrictions have a clear understanding as to what restrictions are likely to reduce risk and why. Placing unnecessary restrictions on personality-disordered sex offenders wastes resources, takes the focus away from more important risk management activities, leads to unnecessary conflict between staff and offenders, and may mitigate against meaningful engagement with the offender.

Although we are a community service, we see a number of individuals in prison. These are cases where community agencies want advice and guidance on whether an offender is ready to move to the community, how an offender should transition to the community, and what management strategies will be required subsequently. These cases have highlighted that often no understanding of an offender's personality or sexual pathology has been factored into management in prison, transition to the community or community planning. All of these aspects of management require an individual case formulation, which is shared by the prison, community agencies, and the offender. There can be tensions between prison and community agencies, and our challenge is to remain objective, be clear about our role, and to try not to get caught in the politics.

An interesting challenge is other agencies deferring to our 'expert opinion' or indeed declining to have an opinion until they have sought an opinion from SOLS. We strive to ensure that our advice and assessments are seen as providing 'an opinion' that is based on the use of specific approaches and skills, i.e. SPJ risk assessment and personality-disorder assessments. We believe other agencies should be able to take our advice and use it to help inform their strategies and thinking, but also enter into a dialogue with us about things with which they may disagree. It would be dangerous to promote ourselves as being 'expert' or 'all-knowing', and when it comes to community risk management, the agencies we work with have their own skills and expertise. It is important that we remain clear about our role and remit, that we do not discourage others from using their skills, and that we maintain good but boundaried working relationships with other agencies.

We have been fascinated to see very recent proposals in England and Wales for the management of personality-disordered offenders (Department of Health, 2011). These proposals suggest that there is a need to identify personality-disordered offenders as they require specialist input, and to delineate a pathway from sentencing, through prison and into the community. The community model stresses the need for specialist psychological consultation to probation staff. We see similarities with our service and watch with interest to see how services develop in England and Wales.

Special groups

We have found some specific groups particularly challenging. We do not aim to cover these groups in detail below, but only to highlight some key issues.

Young people

Children and adolescents who display sexually harmful behaviour can be a particularly difficult group to assess, and assessment and treatment have to be approached differently than for adults (Rich, 2009). Given their developmental level, it is difficult to make definitive statements about the presence of sexual deviancy, personality dysfunction, sexual attitudes, and sexual preoccupation. Relatively few juvenile offenders reoffend, but there may be a concerning small sub-group who start offending early and continue offending into adulthood. Given the differences between adolescents and adult offenders, specific risk assessment tools (e.g. the *Assessment, Intervention and Moving on Project* [AIM], the *Estimate of Risk of Adolescent Sexual Offence Recidivism* [ERASOR], the *Juvenile Sex Offender Assessment Protocol-II* [J-SOAP II]) have been developed (Worling and Långström, 2006; Prentky, et al., 2009). Interventions may send these individuals on very different life paths. Research indicates that intervention with this group should be holistic (focusing on needs across all dimensions of the child's life and development), systemic (involving families and parents to deal with outstanding child protection and parenting concerns) and goal-specific (addressing specific issues related to the child's harmful sexual behaviours). Multi-systemic therapy has been recommended for this group, but is resource intensive (Letourneau, et al., 2009).

We do not specialize in assessing young people. Occasionally we are asked to see a 17-year-old on the cusp of adulthood with a history from early childhood of severe behavioural problems and where there are concerns about the risk of very serious sexual offending. These are individuals with 'emerging' personality disorders, and we assess them but are cautious about applying adult approaches to them.

Sexual sadism and sexual homicide

Sexual sadism is sexual arousal or fantasies involving humiliation, suffering and violence towards another person (Yates, et al., 2008). A minority of sexual offenders are sexually sadistic, but those who are perpetrate some of the most extreme forms of sexual violence and pose a risk of serious harm towards victims. The categorical approach to the diagnosis of sexual sadism in DSM-IV has been criticized, and the reliability of diagnosis by clinicians has been questioned (Marshall and Kennedy, 2003). Marshall and Hucker (2006) have suggested a more dimensional multifaceted approach to assessing sexual sadism (the SSS – see above) looking at behaviours such as strangulation/asphyxiation, abduction, torture, bondage, ritualistic acts, injuries to genitals and breasts. As mentioned above, deviant sexual interest (which includes sexual sadism) is a key risk factor when assessing risk of sexual violence.

Sexual homicide is rare. In most single sexual homicide cases, the perpetrator does not set out to kill, but kills the victim by accident, as a reaction to victim resistance or due to panic. Some perpetrators deliberately kill to prevent victims identifying them. A minority of sexual murderers are intrinsically motivated to meet psychological needs through killing. In these cases, the underlying motivation may be a paraphilia such as sexual sadism or necrophilia, or hatred/rage. Serial sexual murderers are invariably intrinsically motivated to kill. Compared to non-homicidal sexual offenders, sexual killers are more likely to be isolated, not in a relationship, and to have paraphilias. However, most studies have found more similarities than differences, perhaps reflecting that most do not set out to kill. Perpetrators of serial sexual homicide have very high rates of sexual sadism and personality disorders, including psychopathy. For more information on sexual homicide see Purcell and Arrigo (2006), Proulx, et al. (2007), Hill, et al. (2007) and Chan and Heide (2009).

In assessing perpetrators of sexual homicide and sexually sadistic offenders, actuarial approaches are of very limited utility, given the rarity of such cases in development samples (Kingston and Yates, 2008). Structured professional judgment tools for sexual offending and violence should be used, alongside a comprehensive assessment of personality disorder and paraphilia. Assessing sexual sadism, as for other paraphilias, may involve clinical interviews, self-report questionnaires, PPG or assessment of patterns of behaviour at crime scenes. Viewing time measures to assess sexual sadism are in their infancy. Given the potential for very serious harm, detailed consideration should be given to scenarios that may lead to serious injury or fatality to help in guiding risk management strategies. Pharmacological and psychological approaches to treatment may be used, although there is no research on effectiveness in sexually sadistic and/or homicidal offenders. Where there is an ongoing risk of serious harm to others, consideration will need to be given to restrictive measures, such as long-term incarceration.

We have assessed a number of individuals who have committed sexual homicide or other extreme violence in the course of sexual offending. In the rare cases where we identify sexual sadism, we are extremely cautious about community risk management. Given the dearth of evidence, we have sometimes turned to international experts, who are rarely reassuring about managing risk in the community.

Internet offenders

Internet offending is a relatively new form of sexual offending. There are four forms of internet sex offending: (a) downloading indecent images; (b) distributing indecent images; (c) accessing victims through the internet (sometimes called 'online grooming'); and (d) manufacturing indecent images. Images of children being abused can be classified according to the Combating Paedophile Information Networks in Europe or COPINE Scale categories: (1) images depicting erotic posing with no sexual activity; (2) sexual activity between children, or solo masturbation by a child; (3) non-penetrative sexual activity between adults and children; (4) penetrative sexual activity between children and adults; and (5) sadism or bestiality involving children. The COPINE scale has been influential on sentencing in the UK, but there is no evidence that viewing or collecting higher-level images is associated with recidivism or escalation to contact offending. Indeed, the opposite may be the case. Similarly, there is no evidence that the number of images a person has is related to recidivism, and again the opposite may actually be the case.

The main question we are asked in such cases is whether an internet offender will go on to commit a contact offence. Internet offenders who also have a history of contact offending are more likely to commit a contact offence. Similarly, internet-only offenders have a higher risk of going on to commit another internet offence but a lower risk of committing a contact offence. Seto and Eke (2005), in a sample of 201 men, found that only 1 per cent of internet-only offenders went on to commit a contact offence after approximately 30 months. One suggestion is that internet-only offenders have better imaginations and can satisfy their needs through using images on the internet to gain sexual satisfaction (Elliot, et al., 2009). Contact offenders are less able to use the images to meet their sexual needs and therefore go on to commit contact offences to gain sexual satisfaction. Internet offenders have a greater PPG response to visual images of children than contact offenders against children. It may be that sexual deviance (apparently more prevalent in internet than contact child sex offenders) operates differently in these offenders than it does in contact offenders (Quayle, 2008).

The introduction of extreme pornography legislation in the UK, outlawing the possession of material depicting extreme sadism, necrophilia and bestiality, will introduce a new cohort of internet offenders, who may cause concern but where there is little evidence on which to base assessment and management. One of the key anxieties will be potential escalation to serious contact offending.

Female perpetrators

There has been little research into female sex offenders. Although they are a very small percentage of convicted sex offenders, victim surveys suggest women are responsible for between 2–3 per cent of sexual crimes (Cupoli and Sewell, 1988; De Francis, 1969; Kercher and McShane, 1985; Margolin and Craft, 1989; Ramsey-Klawsnik, 1990). Of over 150 cases we have assessed or consulted on, only three have been females. Attempts have been made to develop typologies of female offenders, the best known being by Mathews, et al. (1989):

Predisposed – initiates abuse, motivated by anger and compulsive sexual urges, commits violence/sadistic offences against young victims;

Teacher/lover – victim is adolescent, woman seeking loving sexual relationship, lacks hostility and denies reality of her actions;

Male-coerced/male accompanied – compelled or forced into sexual offending, usually against daughters, motivated by fear and emotional dependency;

Psychologically disturbed – long-standing emotional insecurity, poor self-esteem and social isolation. May be pathologically dependent and willing to participate in abuse.

More recent research on female sexual offenders (Gannon and Cortoni, 2010) suggests that applying assessments and knowledge normally used with male offenders to female sexual offenders is not justified. Gannon, et al. (2008) developed a descriptive model of female sexual offending. This indicated that the majority of female sexual offenders had a significant childhood abuse experience that was more severe and frequent than those experienced by men. They were also highly likely to have experienced domestic abuse prior to the start of their offending. Relationship experiences were found to play a key role in their offence process due to the development of social isolation, maladaptive coping strategies, mental health problems, and so on. Finally, the model incorporates co-offender influences, a factor that is rarely seen in male sexual offender models. It looks at the role of the co-offender in distal planning, goal establishment, and proximal planning. The model has several implications: the strong need for individual case formulation prior to treatment; the need to pay particular attention to both developmental abusive experiences and domestic abuse experiences, and to their relationship to risk factors immediately prior to offending; and the need to differentiate between individuals who reluctantly engage in offending and individuals who actively commit offences to achieve different goals.

Conclusions and practice recommendations

Sex offenders can be a difficult group to work with due to the socio-political context, the ever-developing field of research, and the range and severity of personality and sexual pathology found, particularly in the more unusual, concerning and challenging cases. There is a model of working that can help provide an SPJ formulation-based approach for such cases. Our model involves multi-agency working, which reduces anxiety, demonstrates the role of mental health clinicians through providing consultation and support to criminal justice agencies, and is efficient.

Our experience, supported by the research literature, is that having an understanding of personality disorder is very important when working with sex offenders, particularly in high risk and challenging offenders. If you work with this client group without this knowledge there is a risk that you are focusing on the wrong issues or possibly developing risk management plans that may increase rather than decrease risk. The best way for appropriate input to be provided is for criminal justice agencies to receive support, advice, consultation, and assessments, from mental health professionals (psychologists or psychiatrists), who have expert knowledge of personality disorder and sexual offending and are able to formulate cases through using a structured professional judgment approach. We have developed a service that demonstrates that this joint working approach can be successful. Criminal justice agencies report benefit from the input, it is rewarding work for the clinicians involved, and many cases can benefit from a small resource.

One of the criticisms of the SPJ approach is that it is elitist (requiring specialist psychological skills) and too resource intensive to be of practical use in criminal justice settings (Quinsey, et al., 2006). Actuarial approaches address these issues, but are particularly poor for complex cases. Our approach bridges this gap by making an SPJ formulation-based approach available to criminal justice agencies in the community.

References

Abel, G. G. and Wiegal, M. (2009) 'Visual reaction time: Development, theory, empirical evidence, and beyond', in F. M. Saleh, A. J. Grudzinskas, J. M. Bradford and D. J. Brodsky (eds) *Sex offenders: Identification, risk assessment, treatment and legal issues* (pp. 101–18), Oxford: Oxford University Press.

Alden, A., Brennan, P., Hodgins, S. and Mednick, S. (2007) 'Psychotic disorders and sex offending in a Danish birth cohort', *Archives of General Psychiatry, 64*: 1251–58.

Allen, C. (1991) *Women and men who sexually abuse children: A comparative analysis*, Orwell, VT: The Safer Society Press.

Becker, J. V. and Murphy, W. D. (1998) 'What we know and do not know about assessing and treating sex offenders', *Psychology, Public Policy and Law, 4*: 116–37.

Beech, A. R., Craig, L. and Brown, K. (2009) *Assessment and treatment of sex offenders: A handbook*, London: Wiley-Blackwell.

Beech, A. R., Elliot, I. A., Birdgden, A. and Findlater, D. (2008) 'The internet and child sexual offending: A criminological review', *Aggression and Violent Behavior, 13*: 216–28.

Beech, A. R. and Ward, T. (2004) 'The integration of etiology and risk in sex offenders: A theoretical model', *Aggression and Violent Behaviour, 10*: 31–63.

Blanchette, K. (2002) 'Classifying female offenders for effective intervention: Application of the case-based principles of risk and need', *Forum on Correctional Research, 14*: 31–35.

Blanchette, K. and Brown, S. L. (2006) *The assessment and treatment of women offenders: An integrative perspective*, New York: Wiley.

Boer, D. P., Hart, S. J., Kropp, P. R. and Webster, C. D. (1997) *Manual for the Sexual Violence Risk-20: Professional guidelines for assessing risk of sexual violence*, Vancouver: The Institute Against Family Violence.

Button, D. M., De Michele, M. and Payne, B. K. (2009) 'Using electronic monitoring to monitor sex offenders', *Criminal Justice Policy Review, 20*: 414–36.

Canter, D. V. and Heritage, R. (1989) 'A multivariate model of sexual offence behaviour: Developments in offender profiling (I)', *Journal of Forensic Psychiatry, 1*: 185–212.

Chan, H. C. and Heide, K. M. (2009) 'Sexual homicide: A synthesis of the literature', *Trauma, Violence and Abuse, 10*: 31–54.

Chantry, K. and Craig, R. (1994) 'MCMI typologies of criminal sexual offenders', *Sexual Addiction and Compulsivity, 1*: 215–26.

Coid, J., Yang, M., Ullrich, S., Zhang, T., Roberts, A., Roberts, C., Rogers, R. and Farrington, D. (2007) *Predicting and understanding risk of re-offending: The Prisoner Cohort Study. Research Summary 6*, London: Ministry of Justice.

Cooke, D. (2010) 'More prejudicial than probative?', *Law Society of Scotland: The Journal Online*, http://www.journalonline.co.uk/Extras/1007494.aspx.

Cooke, D. and Michie, C. (2011) 'Violence risk assessment: Challenging the illusion of certainty', in B. McSherry and P. Keyzer (eds) *Dangerous people: Policy, prediction, and practice*, New York: Routledge.

Council of State Governments (2010) *Sex offender management policy in the States. Public Safety Brief*, The Council of State Governments, USA.

Craig, L. A., Browne, K. D. and Beech, A. R. (2008) *Assessing risk in sex offenders: A practitioner's guide*, Chichester: John Wiley and Sons Ltd.

Craissati, J., Minoudis, P., Shaw, J., Chuan, S. J., Simons, S. and Joseph, N. (2011) *Working with personality disordered offenders: A practitioners guide*, London: Ministry of Justice.

Craissati, J., Webb, L. and Keen, S. (2008) 'The relationship between developmental variables, personality disorder and risk in sex offenders', *Sexual Abuse: A Journal of Research and Treatment, 20*: 119–38.

Cupoli, J. M. and Sewell, P. M. (1988) 'One thousand fifty-nine children with a chief complaint of sexual abuse', *Child Abuse and Neglect, 12*: 151–62.

Darjee, R. and Crichton, J. (2003) 'Personality disorder and the law in Scotland: A historical perspective', *Journal of Forensic Psychiatry and Psychology, 14*: 394–425.

—— (2004) 'New mental health legislation', *British Medical Journal, 329*: 634–5.

Darjee, R. and Russell, K. (2011) 'The assessment and sentencing of high risk offenders in Scotland: A forensic clinical perspective', in B. McSherry and P. Keyzer (eds) *Dangerous people: Policy, prediction, and practice*, New York: Routledge.

De Francis, V. (1969) *Protecting the victims of sex crimes committed by adults*, Denver: American Humane Association.

Department of Health (2011) *Consultation on the Offender Personality Disorder Pathway Implementation Plan*, London: Department of Health/NOMS Offender Personality Disorder Team, Department of Health.

Drake, C. R. and Pathé, M. (2004) 'Understanding sexual offending in schizophrenia', *Criminal Behaviour and Mental Health, 14*(2), 108–20.

Duggan, C. (2011) 'Dangerous and severe personality disorder', *British Journal of Psychiatry, 198*: 431–33.

Dunsieth, N. W. Jr., Nelson, E. B., Brusman-Lovins, L. A., Holcomb, J. L., Beckman, D., Welge, J. A., Roby, D., Taylor, Jr., P., Soutullo, C. A. and McElroy, S. L. (2004) 'Psychiatric and legal features of 113 men convicted of sexual offenses', *Journal of Clinical Psychiatry, 65*: 293–300.

D'Silva, K. (2004) 'Does treatment really make psychopaths worse? A review of the evidence', *Journal of Personality Disorders, 18*: 163–77.

Elliot, I. A., Beech, A. R., Mandeville-Norden, R. and Hayes, E. (2009) 'Psychological profiles of internet sexual offenders: Comparisons with contact sexual offenders', *Sexual Abuse: A Journal of Research and Treatment, 21*: 76–92.

Falshaw, L., Friendship, C. and Bates, A. (2003) *Sex offenders: Measuring reconviction, reoffending and recidivism: Findings 183*, London: Home Office.

Fazel, S. and Danesh, J. (2002) 'Serious mental disorders in 23000 prisoners: A systematic review of 62 surveys', *Lancet, 359*: 545–50.

Fazel, S., Sjöstedt, G., Långstrøm, N. and Grann, M. (2007) 'Severe mental illness and risk of sexual offending in men: A case-control study based on Swedish national registers', *Journal of Clinical Psychiatry, 68*: 588–96.

Freund, K. (1990) 'Courtship disorder', in W. L. Marshall, D. R. Laws and H. E. Barbaree (eds) *Handbook of sexual assault: Issues, theories and treatment of the offender* (pp. 195–208), New York: Plenum.

Gannon, T. A. and Cortoni, F. (2010) *Female sexual offenders: Theory, assessment and treatment*, Wiley-Blackwell.

Gannon, T. A., Rose, M. R. and Ward, T. (2008) 'A descriptive model of the offense process for female sexual offenders', *Sexual Abuse: A Journal of Research and Treatment, 20*: 352–74.

Glasgow, D. V. (2009) 'Affinity: The development of a self-report assessment of paedophile sexual interest incorporating a viewing time validity measure', in D. Thornton and D. R. Laws (eds) *Cognitive approaches to the assessment of sexual interest in sexual offenders*, Wiley-Blackwell.

Green, A. and Kaplan, M. (1994, September) 'Psychiatric impairment and childhood victimization experiences in female child molesters', *Journal of American Academy of Child and Adolescent Psychiatry, 33*: 954–61.

Groth, A. N. (1979) *Men who rape: The psychology of the offender*, New York: Plenum Press.

Grubin, D., Wilcox, D. and Madsen, L. (2007) *The use of the polygraph in assessing, treating and supervising sex offenders: A practitioner's guide*, Chichester: John Wiley and Sons.

Hanson, R. K. (2001) *Age and sexual recidivism: A comparison of rapists and child molesters*, Department of the Solicitor General Canada Report.

—— (2002) 'Recidivism and age: Follow-up data from 4,673 sexual offenders', *Journal of Interpersonal Violence, 17*: 1046–62.

Hanson, R. K. and Bussière, M. T. (1998) 'Predicting relapse: A meta-analysis of sexual offender recidivism studies', *Journal of Consulting and Clinical Psychology, 66*: 348–62.

Hanson, R. K. and Harris, A. J. R. (2000) 'Where should we intervene? Dynamic predictors of sexual offence recidivism', *Criminal Justice and Behavior, 27*: 6–35.

Hanson, R. K. and Morton-Bourgon, K. E. (2004) *Predictors of sexual recidivism: An updated meta-analysis* (Corrections User Report No. 2004–02), Ottawa, Ontario, Canada: Public Safety Canada.

— (2005) 'The characteristics of persistent sexual offenders: A meta-analysis of recidivism studies', *Journal of Consulting and Clinical Psychology, 73*: 1154–63.

— (2009) 'The accuracy of recidivism risk assessment for sexual offenders: A meta-analysis of 118 prediction studies', *Psychological Assessment, 21*: 1–21.

Hanson, R. K. and Thornton, D. (1999) '*Static99: Improving actuarial risk assessments for sex offenders*, User Report 1999–02, Department of the Solicitor General of Canada.

Hanson, R. K., Harris, A. J. R., Scott, T-L. and Helmus, L. (2007) *Assessing the risk of sexual offenders on community supervision: The dynamic supervision project*, Public Safety Canada.

Hare, R. D. (2003) *The Revised Psychopathy Checklist, 2nd Edition*, Toronto, Canada: Multi-Health Systems.

Harris, G.T., Rice, M.E., Quinsey, V.L. and Chaplin, T.C. (1996) 'Viewing time as a measure of sexual interest among child molesters and normal heterosexual men', *Behaviour Research and Therapy, 34:* 389–94.

Hart, S.D. and Boer, D.P. (2010) 'Structured professional judgment guidelines for sexual violence risk assessment: The Sexual Violence Risk-20 (SVR-20) and the Risk for Sexual Violence Protocol (RSVP)', in R. K. Otto and K. S. Douglas (eds) *Handbook of Violence Risk Assessment* (pp. 269–94), London: Routledge.

Hart, S. D. and Logan, C. (2011) 'Formulation of violence risk using evidence-based assessments: The structured professional judgment approach', in P. Sturmey and M. McMurran (eds) *Forensic case formulation*, Chichester: Wiley-Blackwell.

Hart, S. D., Kropp, P. R., Laws, D. R., Klaver, J., Logan, C. and Watt, K. A. (2003) *Manual of the Risk for Sexual Violence Protocol (RSVP)*, Vancouver, Canada: Mental Health, Law and Policy Institute, Simon Fraser University.

Heil, P. and Simmons, D. (2008) 'Multiple paraphilias: Etiology, assessment and treatment', in D. R. Laws and W. T. O'Donohue (eds) *Sexual deviance: Theory, assessment and treatment* (2nd edition), (pp. 527–56), New York: Guilford Press.

Hildebrand, M., de Ruiter, C. and de Vogel, V. (2004) 'Psychopathy and sexual deviance in treated rapists: Association with sexual and non-sexual recidivism', *Sexual Abuse: A Journal of Research and Treatment, 16*: 1–24.

Hill, A., Habermann, N., Berner, W. and Briken, P. (2007) 'Psychiatric disorders in single and multiple sexual murderers', *Psychopathology, 40*: 22–28.

Home Office (2001) *Prison Statistics England and Wales, 2001*, London: HMSO.

— (2004) *Home Office Statistical Bulletin: Crime in England and Wales 2003/04*, London: Home Office Research and Statistics Department.

Kafka, M. P. (2003) 'Sex offending and sexual desire: The clinical and theoretical relevance of hypersexual desire', *International Journal of Offender Therapy and Comparative Criminology, 47*: 439–51.

Kercher, G. and McShane, M. (1985) 'Characterizing child sexual abuse on the basis of a multi-agency sample', *Victimology: An International Journal, 9:* 364–82.

Kingston, D. A. and Yates, P. M. (2008) 'Sexual sadism: Assessment and treatment', in D. R. Laws and W. T. O'Donohue (eds) *Sexual deviance: Theory, assessment and treatment* (2nd edition), New York: Guilford Press.

Knight, R. (2010) 'Is a diagnostic category for paraphilic coercive disorder defensible?', *Archives of Sexual Behaviour, 39*: 419–26.

Knight, R. A. and Prentky, R. A. (1990) 'Classifying sexual offenders: The development and corroboration of taxonomic models', in W. L. Marshall, D. R. Laws and H. E. Barbaree (eds) *Handbook of sexual assault: Issues, theories, and treatment of the offender* (pp. 23–52), New York: Plenum.

Kocsis, R. (2010) *Criminal profiling: Principles and practice*, New Jersey: Humana Press.

Kropp, P. R., Hart, S. D. and Lyon, D. R. (2008) *Guidelines for Stalking Assessment and Management (SAM)–Manual*, Toronto, Canada: Multi-Health Systems.

Kropp, P. R., Hart, S. D., Webster, C. D. and Eaves, D. (1999) *Manual for the Spousal Assault Risk Assessment Guide (3rd ed.)*, Toronto, Canada: Multi-Health Systems.

Larson, N. and Maison, S. (1987) *Psychosexual treatment program for female sex offenders: Minnesota Correctional Facility, Shakopee*, St Paul, MN: Meta Resources.

Laws, D. R. and Ward, T. (2011) *Desistance from sexual offending: Alternatives to throwing away the keys*, New York: Guilford Press.

Letourneau, E. J., Bordun, C. M. and Schaeffer, C. M. (2009) 'Multisystemic therapy for youth with problem sexual behaviours', in A. R. Beech, L. A. Craig and K. D. Browne (eds) *Assessment and treatment of sex offenders*, Chichester: Wiley-Blackwell.

Logan, C. and Johnstone, L. (2010) 'Personality disorder and violence: Making the link through risk formulation', *Journal of Personality Disorders, 24*: 610–33.

Loranger, A. W. (1999) *International Personality Disorder Examination: DSM-IV and ICD-10 Interviews*, Odessa, FL: Psychological Assessment Resources, Inc.

Lösel, F. (1998) 'Treatment and management of psychopaths', in D. J. Cooke, A. E. Forth and R. D. Hare (eds) *Psychopathy: Theory, research, and implications for society*, Netherlands: Kluwer Academic Publishers.

Mair, G. (2005) 'Electronic monitoring in England and Wales', *Criminology and Criminal Justice, 5*: 257–77.

Malamuth, N. (1998) 'The confluence model as an organizing framework for research on sexually aggressive men: Risk moderators, imagined aggression and pornography consumption', in R. Geen and E. Donnerstein (eds) *Aggression: Theoretical and empirical reviews* (pp. 229–45), New York: Academic Press.

Mann, R. E., Hanson, R. K. and Thornton, D. (2010) 'Assessing risk for sexual recidivism: Some proposals on the nature of psychologically meaningful risk factors', *Sexual Abuse: A Journal of Research and Treatment, 22*: 191–217.

Margolin, L. and Craft, J. (1989) 'Child sexual abuse by caretakers', *Family Relations, 38*: 450–55.

Marshall, W. L. (2006) 'Clinical and research limitations in the use of phallometric testing with sexual offenders', *Sexual Offender Treatment, 1.* http://www.sexual-offender-treatment.org/marshall.html.

Marshall, W. L. and Hucker, S. (2006) 'Issues in the diagnosis of sexual sadism' *Sexual Offender Treatment, 1.* http://www.sexual-offender-treatment.org/40.html.

Marshall, W. L. and Kennedy, P. (2003) 'Sexual sadism in sexual offenders: An elusive diagnosis', *Aggression and Violent Behaviour, 8*: 1–22.

Marshall, W. L., Kennedy, P., Yates, P. and Serran, G. (2002) 'Diagnosing sexual sadism in sexual offenders: Reliability across diagnosticians', *International Journal of Offender Therapy and Comparative Criminology, 46*: 668–77.

Marshall, W. L., Marshall, L. E., Serran, G. A. and Fernandez, Y. M. (2006) *Treating sexual offenders*, London: Routledge.

Mathews, R., Matthews, J. and Speltz, K. (1989) *Female sexual offenders: An exploratory study*, Vermont: Safer Society Press.

McSherry, B. and Keyzer, P. (2009) *Sex offenders and preventative detention: Politics, policy and practice*, London: Federation Press.

Mercado, C. C. and Ogloff, J. R. P. (2007) 'Risk and the preventive detention of sex offenders in Australia and the United States', *International Journal of Law and Psychiatry, 30*: 49–59.

Middleton, D. (2009) 'Internet sex offenders', in A. R. Beech, L. A. Craig and K. D. Browne (eds) *Assessment and treatment of sex offenders*, Chichester: Wiley-Blackwell.

Miller, H. A., Amenta, A. E. and Conroy, M. A. (2005) 'Sexually violent predator evaluations: Empirical evidence, strategies for professionals, and research directions', *Law and Human Behaviour, 29*: 29–54.

Ministry of Justice (2010a) *Breaking the cycle: Effective punishment, rehabilitation and sentencing of offenders*, Norwich: Her Majesty's Stationery Office.

—— (2010b) *Statistics on race and the criminal justice system 2008/09*, London: Ministry of Justice.

Morin, J. W. and Levenson, J. S. (2008) 'Exhibitionism: Assessment and treatment', in D.R. Laws and W.T. O'Donohue (eds) *Sexual deviance: Theory, assessment and treatment* (2nd edition), (pp. 76–107), New York: Guilford Press.

Murphy, W. D. and Page, I. J. (2008) 'Exhibitionism: Psychopathology and treatment', in D. R. Laws and W. T. O'Donohue (eds) *Sexual deviance: Theory, assessment and treatment* (2nd edition), New York: Guilford Press.

Oliver, C. J., Beech, A. R., Fisher, D. and Beckett, R. (2007) 'A comparison of rapists and sexual murderers on demographic and selected psychometric measures', *International Journal of Offender Therapy and Comparative Criminology, 51*: 298–312.

Page, L., MacLeod, P., Kinver, A., Iliasov, A. and Yoon, P. (2010) *2009/10 Scottish Crime and Justice Survey: Main findings*, Edinburgh: Scottish Government Social Research.

Porter, S., Fairweather, D., Drugge, J., Herve, H., Birt, A. and Boer, D. (2000) 'Profiles of psychopathy in incarcerated sexual offenders', *Criminal Justice and Behavior, 27*: 216–33.

Prentky, R. A., Pimental, A., Cavanaugh, D. J. and Righthand, S. (2009), '*Predicting risk of sexual recidivism in juveniles: Predictive validity of the J-SOAP-II*', in A. R. Beech, L. A. Craig and K. D. Browne (eds) *Assessment and treatment of sex offenders*, Chichester: Wiley-Blackwell.

Proulx, J., Beauregard, E., Cusson, M. and Nicole, A. (2007) *Sexual murderers: A comparative analysis and new perspectives*, Chichester: John Wiley and Sons Ltd.

Purcell, C. E. and Arrigo, B. A. (2006) *The psychology of lust murder: Paraphilia, sexual killing and serial homicide*, Burlington: Academic Press (Elsevier).

Quayle, E. (2008) 'Online sex offending: Psychopathology and theory', in D.R. Laws and W.T. O'Donohue (eds) *Sexual deviance: Theory, assessment and treatment* (2nd edition), New York: Guilford Press.

Quinsey, V. L., Harris, G. T., Rice, M. E. and Cormier, C. A. (2006) *Violent offenders: Appraising and managing risk* (2nd Edition), Washington DC: American Psychological Association.

Ramsey-Klawsnik, H. (1990, April) *Sexual abuse by female perpetrators: Impact upon children,* paper presented at the National Symposium on Child Victimisation: 'Keepers of the children', Atlanta. GA.

Raymond, N., Coleman, E., Ohlerking, F., Christenson, G. A. and Miner, M. (1999) 'Psychiatric comorbidity in pedophilic sex offenders', *American Journal of Psychiatry, 156*: 786–88.

Rich, P. (2009) 'Understanding the complexities and needs of adolescent sex offenders', in A. R. Beech, L. A. Craig and K. D. Browne (eds) *Assessment and treatment of sex offenders*, Chichester: Wiley-Blackwell.

Seto, M. C. and Eke, A. W. (2005) 'The criminal histories and later offending of child pornography offenders', *Sexual Abuse: A Journal of Research and Treatment, 17:* 201–10.

Seto, M. C. and Lalumière, M. L. (2001) 'A brief screening scale to identify pedophilic interests among child molesters', *Sexual Abuse: A Journal of Research and Treatment, 13*: 15–25.

Siegert, R. J., Ward, T., Levack, W. M. and McPherson, K. M. (2007) 'A Good Lives Model of clinical and community rehabilitation', *Disability and Rehabilitation, 29*: 1604–15.

Thornton, D. (2010) *Scoring guide for Risk Matrix 2000 10/SVC*. David Thornton.

Thornton, D., Mann, R., Webster, S., Blud, L., Travers, R., Friendship, C. and Erikson, M. (2003) 'Distinguishing and combining risks for sexual and violent recidivism', *Annals of New York Academy of Sciences, 989*: 225–35.

Turner, K., Miller, H. A. and Henderson, C. E. (2008) 'Latent profile analyses of offense and personality characteristics in a sample of incarcerated female sexual offenders', *Criminal Justice and Behaviour, 35*: 879–94.

Tyrer, P., Duggan, C., Cooper, S., Crawford, M., Seivewright, M., Rutter, D., Maden, T., Byford, S. and Barratt, B. (2010) 'The successes and failures of the DSPD experiment: The assessment and management of severe personality disorder', *Medicine, Science and the Law, 50*: 95–99.

Walker, A., Kershaw, C. and Nicholas, S. (2009) *Crime in England and Wales 2008/09*, London: Home Office Statistical Bulletin.

Walker, A., Flatley, J., Kershaw, C. and Moon, D. (2009) *Crime in England and Wales 2008/09: Home Office Statistical Bulletin 11/09*, London: Home Office, available at http://www.homeoffice.gov.uk/rds/pdfs09/hosb1109vol1.pdf.

Ward, T. and Beech, A. (2006) 'An integrated theory of sexual offending', *Aggression and Violent Behaviour, 11*: 44–63.

Ward, T., Polaschek, D. and Beech, A. R. (2005) *Theories of sexual offending*, Chichester: Wiley-Blackwell.

Ward, T. and Siegert, R. (2002) 'Toward a comprehensive theory of child sexual abuse: A theory knitting perspective', *Psychology, Crime and Law, 8*: 319–51.

Webb, L., Craissati, J. and Keen, S. (2007) 'Characteristics of internet child pornography offenders: A comparison with child molesters', *Sexual Abuse: A Journal of Research and Treatment, 19*: 449–65.

Widiger, T. A., Huprich, S. and Clarkin, J. (2011) 'Proposals for DSM-5: Introduction to Special Section of *Journal of Personality Disorders*', *Journal of Personality Disorders, 2*: 135.

Wong, S. C. P. and Olver, M. E. (2010) 'Two treatment- and change- oriented risk assessment tools: The Violence Risk Scale and Violence Risk Scale-Sex Offender Version', in R. K. Otto and K. S. Douglas (eds) *Handbook of violence risk assessment* (pp. 121–46), New York: Routledge.

Worling, J. R. and Långström, N. (2006) 'Risk of sexual recidivism in adolescents who offend sexually: Correlates and assessments', in H. E. Barbaree and W. L. Marshall (eds) *The juvenile sexual offenders*, New York: Guilford Press.

Yates, P. M., Hucker, S. J. and Kingston, D. A. (2008) 'Sexual sadism: Psychopathology and theory', in D. R. Laws and W. T. O'Donohue (eds) *Sexual deviance: Theory, assessment and treatment* (2nd edition), New York: Guilford Press.

5   Suicide and self-harm

Clinical risk assessment and management using a structured professional judgement approach

Caroline Logan

Introduction

Suicide and self-harm are the daily concerns of practitioners in mental health and correctional facilities all over the world (Hawton and van Heeringen, 2000). Wherever there exist people in distress – for example, as a result of mental health problems of a variety of different kinds, traumatic experiences, excessively demanding social circumstances, or chronic or serious physical illness – there is the potential for some to harm themselves as a way of responding to the distress that they feel. Some will seek an end to all that they know and will act with the explicit intention of terminating their lives by the act of suicide. In others, the purpose of self-harmful behaviour may be less clear and death or serious injury may result from acts that suggest an ambivalence about living or a reckless disregard for their own safety, and sometimes for the safety of others as well. And in others still, the intention may not be to die at all but instead to feel pain or to see blood or injury as a means of expressing emotions, releasing fears or internal distress, communicating, or controlling others or the situations that they are in.

The consequences for practitioners and organizations of a client in their care completing suicide are enormous. Consequences include the distressing emotions it generates, such as guilt for not having prevented the death, and the financial cost of the time spent subsequently accounting for decisions made and action taken in the inevitable investigations into root causes (Anderson and Jenkins, 2005). This is because people who are in the care of organizations like psychiatric hospitals and prisons because of problems in their lives have a right to expect to be cared for and a completed suicide implies – but does not always mean – a neglect of that right (World Health Organization, 2007). Investigations are necessary for that reason, but are demanding and distressing for all involved and can have repercussions lasting years.

Non-fatal self-harm, though generally less devastating in its consequences for the client, the practitioners who care for him or her, and the organizations governing them, is a challenge to the whole transaction of ongoing care. That is, the practitioner provides care to a person in need but in response to its delivery, the person elects to direct violence towards him or herself, negating the effort of care and seemingly rejecting its purpose. Practitioners can feel bad as a consequence – guilty, incompetent, angry, rejecting (Alexander, Klein, Gray, et al., 2000; Whittle, 1997). Further, they and the clinical teams to which they belong or the prison wings on which they work can over time become dominated by this self-harmful behaviour, by the desire to control it, often overlooking its purpose and function in the process. In the event of the death of a self-harming client, whether by accident or design, the consequences can be severe for all involved because the risks were known and ostensibly being managed yet the client still died.

For these reasons, practitioners in mental health and correctional facilities – mainly nurses, prison officers, psychiatrists, psychologists, and occupational therapists – spend a great deal of time trying to manage and ultimately prevent acts of suicide and self-harm. Their prevention is the subject of this chapter, and their prevention in forensic facilities its special focus. The chapter will begin with a brief overview of the topics of suicide and self-harm, which will highlight their causes and the critical links between them as well as the differences. There will then follow a review of current practice in respect of suicide and self-harm risk assessment and a discussion of options for its development using the structured professional judgement approach. A new guide to suicide and self-harm risk assessment and management will be introduced. The chapter will conclude with a summary of key points and recommendations for future practice.

Suicide and self-harm: an overview

Introduction

It stands to reason that the management of suicide and self-harm risk – ultimately leading to their prevention – is most likely to be successful if there is consistency in the terms used to describe the behaviours of concern. However, the literature on suicide and self-harm contains many examples of studies and practice in which the same terms are used to mean different things (Goldney, 2008; Leitner, Barr and Hobby, 2008; Leitner and Barr, 2011; Lohner and Konrad, 2007). This is a problem because expressions used with no real understanding of their meaning and terms used inconsistently among practitioners and researchers will promote rather than discourage confusion and disagreement. Therefore, this section will begin by clarifying terms. The prevalence of suicide and self-harm will then be discussed, followed by what we understand now about its most critical determinants and triggers.

Definitions of key terms

In 2008, the Scottish Development Centre for Mental Health, in partnership with the Universities of Edinburgh and Stirling, completed a literature review commissioned by the then Scottish Executive into risk and protective factors for suicide and suicidal behaviour (McLean, Maxwell, Platt, Harris and Jepson, 2008).

To ensure clarity, focus and consistency in their work, the authors of the review offered the following definitions of key terms.

Suicidal behaviour is an all-encompassing term that refers to both completed suicide and to self-harmful acts that do not have a fatal outcome. Thus, the term suicidal behaviour can be used to refer to the whole range of activities indicative of self-inflicted harm, including suicide, attempted suicide, intentional self-harm, and parasuicide.

Completed suicide is death resulting from an intentional, self-inflicted act, with evidence (either explicit, such as a note that clearly communicates the person's expectation of death, or implicit, such as the mode of death, as when a person is found hanging in their locked home) that the person intended to die by his or her own hand. Sometimes, however, the evidence is not clear or is disputed because suicidal intent appeared absent or was ambiguous (e.g., Baker, 2007; Blake, 2006).

Attempted suicide, a term used more in American research than in research in the UK, refers to self-injurious behaviour with a non-fatal outcome accompanied by evidence (either explicit or implicit) that the person intended to die. Why the person failed to die when this was their intention should be the subject of inquiry. It is this group of people who are a necessary focus of concern regarding the prevention of future attempts.

Self-harm – or *parasuicide* – is a very broad term used to refer to the intentional self-inflicting of painful, destructive, or injurious (but non-fatal) acts, generally without intent to die. The National Collaborating Centre for Mental Health uses the term self-harm to refer to any intentional 'self-poisoning or self-injury, irrespective of the apparent purpose of the act' (p.16, NCCMH, 2004; see also Hawton, et al., 2003a). This means the term self-harm can be used to refer to behaviour as serious as cutting and ligature-tying and more ambiguously self-hurtful activities like smoking or hazardous eating or drinking patterns, which may be less explicitly or intentionally self-harmful. This wide range of interpretation can make the term self-harm not particularly helpful and the term *self-injury* has been used to refer to self-harmful acts that clearly lack any intention to die. Thus McLean, et al. (2008) propose that non-fatal self-harm be subdivided into behaviour with a high level of suicidal intent, which could also be referred to as attempted suicide, and behaviour with mixed/ambivalent or no suicidal intent, which could also be referred to as *self-injury*.

Suicidal intent is a term used to refer to the subjective desire and expectation for a self-destructive act to end in death; it refers to the presence of a purpose in causing self-harm where that purpose is the ending of the person's life. Finally, the term *suicidal ideation* refers to thoughts of serving as the agent of one's own death. Suicidal ideation may vary in seriousness depending on how specific or detailed the person's plans are to end their life and the degree of suicidal intent underpinning or driving them. Suicidal ideation can be present without the person taking any overt action to bring about their death but its very presence is regarded as an indicator of the potential for that action to come about in the event of change – a deterioration – in personal circumstances.

The prevalence of suicide and self-harm

Suicide

Suicide is an extremely important component of public health policy in most if not all developed nations (Anderson and Jenkins, 2005), increasingly so because of worrying changes in trends such as an increase in the suicide rate among young people, in particular, young men (Goldney, 2008). The World Health Organization estimates that approximately one million people die as a result of suicide every year, suggesting a global suicide rate of 16 per 100,000 people. There is considerable national variation in suicide rates. Suicide rates are very high in the Baltic States and in the countries of the Russian Federation (Goldney, 2008); presently, the country with the highest reported suicide rate in the world is Lithuania, with a total of 31.5 suicides per 100,000. Japan also reports a high suicide rate (25.5) as does rural (22.5) but not urban (6.7) China (Goldney, 2008). In Europe, the highest suicide rates are reported in Belgium (21.1) and Finland (20.3) and the lowest in Greece (3.4) and the United Kingdom (6.9) (Goldney, 2008). In the USA, the suicide rate is 11.1 and it is 11.6 in Canada. Australia has a slightly lower suicide rate (10.3) and New Zealand somewhat higher (13.1). The countries with the lowest reported suicide rates are in Central and South America and in the Middle East, although these data may be questionable due to the stigma surrounding suicide in these areas and the possibility of incorrect recording of cause of death. Everywhere but in rural China, the suicide rate among men exceeds that among women.

For reasons that will become clear in the third section of this chapter, suicide among the users of mental health services is a critical consideration and a risk evaluated and monitored frequently and as a matter of priority – and with good reason. In the UK, the National Confidential Inquiry into Suicide and Homicide (NCISH), based at the University of Manchester, examines the deaths of all users of mental health services (e.g., NCISH, 2010). Twenty-seven per cent of the deaths of people in contact with mental health services in the preceding 12 months were by suicide (Windfuhr and Swinson, 2011). The majority of these deaths – 74 per cent – were among males and suicide was the most common cause of death in the 25 to 44 year old age group. The most common methods of death were hanging/strangulation (52 per cent), self-poisoning (35 per cent), and jumping or multiple injuries (13 per cent). Fourteen per cent of mental health service users were inpatients at the time, and the majority of these died by hanging or strangulation (75 per cent). Fifteen per cent of suicides took place during the first week of inpatient admission and 35 per cent during the period of discharge planning, towards the end of their inpatient stay. Twenty-two per cent took place while the inpatient was under some form of non-routine observations (including 3 per cent who were on one-to-one observations), and 27 per cent absconded from an inpatient setting prior to their suicide.

The death by suicide of users of mental health services living in the community was associated with recent discharge from an inpatient service – 20 per cent of all those examined in the NCISH had been discharged from inpatient services in the three months prior to their suicide, a third in the preceding three weeks (Windfuhr and Swinson, 2011). A total of 46 per cent of those who committed suicide died prior to their first follow-up visit in the community from mental health services based there. These early discharge deaths were more likely to have discharged themselves from the inpatient unit, and the cause of death was more likely to be jumping or multiple injuries. Non-compliance with treatment (e.g. missed appointments) was identified in 14 per cent of those former patients who committed suicide and a dual diagnosis – major mental illness and a comorbid substance-use disorder – was detected in 27 per cent of all NCISH cases (Windfuhr and Swinson, 2010). The majority of the users of mental health services who completed suicide were judged to be at low or no immediate risk of doing so (86 per cent).

In prisons, well-known repositories for vulnerable and damaged people, suicide (meaning all self-inflicted deaths regardless of evidence of intent; Borrill, 2008) accounts for around half of all deaths in the UK (Natale, 2010) and is the leading cause of death in prisoner populations in the majority of developed countries (Konrad, et al., 2007). The three-year average annual rate of suicide in England and Wales was 71 deaths per 100,000 prisoners in 2010 (Ministry of Justice, 2010). In the US, the state prison suicide rate in 2002 was 14 deaths per 100,000 prisoners (Mumola, 2005) and the suicide rate for local prisons was 36 per 100,000 prisoners in 2007 (Noonan, 2010).

The overall suicide rate for men in prison is estimated to be five times greater than among men in the community (Natale, 2010; Rivlin, Hawton, Marzano et al., 2010). In pretrial facilities housing short-term, often young inmates, the suicide rate is higher – around 7.5 times the rate of male suicides in the community (Jenkins, Bhugra, Meltzer et al., 2005); unsentenced prisoners comprised 50 per cent of self-inflicted deaths in prisons in England and Wales in 2009 (HM Chief Inspector of Prisons, 2010). Children in custody are 18 times more likely to complete suicide than boys the same age in the community (Frühwald and Frottier, 2005) and women in custody are 20 times more likely to die by suicide than women of the same age in the general population (Fazel and Benning, 2009).

Almost three quarters of prisoners who take their own lives suffer from some form of mental health problem (Shaw, Baker, Hunt, et al., 2004). Shaw and colleagues observed that two thirds had a history of drug misuse problems and a third had a history of alcohol misuse (Shaw, et al., 2004). Almost one third of suicides occur within the prisoner's first week in custody – 11 per cent in the first 24 hours (Shaw, et al., 2004). A link between overcrowding and suicide has been noted in a number of publications in the UK and the US (e.g., Huey and Mcnulty, 2005; Romilly and Bartlett, 2010; Sharkey, 2010): 75 per cent of those who committed suicide in prison in the UK between 2000 and 2004 did so in overcrowded prisons (Natale, 2010). The most common method of suicide in prison is asphyxiation (usually by hanging) and usually at night (Royal College of Psychiatrists, 2002). Just over half of prisoners completing suicide had a history of self-harm (Shaw, et al., 2004) and an elevated rate of completed suicide has been noted in recently released prisoners also (Pratt, Piper, Appleby, et al., 2006).

Self-harm

Data regarding suicidal behaviours other than completed suicide are sparse, which is problematic given its very strong association with subsequent completed suicide (Cooper, Kapur, Webb, et al., 2005; Haw, Bergen, Casey, et al., 2007; Kerr, Mühlenkamp and Turner, 2010; Leitner and Barr, 2011). The majority of data on the subject come from studies of hospital attendance and admissions, especially from accident and emergency departments, and to a lesser degree from studies of psychiatric services and general population surveys. This rather narrow range of data can produce misleading findings because those who self-poison tend to seek help more readily than those who cut (Hawton, Rodham, Evans, et al., 2002; Meltzer, Lader, Corbin, et al., 2002). In addition, it ignores those who seek help from their general practitioners or other care facilities, or who don't seek help at all (Horrocks and House, 2002). Such limitations are likely to lead not only to an underestimation of the scale of the problem but possibly also to a too-narrow focus on certain kinds and precipitants of self-harm. With these limitations in mind, what do we know about the prevalence of self-harm?

The UK appears to have one of the highest rates of self-harm in Europe – estimated at approximately 400 per 100,000 per year (Hawton and Fagg, 1992). A more recent survey observed a lifetime prevalence of 4.9 per cent for self-harm (5.4 per cent in women and 4.4 per cent in men) and a lifetime prevalence of 5.6 per cent for suicide attempts (6.9 per cent of women and 4.3 per cent of men; McManus, Meltzer, Brugha, et al., 2009). Studies of US samples suggest comparable figures (e.g., Kerr, Mühlenkamp and Turner, 2010) – there, it is estimated that 5 per cent have a history of self-harm, and approximately 1 per cent of the population engages in self-harmful activity at a chronic or severe level.

In England and Wales, intentional self-harm is one of the most common reasons for attendance at accident and emergency services (Gunnell, Bennewith, Peters, et al., 2005). More women than men self-harm – at a ratio estimated to be 1.6 to 1 (Horrocks and House, 2002) – although Kerr and colleagues propose a higher level of parity between the sexes than has been suggested before, especially if self-harm is more broadly defined to include self-injury (Kerr, et al., 2010). In addition, a notable proportion of adolescents and young adults self-harm (Olfson, Gameroff, Marcus. et al., 2005; Whitlock, Eckenrode and Silverman, 2006); among young people in general, 12 to 15 per cent report some form of self-injury (Hawton, Rodham and Evans, 2006; Madge, Hewitt, Hawton, et al., 2008) and self-harm is more than twice as common among young females than young males (Madge, et al., 2008). Cutting appears to be a preferred method among young people (Madge, et al., 2008) – following a mostly impulsive decision to do so for which professional medical assistance is rarely sought, and in over half of whom it represents a repeated pattern of behaviour. Only a small proportion of all episodes of self-harm occur in older people over the age of 65 (Draper, 1996; Harwood and Jacoby, 2000). However, one in five older people who self-harm go on to complete suicide suggesting that suicidal intent may be more prevalent in this group or more easily acquired in those who previously self-harmed (NCCMH, 2004).

Research suggests that self-harm is common among primary care patients (NCCMH, 2011), estimated to be as high as 22 per cent (Kerr, et al., 2010). Beautrais (2003) conducted a prospective study of 302 people who had made a serious attempt on their life – one in 11 died during the following five years, over half as a consequence of suicide. Between 13 and 15 per cent of people who attend an accident and emergency department for treatment for a self-inflicted injury will self-harm again in the following 12 months (Kapur, Cooper, King-Hele, et al., 2006; Owens, Horrocks and House, 2002). The rate of suicide increases to between 50 and 100 times the rate of suicide in the general population following an act of self-harm (Hawton, et al., 2003a; Owens, et al., 2002). Men who have self-harmed are more than twice as likely to complete suicide as women – and the risk of suicide increases with age for both men and women (Hawton, et al., 2003b). It has been proposed that the more serious the method of self-harm – for example, attempted hanging – the greater the increase in risk of completed suicide (Runeson, Tidemalm, Dahlin, et al., 2010).

Studies of the prevalence of self-harm in prison and forensic mental health facilities confirm that the practice is common in these settings. Singleton, et al., (1998) reported that 15 per cent of male remand prisoners and 27 per cent of female remand prisoners had made a suicide attempt in the 12 months prior to assessment. Among sentenced prisoners, 5 per cent of men and 9 per cent of women reported that they had self-harmed during their current sentence. Singleton and colleagues concluded that a prisoner had a sevenfold risk of suicide compared with a person in the community. More recent studies suggest that around 30 per cent of prisoners engage in some kind of self-injurious behaviour during their time in custody (Borrill, Burnett, Atkins, et al., 2003; Brooker, Repper, Beverley, et al., 2003).

Looking at the genders separately, Völlm and Dolan (2009) reported that 46 per cent of a sample of imprisoned women had ever self-harmed or attempted suicide, the majority by acts of cutting, and just under half of this number made their first attempt to harm themselves after they were sentenced to a period of imprisonment. In this study, women with a history of self-harm had significantly higher rates of violent offending (including arson), complex psychopathologies and needs, and the needs of around a third were undetected by the prison authorities. As in the general population, Völlm and Dolan (2009) noted a trend towards self-harming behaviour being more common among young compared to adult female prisoners. In imprisoned men, the rate of self-harming is lower than in women. In a sample of young male offenders, Kenny, Lennings and Munn (2008) reported that 8.4 per cent had attempted suicide (44 per cent in detention), and 9.1 per cent had inflicted self-harm in the past 12 months (75 per cent in detention). Kenny and colleagues also observed that the lifetime prevalence for suicidal ideation was 19.2 per cent and for self-harm ideation, it was 18.2 per cent.

Causes and triggers of suicide and self-harm

Most studies have looked at the variables associated with suicidal behaviours in samples of individuals who have a history of such activity. Key risk and protective factors for suicide and self-harm are now described.

Key risk factors

MENTAL HEALTH PROBLEMS

The majority of those dying by suicide have a mental health disorder of some kind (Arsenault-Lapierre, Kim and Turecki, 2004; Fleischmann, Bertolote, Belfer, et al., 2005). Arsenault-Lapierre and colleagues conducted a meta-analysis of psychiatric diagnoses in studies of completed suicides. They noted that, overall, 87.3 per cent of those who completed suicide were diagnosed with a mental disorder prior to death. Some geographical variation was noted by these authors: mental disorder was diagnosed prior to death in 89.7 per cent of the suicides discussed in American studies, 88.8 per cent of the European studies, 83 per cent of the Asian studies, and 78.9 per cent of the Australian suicides.

The most common mental disorders identified in those who complete suicide are mood or affective disorders, in particular depression (Fleischmann, et al., 2005; Windfuhr and Swinson, 2011; Wulsin, Vaillant and Wells, 2005), and substance-misuse disorders (Windfuhr and Swinson, 2011). Fleischmann and colleagues noted that alcohol-misuse disorders were more common in the 894 completed suicides they examined than other substance-misuse conditions; where any substance misuse was diagnosed, alcohol misuse was present in 53.7 per cent of cases. For bipolar disorder and schizophrenia, the risk of suicide is exacerbated if accompanied by a history of suicide attempts, other comorbid psychiatric diagnoses, drug or alcohol misuse, anxiety, recent bereavement, severity of symptoms and hopelessness (McLean, et al., 2008). Schizophrenia – especially around the time of first diagnosis – childhood disorders, and a history of psychiatric treatment in general have also been implicated in completed suicide (McLean, et al., 2008). Palmer, Pankratz and Bostwick (2005) reported that the lifetime suicide prevalence rate for individuals followed up from the time of first diagnosis of schizophrenia or first hospital admission was 5.6 per cent. Overall, the lifetime suicide risk for schizophrenia is 10 per cent (van Velsen, 2010).

Hawton, Sutton, Haw, et al. (2005a) reported an inverse relationship between acute symptoms of schizophrenia, specifically hallucinations, and the likelihood of suicidal behaviour in people with schizophrenia. Hawton, et al. (2005b) identified a number of characteristics of bipolar disorder associated with the likelihood of completed suicide, including prior suicide attempts and hopelessness. Risk of completed suicide in those with bipolar disorder appears higher in men than in women (Hawton, et al., 2005b). Risk factors for non-fatal suicidal behaviour in this population were identified as family history of suicide, early onset of bipolar disorder, the extent of depressive symptoms, increasing severity of affective episodes, the presence of mixed affective states, rapid cycling, comorbid Axis

I disorders, and alcohol and drug misuse. Hawton and colleagues reported no gender effect on risk of attempted suicide or other suicidal behaviours (Hawton, et al., 2005b).

Personality traits (neuroticism and extroversion; Brezo, Paris and Turecki, 2006) and personality disorder have been associated with suicidal behaviour in a number of studies (MacLean, et al., 2008). The principal personality disorder associated with suicidal behaviour is borderline personality disorder (BPD) (Pompili, Girardi, Ruberto, et al., 2005a). However, the association is circular – a diagnosis made in part on the presence of suicidal behaviour does not offer any understanding or coherent explanation for why a person with this condition self-harms. Poor impulse control affecting behaviour and cognition and labile mood affecting subjective wellbeing and perceptions of control, in addition to fearful and emotionally dependent relationships with others, are likely to be important contenders for the link between BPD and suicidal behaviour.

Personality disorders, substance-use disorders, and childhood and disruptive behaviour disorders (conduct disorder, attention-deficit hyperactivity disorder) (see also James, Lai and Dahl, 2004), oppositional disorder and identity disorder appear more common among male suicides than female suicides – and affective disorders less common among male than female suicides (Arsenault-Lapierre, et al., 2004). A relationship between suicide and eating disorders has also been noted (Pompili, Girardi, Tatarelli, et al., 2006); higher numbers of suicide attempts and instances of self-harm were noted among anorexic and bulimic patients who exhibited purging behaviour and suicide risk is higher still when eating disorders are comorbid with other conditions such as major depression and substance misuse. In one study, individuals with a personality disorder, a psychiatric history, schizophrenia, bipolar disorder, neurosis or depression were noted to be 6.1 to 19.7 times more likely to die by suicide than someone without any of these diagnoses, and depression and bipolar were the most risky conditions (Neeleman, 2001).

PRIOR SUICIDE ATTEMPTS

The lifetime prevalence of suicide among affective disordered patients who have been hospitalized for suicidal behaviour is estimated at 8.6 per cent compared to 4.0 per cent among those hospitalized with affective disorders but who have no history of suicidal behaviour (Bostwick and Pankratz, 2000). A history of suicide attempts elevates risk of completed suicide in individuals with a diagnosis of schizophrenia (Hawton, et al., 2005a) and bipolar disorder (Hawton, et al., 2005b).

SUBSTANCE MISUSE

Rates of completed suicide are high among those abusing alcohol. There are more than nine times the expected rate of suicide deaths among problem drinkers (Neeleman, 2001; Wilcox, Conner and Caine, 2004), a link thought to be stronger in women than in men (Cherpitel, Borges and Wilcox, 2004; Wilcox, et al., 2004).

Intoxication is thought to be the trigger – the proximal risk factor for suicide – rather than the consequences of alcohol-free periods. Higher rates of suicide have been observed in populations with opioid disorder, intravenous drug use, and mixed drug use (Wilcox, Conner and Caine, 2004). Neeleman (2001) reported that the standardized mortality ratios (the ratio of observed to expected deaths) for death by suicide among those who abuse drugs are 10.1 times higher than that among non-drug abusers. However, there is a problem determining the direction of effect here: does intoxication cause suicidal behaviour or does a person become intoxicated in order to disinhibit them, thus enabling suicide?

PRIOR SELF-HARM

Prior self-harm is a very strong predictor of both future self-harm and completed suicide (Haw, et al., 2007; Kapur, et al., 2006; Neeleman, 2001; Windfuhr and Swinson, 2011). Neeleman (2001) conducted a review of the standardized mortality ratios for death by suicide, death by natural causes, and accidental death in 146 published studies of over one million participants and found that those who self-harm (suicidal intent not known) are 24.7 times more likely to die by suicide than those who do not self-harm.

EMPLOYMENT

Work and unemployment have also been studied for their relationship to completed suicide and self-harm (e.g., Kapur, et al., 2006; Platt and Hawton, 2000). Unemployment – and relative low socioeconomic status (Neeleman, 2001) – show an association with the likelihood of suicide and self-harm at a population level. Individual longitudinal studies show a double or triple rate of suicide in the unemployed but only inconsistent evidence for self-harm. Evidence suggests that it is relative rather than absolute poverty that appears to be the driver in this association (Rehkopf and Buka, 2006). Certain professions have higher than expected levels of suicide: medical and allied, where rates exceed four times those in the general population, and where it is highest among women (Lindeman, Laara, Hakko, et al., 1996); male (but not female) farmers; nurses; health and education professionals; welfare workers; and personal service workers. Elevated rates among medical and allied workers could be a reflection of the easy access to means as well as frequent exposure to death. The police appear to have one of the lowest occupational suicide rates (Hem, Berg, and Ekeberg, 2001).

PHYSICAL CONDITIONS AND ILLNESS

Terminal illness (Kleespies, Hough and Romeo, 2009), epilepsy (Pompili, et al., 2005b), the menstrual cycle (Saunders and Hawton, 2006), pregnancy (Shadigian and Bauer, 2005), and deficits in social problem-solving skills (Speckens and Hawton, 2005) have also been linked to higher rates of completed and attempted suicide. However, the general association between physical conditions and suicide risk is not always strong or consistent across studies (Kleespies, et al., 2009; McLean, et al., 2008). There is no strong evidence to support a genetic link to suicide or attempted suicide, although one study reported a link between one poly-morphism at the H-5T2A locus and suicidal behaviour (Li, Duan and He, 2006).

Protective factors

How protective factors operate to mitigate the functioning of risk factors and risk overall is not entirely clear (de Vogel, de Ruiter, Bouman, et al., 2009; de Vries Robbé and de Vogel, this volume). However, a number of factors have been identi-fied with demonstrable positive effects. Coping strategies enhancing self-control appear to be critical (McLean, et al., 2008). The application of problem-focused coping strategies to situations engendering hopelessness appears to act in a protective way in those at risk of suicide and serious self-harm (Elliott and Frude, 2001), although their effectiveness is likely to be dependent upon the amenability of the situation the person is in to change. In addition to problem-focused coping strategies, believing in one's ability to survive and cope with adversity has also been highlighted for its protective effect on suicidal behaviour in a study of female prison inmates (Chapman, Specht and Cellucci, 2005), although in this study it appeared the level of hopelessness mediated (against) the protective effects of problem-focused coping strategies in this sample. In a qualitative study of previously suicidal adolescent females (Everall, Altrows and Paulson, 2006), resilience to suicidal behaviour was thought to be linked to (a) cognitive processes enabling increased perspective on their lives and increased attention to positives, (b) purposeful and goal-directed action, that is, a sense of control and self-efficacy, and (c) the willingness to confront difficult emotions or situations – effortful coping (Piquet and Wagner, 2003) – and make progress towards their improvement.

Reasons for living (Malone, Oquendo, Haas, et al., 2000) and hope (Meadows, Kaslow, Thompson, et al., 2005) for the future are also critical protective factors, which appear to act as buffers between stressors and response. Reasons for living include responsibilities towards family members, especially dependents, fear of disapproval, moral or religious objections to suicide, and fear of suicide. Personal relationships and professional help have also been identified as protective in a number of studies, as has religion (for a review, see McLean, et al., 2008).

Concluding comments

In this section, fundamental issues of definition have been considered and the scale of the problem of suicide and self-harm has been examined. Important and commonly observed risk and protective factors have also been identified and described. However, risk and protective factors identified in large samples of people who have completed or attempted suicide or who have harmed themselves tell us little about the interactions among these variables or about their relevance to the individual. Professional judgement is required therefore alongside the opinions of the client to identify from those factors present the ones that are most relevant to risk and why. It is to risk assessment practice that we will now turn.

Suicide and self-harm: risk assessment practice today

Introduction

The practice of suicide risk assessment is extensive, yet complicated by the lack of very clear evidence about the efficacy of the different procedures available to support it. What does appear clear is that subjective judgements about suicide and self-harm risk are less reliable than judgements based on evidence (Department of Health, 2002, 2007). What procedures are available to support evidence-based judgements about the risk of these outcomes?

Existing tools to aid suicide and self-harm risk assessment

In the UK, recent Department of Health (DH) guidance on best practice in clinical risk assessment and management identified only six structured assessment tools that had an evidence base confirming their efficacy in suicide prevention (DH, 2007), and none that could be recommended without caution (Leitner and Barr, 2011). At the time of writing, the best-evidenced tools available to assist with risk assessment are the *Beck Hopelessness Scale* (BHS) and the *Beck Scale for Suicide Ideation* (BSS) (Leitner and Barr, 2011).

The BHS (Beck and Steer, 1993) is a self-report scale consisting of 20 items assessing the client's feelings about the future, loss of motivation and expectations. It can take less than 10 minutes to complete. Each item on the BHS is a true/false statement and scored 0 or 1 depending on whether the response gives cause for concern. Scores on the BHS – out of 20 – have no explicit link to risk because hopelessness is only one of several risk factors for suicide. However, ratings on the BHS have been demonstrated to correlate well with changes in clinical symptoms in randomized controlled trials of interventions for high risk or suicidal patients (e.g., McMillan, et al., 2007).

The BSS (Beck, 1991) is a 21-item assessment tool that can be completed either by self-report or through an interview with the client. It is intended as an evaluation of the client's suicidal thinking – the intensity of their attitudes accepting of suicide and their behaviours and plans in the past week in relation to suicide. Nineteen of the items are rated between 0 and 2 and they add together to produce a total score ranging from 0 to 38. Two additional items enquire about previous suicide attempts and the seriousness of intent in the most recent attempt. A higher score on the BSS is associated with a higher risk but there are no specific cutoffs and a positive response to any of the items should be regarded as a cause for concern. Brown, Beck, Steer, et al. (2000) found evidence of an association between scores on the interview version of this scale and completed suicide in outpatients.

The other tools or procedures identified in the DH guidance as having an evidence base in suicide risk assessment include *Applied Suicide Intervention*

Skills Training (ASIST) (Rodgers, 2010), the *Skills-based Training on Risk Management* (STORM) (Hayes, Shaw, Lever-Green, et al., 2008), SADPERSONS (e.g., Kripalani, Nag, Nag, et al., 2010), and the *Suicide Intent Scale* (SIS) (Beck, Morris and Beck, 1974; Harriss and Hawton, 2005). In addition, a number of instruments or procedures are available to assess the risks presented by clients in multiple areas, including suicide and self-harm, such as the promising *Short-Term Assessment of Risk and Treatability* (START) (Doyle, Lewis, and Brisbane, 2008; Nicholls, Brink, Desmarais, et al., 2006; Webster, Martin, Brink, et al., 2004).

In addition to the instruments listed above, there are a small number of tools or frameworks available to support a more comprehensive evaluation of risk of suicide. These tools represent promising developments in the suicide and serious self-harm arena and they have applications to practitioners working in diverse areas. However, they have particular application to practitioners working in forensic mental health and correctional settings because of their structured approach to risk assessment.

The *Estimate of Suicide Risk* (ESR) (Polvi, 1997) aims to facilitate the assessment and prediction of suicide in correctional settings. Based on an extensive review of the literature on suicide prediction in prisoners, suicide risk in individual prisoners is assessed through the evaluation of 20 items. There are nine historical items, evaluating psychiatric problems, impulsive behaviour, substance misuse, suicide attempts, experience of suicide within the family, age, marital status, length of prison sentence and time served to date. In addition, there are 11 clinical items evaluating hopelessness, suicidal ideation, intent and planning, recent change in psychological functioning, stress vulnerability, acute symptoms of depression or psychosis, current abuse of alcohol or drugs, physical and psychosocial isolation. Practitioners evaluate their clients through interview and file review and then rate them on each of the 20 items of the ESR, where a rating of 2 is given for each item judged to be definitely present, a rating of 1 is given for each item partially or possibly present, and a rating of 0 is given if the item is not present at all. Ratings are summed to produce a total out of 40, where this number represents the 'amount' of risk based on the number of risk factors present in the individual. Risk management is addressed in terms of minor monitoring and notification tasks.

Like the ESR, the *Suicide Assessment Manual for Inmates* (SAMI) (Zapf, 2006) was also designed for use in correctional settings. It also consists of 20 items covering such risk factors as marital status, history of substance misuse, psychiatric problems, prior suicide attempts, including while in custody, family history of suicide, arrest history, poor impulse control, high-profile crime, hopelessness, suicidal ideation, intent and planning, recent loss, depressive symptomatology and so on. As with the ESR, practitioners evaluate each of the items and determine whether each is definitely, possibly or partially, or not present in the client, rating 2, 1 or 0 accordingly. Ratings are summed for a grand total out of 40 and imminent risk of suicide is rated high, medium or low. Also like the ESR, risk management is addressed in terms of monitoring and notification tasks.

Finally, the *Suicide Risk Assessment and Management Manual* (S-RAMM) provides a comprehensive guide to support suicide risk assessment and management planning by supporting practitioners in the examination of 22 historical, current clinical and future risk management characteristics. Historical risk factors include history of self-harm, seriousness of previous suicidality, previous hospitalization, mental disorder, personality problems, substance abuse, childhood adversity, family history of suicide, and age, gender and marital status. Current clinical factors include suicidal ideation, communication and intent, hopelessness, acute symptoms of distress, treatment non-adherence, current substance abuse, recent or imminent psychiatric admission or discharge, stress and problem-solving deficits. Future risk management items include access to preferred method of committing suicide, service contact, treatment response, response to interventions more generally, and stress. As with the ESR and the SAMI, clients are rated on each risk factor and given a score of 2, 1 or 0. Ratings are summed and level of risk determined depending on the number of risk factors present – for example, a client would be considered a very high risk of suicide if he or she scored 34 or more on the S-RAMM items. Some guidance is offered on the management of the suicide risks observed. The S-RAMM appears to have acceptable characteristics for use as a clinical and research tool (Ijaz, Papaconstantinou, O'Neill, et al., 2009).

Concluding comments

It is positive that there is guidance available for practitioners to use in their efforts to structure and make more transparent their decision-making about the suicide risk of clients in their care. However, less positive are (a) the limited amount of research that has been carried out into the guidance available, especially those suitable for use on forensic mental health and correctional settings, (b) the relatively limited applications of those with the most research (e.g., the BHS), and (c) the emphasis on risk prediction over risk prevention. To date, there is no structured professional judgement approach to the assessment and management of risk of suicide and serious self-harm, which is regrettable given the strength of its applications elsewhere (e.g., violence, Hart and Logan, 2011). However, in the following section, a structured professional judgement approach for use with clients who are at risk of completing suicide will be introduced.

Suicide and serious self-harm: a structured professional judgement approach

The structured professional judgement approach to clinical risk assessment and management

In the last twenty years, general practice in clinical risk assessment has advanced a great deal, largely because of the development of instruments or guides intended to structure the judgement of practitioners – and researchers – on complex issues where bias may otherwise influence the opinions formed. Such guides are based on research identifying the variables most frequently or strongly associated with the harmful outcome of interest (Otto and Douglas, 2010). For example, affective disorders are very strongly associated with suicide risk and with self-harm (e.g., Fleischmann, et al., 2005; Windfuhr and Swinson, 2011; Wulsin, et al., 2005). Therefore, problems with mood feature in all risk assessments for these outcomes (e.g., ESR, SAMI, S-RAMM). In essence, practitioners are required to examine their client in relation to all the risk factors listed in the guide they have elected to use and to denote through a rating whether the factor is present or not and, if present, the extent to which it is present (e.g., partially, definitely).

Once all risk factors have been examined, some form of risk estimate or judgement – generally an indication of level of risk, expressed as high, medium/ moderate or low risk – is then derived. This risk estimate may be based on the number of risk factors present in the client's past or recent history; scores given to present risk factors are summed and the total score related to a level of risk derived from data from similar others (e.g., people who have completed suicide) measured on the same risk factors. Thus, clients who have lots of risk factors that the research suggests are also present in those who complete suicide are generally regarded as at more risk than those with fewer risk factors.

However, an alternative way of deriving a risk estimate is to make a structured judgement about the individual's potential to be harmful in the future based on an appraisal of all the present factors (see Douglas, et al., this volume). This judgement may be substantially structured by involving a formal process of formulation (Hart and Logan, 2011; Logan, Nathan and Brown, 2011), which organizes the information derived about prior self-harmful conduct into an explanation for why it happened as it did and when, and therefore the circumstances in which it could potentially happen again. In such structured formulations, risk estimates or judgements (high, medium or low risk) are obsolete because what are prepared are an understanding about individual risk and a plan of action for continuously monitoring risk and adjusting risk management. This is structured professional judgement.

As stated above, the ultimate goal of risk assessment is the prevention of harmful outcomes. The very fact of doing a risk assessment of any kind heightens the awareness of practitioners about the possible risks posed by an individual client. It also demonstrates to others that risk has been considered; it forms evidence of attention to risk in the event that disaster does happen and the post-incident review or subsequent litigation proceedings search for oversights and omissions on which to blame the unprevented suicide. However, risk assessments that produce risk judgements based on summed scores or on an appraisal based on the risk factors that are present have only a broad link to risk management; assessments generating conclusions about level of risk – high, medium, low – imply a volume of risk management, although not necessarily its focus. In many circumstances, this blunt matching of risk assessment findings to risk management interventions is all that is required – or possible. However, there are some circumstances where a closer link is required between risk assessment findings and risk management interventions; for example, where a practitioner is required to make a decision about restricting the person's liberty as a way of managing risk. Structured professional judgement forms of risk assessment produce a detailed evaluation in which assessment findings are linked directly to often long-term prevention strategies, namely risk management. This is structured professional judgement at its most refined.

Operationalizing SPJ in risk assessment and management

The application of SPJ guidelines for risk assessment and management involves six discrete steps. In the first step, information is gathered from a variety of sources, including the client, if he or she chooses to collaborate in the assessment. The information gathered pertains to the past self-harmful behaviour and lifestyle of the client and its identification is prompted and its interpretation framed by the risk factors described in the guidelines. In the second step, practitioners determine whether and to what extent each of the risk factors identified in the guidance being used is present in the client. In the third step, practitioners determine whether and to what extent in their opinion those risk factors that are present are also *relevant* to the client's potential to be harmful again in the future. (For example, one client may only have attempted suicide when they have been intoxicated, making substance abuse both present and potentially relevant to any future self-harm. However, another client may have a history of substance abuse but his or her self-harm post-dates his hospitalization or imprisonment, making it not relevant to future potential. A risk factor can, therefore, be present in a client's history but not be relevant to self-harm. This judgement of relevance is what is required at this step.)

In the fourth step, the risk factors identified as relevant are added to with clinical judgements about potential protective factors (e.g., attitudes demonstrating a commitment to living) and all are woven together into a formulation – an understanding based on the decisions to self-harm that have been made in the past and the scenarios in which the same decision could be made again in the future – about future potential for harm (Hart and Logan, 2011). In the fifth step, risk management strategies are identified. Strategies – covering the main areas of treatment, supervision, and monitoring – are linked directly to the risk formulation derived from the identification of the most relevant risk and protective factors.

Specifically, treatment strategies for risk management are those active interventions that are intended to repair or restore deficits in functioning linked to risk (e.g., psychotropic medication for a severe affective disorder; see Leitner, Barr and Hobby, 2008). Supervision strategies target the environment or the setting in which the client is currently based, or likely to be based in the future, in order to limit the potency of risk factors and enhance the effectiveness of protective factors to diminish risk potential (e.g., regular contact between the client and practitioners in his or her clinical team in the run up to and immediately following discharge from an inpatient facility). Finally, monitoring as a risk management activity involves, first, the identification of early warning signs of a relapse to suicidal behaviour, ideally derived from the client through their engagement with treatment and supervision. Second, monitoring refers to the preparation and implementation of plans to be vigilant for evidence of the presence of these early warning signs.

These risk management strategies – hypotheses for ensuring the prevention of future self-harmful conduct by the client – are intended to influence the operation of relevant risk and protective factors on overall risk potential, diminishing it in the short term. Finally, in the last step, summary judgements are made regarding the urgency of action or case prioritization, risks in other areas (e.g. violence), any immediate action required, and the date for next case review, including reassessment of risk.

The Suicidal Behaviours Risk Evaluation *(SBRE)*

The SBRE is a structured professional judgement guide to risk assessment and management with clients at risk of suicide or serious self-harm. It was developed for use with clients in mental health settings, including forensic mental health and correctional settings, whose risk of suicide is chronic and with whom complex (restrictive) risk management is likely to be required, which will necessitate justification to the client, his or her carer and to others. It is also intended for use with those service users whose risk of suicide is unclear or not well understood, as a means of achieving an understanding and determining proportionate risk management plans. The SBRE was developed for use as an advanced tool – one to be used when something more than the BHS or the START or even the S-RAMM is required to understand risk in the long term – for use with long-stay inpatients or with those whose suicide risk is chronic or recurrent.

The SBRE comprises a selection of risk and protective factors drawn from the current empirical and clinical research literatures on suicide and self-harm and listed in a worksheet. The worksheet exemplifies the six steps of the structured professional judgement approach described above. Therefore, the practitioner determines the presence of risk and protective factors, rating each one as *definitely present, possibly or partially present*, or *not present*. The practitioner then determines the relevance of the factor to future suicidal behaviour using the same three-point rating – *definitely, partially/possibly* or *not relevant*. Once the most relevant factors have been identified, the practitioner moves to consider the risk formulation by examining the role of those factors relevant to past instances of self-harm and the scenarios in which future self-harm may occur. The formulation is then prepared as an explanation for the client's risk, presented to the client and colleagues in the form of a narrative written in natural – comprehensible – language. This formulation then becomes the basis of decision-making around the most practically useful treatment, supervision and monitoring strategies. Table 5.1 lists the risk and protective factors in the SBRE. The final written communication about the risks posed by the client comprises the formulation and risk management plan.

The SBRE consists of a set of guidelines for use (a manual) and a worksheet on which to plot and record thinking on risk. (Materials are available from the author

Table 5.1 Risk and protective factors in the *Suicidal Behaviours Risk Evaluation* (SBRE)

Factor	Description
	Experience of suicide and preparation
E1	Previous and serious attempts at suicide
E2	History of self-harming behaviour
E3	Family history of suicide (including attempts)
E4	Easy access to lethal means
E5	Suicide ideation/planning
E6	Attitudes and beliefs tolerant of suicide
	Psychological adjustment
P7	Hopelessness
P8	Problems with stress and coping
P9	Impulse-control problems
P10	Problems with making and carrying out plans
P11	Problems with thinking
P12	Unstable mood
P13	Problems with self-awareness
P14	Problems with child abuse
P15	Experience of loss or other acute distress
	Social adjustment
A16	Difficulties with rule adherence
A17	Socially isolated
	Mental and physical health needs
M18	Serious mental illness with incapacitation
M19	Substance use problems
M20	Serious mood episode
M21	Physical illness with incapacitation
M22	Problems with adherence to treatment (including medication)
M23	Poor response to treatment
M24	Recent change in care arrangements
	Strengths
S25	Attitudes demonstrating a commitment to living
S26	Negative attitude to suicide
S27	Presence of close social relationships
S28	Presence of a supportive therapeutic relationship with a care provider

on request). The guidelines have been subject to several stages of development. First, an extensive literature review was carried out. Second, the findings of this review and a prototype list of risk and protective factors were presented to a panel of service managers, practitioners and service users and carers. Feedback from this presentation was used to refine the prototype. Third, the first version of the guidelines and the SBRE worksheet were then prepared in order that it could be subject to preliminary field testing as an adjunct to existing practice with clients in general mental health and forensic mental health settings who were at risk of suicide or serious self harm. Fourth, the SBRE was distributed more widely to practitioners working in a variety of settings and feedback was sought on its application and clinical utility. Fifth, a series of research projects have been prepared and some are underway to establish the reliability of risk assessment using the SBRE and the validity of the instrument in terms of its comparison with instruments intended to do the same job (e.g. the BHS, the ESR-20 and the S-RAMM) and its ability to distinguish among those at risk of completing suicide, those who self-harm without suicidal intent, and those who have mental health needs but who are not suicidal. This latter research stage is ongoing.

Concluding comments

There are a number of guides available to assist practitioners in their assessment of risk of suicide and self-harm in the clients with whom they work. However, many cover only aspects of suicide risk and few assist the practitioner with a set of clinical guidelines towards an understanding of the function of suicidal behaviour for the client, represented in a risk formulation, and a risk management plan tailored to the needs and circumstances of the individual client. The SBRE is a step towards this end, but further work is required to verify it as a clinically useful instrument in the practitioner's toolkit of risk assessment and management guides.

Conclusions and recommendations

Understanding suicidal behaviour has been the focus of this chapter. The chapter began with a brief overview of the topics of suicide and self-harm, which highlighted what we understand about the links between these outcomes as well as the important differences. There followed a review of current practice in respect of suicide and self-harm risk assessment and a discussion of options for the development of current practice using the structured professional judgement approach, and a new guide to suicide and self-harm risk assessment and management, the *Suicidal Behaviours Risk Evaluation*, was introduced. It is clear that there exists a great deal of research examining the associations between individual and situational variables and risk of suicide and self-harm. Publications by Leitner and Barr (2011), Leitner, et al. (2008) and McLean, et al. (2008) offer recent reviews of risk assessment and of strategies that might be used to manage these risks with some degree of efficacy. However, much work remains to be done to improve the current limited practice in terms of risk assessment and management, especially in forensic mental health and correctional settings. What should practitioners do in the meantime to ensure the standard of their practice is good?

1. *If possible, supplement a good clinical interview of a suicidal client with a structured form of assessment.* Bolstering clinical judgement with an evidence-based form of assessment of either a critical risk factor (e.g., hopelessness using the BHS) or risk in general (such as with the ESR-20, the SAMI, S-RAMM, or even the SBRE) will ensure the anchoring of judgement in empirical evidence. With the use of a comprehensive measure of risk, a detailed assessment is more likely to have significant implications for the scale and thoroughness of risk management. Best practice in clinical risk

assessment and management involves making decisions based on knowledge of the research evidence, knowledge of the client and their social context, knowledge of the client's own experience of disorder and distress, and clinical judgement (DH, 2007).

2. *Practitioners should endeavour to proactively engage clients in assessments of risk and in its subsequent and ongoing management.* Regardless of how the assessment is carried out – what guides are used to structure judgement, if any – the client's point of view should be sought and their collaboration in evaluation sought as a matter of necessity.

3. *The structured professional judgement approach offers the potential to help practitioners think through complex cases in which suicidal intent is chronic, recurrent, or difficult to access yet where they are required to be accountable to their clients and to those who manage their services as to the costly actions they might recommend to manage risk.* The structured professional judgement approach does not offer a quick assessment but its capacity to influence risk management is enduring, more so than the outcomes of brief and speedy assessments of suicide risk based on a small number of mainly static variables. Therefore, structured professional judgement approaches offer practitioners the opportunity to be flexible, dynamic and responsive to the needs of their clients.

4. *Careful forward planning should be the point of clinical risk assessment and management, especially in relation to risk of suicide and self-harm.* The purpose of risk assessment is to manage the future in order to prevent harm based on an understanding of the purpose of past harmful acts. A formulation of future risk should feature in every risk assessment and scenario planning should always be a component of risk formulation. Risk management recommendations should be derived from an understanding of risk represented in the formulation.

5. *The best risk assessments are undertaken, and the best risk management plans are implemented, by a group of practitioners working from different professional perspectives, even if one practitioner representing one profession takes the lead in the preparation of the assessment and the subsequent plan.* Multidisciplinary teamwork is essential in the assessment and management of clinical risk in all areas.

6. *Finally, risk management plans should address individual factors – mental disorder, emotional distress, and so on – but also structural, procedural and organizational factors in the environment in which the individual resides where those factors make a contribution to risk.* Altering risk and protective factors in the individual – internal variables – is only one aspect of risk management. Changing environments is often necessary to support individual and sustained change.

Notes

1   The *Suicidal Behaviours Risk Evaluation* worksheet and manual described in this chapter are based on the *Risk for Sexual Violence Protocol* (RSVP, Hart, Kropp, Laws, et al.,

2003) worksheet and manual, the copyright owner of which is the Mental Health, Law, and Policy Institute at Simon Fraser University in Vancouver, Canada. The RSVP worksheet and manual format were adapted with the kind permission of the copyright owner.

2 I would like to thank Dr Jayne Cooper and Dr Jane Senior of the Department of Community Based Medicine at the University of Manchester, and Dr Rabia Zeb of Greater Manchester West Mental Health NHS Foundation Trust, for their comments on an early draft of this chapter.

References

Alexander, D. A., Klein, S., Gray, N. M., Dewar, I. G. and Eagles, J. M. (2000) 'Suicide by patients: Questionnaire study of its effect on consultant psychiatrists', *British Medical Journal, 320*: 1571.

Anderson, M. and Jenkins, R. (2005) 'The challenge of suicide prevention: An overview of national strategies', *Disease Management and Health Outcomes, 13*: 245–53.

Arsenault-Lapierre, G., Kim, C. and Turecki, G. (2004) 'Psychiatric diagnoses in 3275 suicides: A meta-analysis', *BMC Psychiatry, 4*: 37.

Baker, N. (2007) *The Strange Death of David Kelly*, London: Methuen Publishing.

Beautrais, A. (2003) 'Subsequent mortality in medically serious suicide attempts: A five-year follow-up', *Australian and New Zealand Journal of Psychiatry, 37*: 595–99.

Beck, A. T. (1991) *Manual for the Beck Scale for Suicide Ideation*, San Antonio, Texas: Psychological Corporation.

Beck, A. T. and Steer, R. A. (1993) *Manual for the Beck Hopelessness Scale*, San Antonio, Texas: Psychological Corporation.

Beck, R. W., Morris, J. B. and Beck, A. T. (1974) 'Cross-validation of the *Suicidal Intent Scale*', *Psychological Reports, 34*: 445–46.

Blake, N. (2006) *The Deepcut Review: A Review of the Circumstances Surrounding the Deaths of Four Soldiers at Princess Royal Barracks, Deepcut Between 1995 and 2002*, Report: House of Commons Papers 2005–6, London: HM Stationery Office.

Borrill, J. (2008) '*Suicide*', in G. J. Towl, D. P. Farrington, D. A. Crighton and G. Hughes (eds) *Dictionary of Forensic Psychology*, Collumpton, Devon: Willan Publishing.

Borrill, J., Burnett, R., Atkins, R., Miller, S., Briggs, D., Weaver, T. and Maden, A. (2003) 'Patterns of self-harm and attempted suicide among white and black/mixed race female prisoners', *Criminal Behavior and Mental Health, 13*: 229–40.

Bostwick, J. M. and Pankratz, V. S. (2000) 'Affective disorders and suicide risk: A re-examination', *American Journal of Psychiatry, 157*: 1925–32.

Brezo, J., Paris, J. and Turecki, G. (2006) 'Personality traits as correlates of suicidal ideation, suicide attempts, and suicide completions: A systematic review', *Acta Psychiatrica Scandanavica, 113*: 180–206.

Brooker, C., Repper, J., Beverley, C. and Ferriter, M. (2003) *Mental Health Services and Prisoners: A Review for the Department of Health*, Sheffield: University of Sheffield. Accessed at www.dh.gov.uk/assetRoot/04/06/43/78/04064378.pdf.

Brown, G. K., Beck, A. T., Steer, R. A. and Grisham, J. R. (2000) 'Risk factors for suicide in psychiatric out-patients: A 20-year prospective study', *Journal of Consulting and Clinical Psychology, 68*: 371–77.

Chapman, A. L., Specht, M. W. and Cellucci, T. (2005) 'Factors associated with suicide attempts in female inmates: The hegemony of hopelessness', *Suicide and Life-Threatening Behavior, 35*: 558–69.

Cherpitel, C. J., Borges, G. L. G. and Wilcox, H. C. (2004) 'Acute alcohol use and suicidal behavior: A review of the literature', *Alcoholism: Clinical and Experimental Research, 28*: 18S–28S.

Cooper, J., Kapur, N., Webb, R., Lawlor, M., Guthrie, E., Mackway-Jones, K. and Appleby, L. (2005) 'Suicide after deliberate self-harm: A 4-year cohort study', *American Journal of Psychiatry, 162*: 297–303.

Department of Health (2002) *Mental Health Policy Implementation Guide: Adult Acute Inpatient Care Provision*, Department of Health, London. Accessed at www.dh.gov.uk/en/ Publicationsandstatistics/Publications/PublicationsPolicyAndGuidance/DH_4009156.

— (2007) *Best Practice in Managing Risk: Principles and Evidence for Best Practice in the Assessment and Management of Risk to Self and Others in Mental Health Services*, Department of Health, London. Accessed at webarchive.nationalarchives.gov.uk/+/www. dh.gov.uk/en/Publicationsandstatistics/Publications/PublicationsPolicyAndGuidance/ DH_076511.

Doyle, M., Lewis, G. and Brisbane, M. (2008) 'Implementing the *Short-Term Assessment of Risk and Treatability* (START) in a forensic mental health service', *The Psychiatrist, 32*: 406–8.

Draper, B. (1996) 'Attempted suicide in old age', *International Journal of Geriatric Psychiatry, 11*: 577–87.

Elliott, J. L. and Frude, N. (2001) 'Stress, coping styles, and hopelessness in self-poisoners', *Crisis: Journal of Crisis Intervention and Suicide Prevention, 22*: 20–26.

Everall, R. D., Altrows, K. J. and Paulson, B. L. (2006) 'Creating a future: A study of resilience in suicidal female adolescents', *Journal of Counseling and Development, 84*: 461–71.

Fazel, S. and Benning, R. (2009) 'Suicides in female prisoners in England and Wales 1978–2004', *British Journal of Psychiatry, 194*: 183–84.

Fleischmann, A., Bertolote, J. M., Belfer, M. and Beautrais, A. (2005) 'Completed suicide and psychiatric diagnoses in young people: A critical examination of the evidence', *American Journal of Orthopsychiatry, 75*: 676–83.

Frühwald, S. and Frottier, P. (2005) 'Suicide in prison', *The Lancet, 366*: 8.

Goldney, R. D. (2008) *Suicide Prevention*, Oxford: Oxford University Press.

Gunnell, D., Bennewith, O., Peters, T. J., House, A. and Hawton, K. (2005) 'The epidemiology and management of self-harm amongst adults in England', *Journal of Public Health, 27*: 67–73.

Harriss, L. and Hawton, K. (2005) 'Suicidal intent in deliberate self-harm and the risk of suicide: The predictive power of the *Suicide Intent Scale'*, *Journal of Affective Disorders, 86*: 225–33.

Hart, S. D. and Logan, C. (2011) 'Formulation of violence risk using evidence-based assessments: The structured professional judgment approach', in P. Sturmey and M. McMurran (eds) *Forensic Case Formulation*, Chichester: Wiley-Blackwell.

Hart, S. D., Kropp, P. K., Laws, D. R., Klaver, J., Logan, C. and Watt, K. A. (2003) *The Risk for Sexual Violence Protocol: Structured Professional Guidelines for Assessing Risk of Sexual Violence*, Mental Health, Law and Policy Institute, Vancouver, Canada: Simon Fraser University.

Harwood, D. and Jacoby, R. (2000) 'Suicidal behavior among the elderly', in K. Hawton and K. van Heeringen (eds) *The International Handbook of Suicide and Attempted Suicide*, Chichester: John Wiley and Sons Ltd.

Haw, C., Bergen, H., Casey, D. and Hawton, K. (2007) 'Repetition of deliberate self-harm: A study of the characteristics and subsequent deaths in patients presenting to a general hospital according to extent of repetition', *Suicide and Life-Threatening Behavior, 37*: 379–96.

Hawton, K. and Fagg, J. (1992) 'Trends in deliberate self-poisoning and self-injury in Oxford, 1976–90', *British Medical Journal, 304*: 1409–11.

Hawton, K. and van Heeringen, K. (eds) (2000) *The International Handbook of Suicide and Attempted Suicide*, Chichester: Wiley.

Hawton, K., Fagg, J., Simkin, S., Bale, E. and Bond, A. (1997) 'Trends in deliberate self-harm in Oxford, 1985–95, and their implications for clinical services and the prevention of suicide', *British Journal of Psychiatry, 171*: 556–60.

Hawton, K., Harriss, L., Hall, S., Simkin, S., Bale, E. and Bond, A. (2003a) 'Deliberate self-harm in Oxford, 1990–2000: A time of change in patient characteristics', *Psychological Medicine, 33:* 987–95.

Hawton, K., Rodham, K., Evans, E. and Weatherall, R. (2002) 'Deliberate self-harm in adolescents: Self-report survey in schools in England', *British Medical Journal, 325*: 1207–11.

Hawton, K., Rodham, K. and Evans, E. (2006) *By Their Own Young Hand: Deliberate Self-harm and Suicidal Ideas in Adolescents*, London: Jessica Kingsley Publishers.

Hawton, K., Sutton, L., Haw, C., Sinclair, J. and Deeks, J. J. (2005a) 'Schizophrenia and suicide: Systematic review of risk factors', *British Journal of Psychiatry, 187*: 9–20.

Hawton, K., Sutton, L., Haw, C., Sinclair, J. and Harriss, L. (2005b) 'Suicide and attempted suicide in bipolar disorder: A systematic review of risk factors', *Journal of Clinical Psychiatry, 66*, 693–704.

Hawton, K., Zahl, D. and Wetherall, R. (2003b) 'Suicide following deliberate self-harm: Long-term follow-up of patients who presented to a general hospital', *British Journal of Psychiatry, 182*: 537–42.

Hayes, A. J., Shaw, J. J., Lever-Green, G., Parker, D. and Gask, L. (2008) 'Improvements to suicide prevention training for prison staff in England and Wales', *Suicide and Life-Threatening Behavior, 38*: 708–13.

Hem, E., Berg, A. M. and Ekeberg, Ø. (2001) 'Suicide in police: A critical review', *Suicide and Life-Threatening Behavior, 31*: 224–33.

Her Majesty's Chief Inspector of Prisons for England and Wales (2010) *Annual Report 2008–09*, London: The Stationery Office. Accessed at www.justice.gov.uk/inspectorates/hmi-prisons/docs/HMIP_AR_2008-9_web_published_rps.pdf.

Horrocks, J. and House, A. (2002) 'Self-poisoning and self-injury in adults', *Clinical Medicine, 2*: 509–12.

Huey, M. P. and Mcnulty, T. L. (2005) 'Institutional conditions and prison suicide: Conditional effects of deprivation and overcrowding', *The Prison Journal, 85*: 490–514.

Ijaz, A., Papaconstantinou, A., O'Neill, H. and Kennedy, H. G. (2009) 'The Suicide Risk Assessment and Management Manual (S-RAMM) validation study 1', *Irish Journal of Psychological Medicine, 26*: 54–58.

James, A., Lai, F. H. and Dahl, C. (2004) 'Attention deficit hyperactivity disorder and suicide: A review of possible associations', *Acta Psychiatrica Scandanavica, 110*: 408–15.

Jenkins, R., Bhugra, D., Meltzer, H., Singleton, N., Bebbington, P., Brugha, T., Coid, J., Farrell, M., Lewis, G. and Paton, J. (2005) 'Psychiatric and social aspects of suicidal behaviour in prisons', *Psychological Medicine, 35*: 257–69.

Kapur, N., Cooper, J. B., King-Hele, S., Webb, R., Lawlor, M., Rodway, C. and Appleby, L. (2006) 'The repetition of suicidal behavior: A multicenter cohort study', *Journal of Clinical Psychiatry, 67*: 1599–1609.

Kenny, D. T., Lennings, C. J. and Munn, O. A. (2008) 'Risk factors for self-harm and suicide in incarcerated young offenders: Implications for policy and practice', *Journal of Forensic Psychiatry and Psychology, 8*: 358–82.

Kerr, P. L., Mühlenkamp, J. J. and Turner, J. M. (2010) 'Non-suicidal self-injury: A review of current research for family medicine and primary care physicians', *Journal of the American Board of Family Medicine, 23*: 240–59.

Kleespies, P. M., Hough, S. and Romeo, A. M. (2009) 'Suicide risk in people with medical and terminal illness', in P. M. Kleespies (ed.) *Behavioral Emergencies: An Evidence-based Resource for Evaluating and Managing Risk of Suicide, Violence, and Victimization*, pp. 103–21, Washington DC, US: American Psychological Association.

Konrad, N., Daigle, M. S., Daniel, A. E., Dear, G. E., Frottier, P., Hayes, L. M., Kerkhof, A. and Sarchiapone, M. (2007) 'Preventing suicides in prisons, Part 1: Recommendations from the international association for suicide prevention task force on suicide in prisons', *Crisis, 28*: 113–21.

Kripalani, M., Nag, S., Nag, S. and Gash, A. (2010) 'Integrated care pathway for self-harm: Our way forward', *Emergency Medicine Journal, 27*: 544–46.

Leitner, M. and Barr, W. (2011) 'Understanding and managing self-harm in mental health services', in R. Whittington and C. Logan (eds) *Self-harm and Violence: Towards Best Practice in Managing Risk in Mental Health Services*, pp. 55–78, Chichester: Wiley-Blackwell.

Leitner, M., Barr, W. and Hobby, L. (2008) *Effectiveness of Interventions to Prevent Suicide and Suicidal Behaviour: A Systematic Review*, Edinburgh: Scottish Government Social Research. Accessed at www.scotland.gov.uk/Resource/Doc/208329/0055247.pdf.

Li, D., Duan, Y. and He, L. (2006) 'Association study of serotonin 2A receptor (5-HT2A) gene with schizophrenia and suicidal behaviour using systematic meta-analysis', *Biochemical and Biophysical Research Communications, 340*: 1006–15.

Lindeman, S., Laara, E., Hakko, H. and Lonnqvist, J. (1996) 'A systematic review on gender-specific suicide mortality in medical doctors', *British Journal of Psychiatry, 168*: 274–79.

Logan, C., Nathan, R. and Brown, A. (2011) 'Formulation in clinical risk assessment and management', in R. W. Whittington and C. Logan (eds) *Self-harm and Violence: Towards Best Practice in Managing Risk in Mental Health Services*, Chichester, England: Wiley-Blackwell.

Lohner, J. and Konrad, N. (2007) 'Risk factors for self-injurious behaviour in custody: Problems of definition and prediction', *International Journal of Prisoner Health, 3*: 135–61.

McLean, J., Maxwell, M., Platt, S., Harris, F. and Jepson, R. (2008) *Risk and Protective Factors for Suicide and Suicidal Behaviour: A Literature Review*, Edinburgh: Scottish Government Social Research. Accessed at www.scotland.gov.uk/publications/2008/11/28141444/0.

McManus, S., Meltzer, H., Brugha, T., Bebbington, P. and Jenkins, R. (2009) *Adult Psychiatric Morbidity in England, 2007: Results of a Household Survey*, The NHS Information Centre for Health and Social Care. Accessed at www.ic.nhs.uk/pubs/.

McMillan, D., Gilbody, S., Beresford, E. and Neilly, L. (2007) 'Can we predict suicide and non-fatal self-harm with the Beck Hopelessness Scale? A meta-analysis', *Psychological Medicine, 37*: 769–78.

Madge, N., Hewitt, A., Hawton, K., de Wilde, E. J., Corcoran, P., Fekete, S., van Heeringen, K., de Leo, D. and Ostgaard, M. (2008) 'Deliberate self-harm within an international community sample of young people: Comparative findings from the Child and Adolescent Self-harm in Europe (CASE) Study', *Journal of Child Psychology and Psychiatry, 49*: 667–77.

Malone, K. M., Oquendo, M. A., Haas, G. L., Ellis, S. P., Li, S. and Mann, J. J. (2000) 'Protective factors against suicidal acts in major depression: Reasons for living', *American Journal of Psychiatry, 157*: 1084–88.

Marzano, L., Fazel, S., Rivlin, A. and Hawton, K. (2010) 'Psychiatric disorders in women prisoners who have engaged in near-lethal self-harm: Case-control study', *British Journal of Psychiatry, 197*: 219–26.

Meadows, L. A., Kaslow, N. J., Thompson, M. P. and Jurkovic, G. J. (2005) 'Protective factors against suicide attempt risk among African American women experiencing intimate partner violence', *American Journal of Community Psychology, 36*: 109–21.

Meltzer, H., Lader, D., Corbin, T., Singleton, N., Jenkins, R. and Brugha, T. (2002) *Non-fatal Suicidal Behavior among Adults aged 16 to 74 in Great Britain*, London: The Stationery Office.

Ministry of Justice (2010) *Deaths in Prison Custody 2010*. News Release. Accessed at www.justice.gov.uk/news/press-release-020111a.htm.

Mumola, C. J. (2005) *Suicide and Homicide in State Prisons and Local Jails*. Special Report, US Department of Justice. Accessed at bjs.ojp.usdoj.gov/content/pub/ascii/shsplj.txt.

Natale, L. (2010) *Factsheet: Prisons in England and Wales*. CIVITAS Institute for the Study of Civil Society. Accessed at www.civitas.org.uk/crime/factsheet-Prisons.pdf.

National Collaborating Centre for Mental Health (2004) *Self-harm: The Short-term Physical and Psychological Management and Secondary Prevention of Self-harm in Primary and Secondary Care*, Leicester: The British Psychological Society and the Royal College of Psychiatrists. Accessed at www.nice.org.uk/nicemedia/live/10946/29424/29424.pdf.

— (2011) *Self-harm: Longer-term Management in Adults, Children and Young People*. Draft guidance for consultation. Accessed at www.nccmh.org.uk/downloads/Self_harm_LTM/cons_nice_54071.pdf?id = 44B45E71–19B9-E0B5-D418F2D847979E8C.

National Confidential Inquiry into Suicide and Homicide by People with Mental Illness (2010) *Annual Report*. July. Accessed at www.medicine.manchester.ac.uk/mentalhealth/research/suicide/prevention/nci/inquiryannualreports/AnnualReportJuly2010.pdf.

Neeleman, J. (2001) 'A continuum of premature death: Meta-analysis of competing mortality in the psychosocially vulnerable', *International Journal of Epidemiology, 30*: 154–62.

Nicholls, T. N., Brink, J., Desmarais, S. L., Webster, C. D. and Martin, M. L. (2006) 'The *Short-Term Assessment of Risk and Treatability* (START): A prospective validation study in a forensic psychiatric sample', *Assessment, 13*: 313–27.

Noonan, M. (2010) *Deaths in Custody Reporting Programme: Mortality in Local Jails, 2000–2007*. Special Report, US Department of Justice. Accessed at bjs.ojp.usdoj.gov/content/pub/ascii/mlj07.txt.

Olfson, M., Gameroff, M. J., Marcus, S. C., Greenberg, T. and Shaffer, D. (2005) 'National trends in hospitalization of youth with intentional self-inflicted injuries', *American Journal of Psychiatry, 162*: 1328–35.

Otto, R. K. and Douglas, K. S. (2010) *Handbook of Violence Risk Assessment*, New York: Routledge.

Owens, D., Horrocks, J. and House, A. (2002) 'Fatal and non-fatal repetition of self-harm: Systematic review', *British Journal of Psychiatry, 181*: 193–99.

Palmer, B. A., Pankratz, V. S. and Bostwick, J. M. (2005) 'The lifetime risk of suicide in schizophrenia: A re-examination', *Archives of General Psychiatry, 62*: 247–53.

Piquet, M. L. and Wagner, B. M. (2003) 'Coping responses of adolescent suicide attempters and their relation to suicidal ideation across a 2-year follow-up: A preliminary study', *Suicide and Life-Threatening Behavior, 33*: 288–301.

Platt, S. and Hawton, K. (2000) 'Suicidal behaviour and the labour market', in K. Hawton and K. van Heeringen (eds) *The International Handbook of Suicide and Attempted Suicide*, Chichester: John Wiley and Sons Ltd.

Polvi, N. (1997) 'Assessing risk of suicide in correctional settings', in C. D. Webster and M. A. Jackson (eds) *Impulsivity: Theory, Assessment, and Treatment*, pp. 278–300, New York: Guilford Press.

Pompili, M., Girardi, P., Ruberto, A. and Tatarelli, R. (2005a) 'Suicide in borderline personality disorder: A meta-analysis', *Nordic Journal of Psychiatry, 59*: 319–24.

— (2005b) 'Suicide in the epilepsies: A meta-analytic investigation of 29 cohorts', *Epilepsy and Behavior, 7*: 305–10.

Pompili, M., Girardi, P., Tatarelli, G., Ruberto, A. and Tatarelli, R. (2006) 'Suicide and attempted suicide in eating disorders, obesity and weight-image concern', *Eating Behaviors, 7*: 384–94.

Pratt, D., Piper, M., Appleby, L., Webb, R. and Shaw, J. (2006) 'Suicide in recently released prisoners: A population-based cohort study', *The Lancet, 368*: 119–23.

Rehkopf, D. H. and Buka, S. L. (2006) 'The association between suicide and the socio-economic characteristics of geographical areas: A systematic review', *Psychological Medicine, 36*: 145–57.

Rivlin, A., Hawton, K., Marzano, L. and Fazel, S. (2010) 'Psychiatric disorders in male prisoners who made near lethal suicide attempts: Case-control study', *British Journal of Psychiatry, 197*: 313–19.

Rodgers, P. (2010) *Review of the Applied Suicide Intervention Skills Training Program (ASIST): Rationale, Evaluation Results, and Directions for Future Research*, Calgary, Canada: LivingWorks Education. Accessed at www.livingworks.net/userfiles/file/ASIST_review2010.pdf.

Romilly, C. and Bartlett, A. (2010) 'Prison mental health care', in A. Bartlett and G. McGauley (eds) *Forensic Mental Health: Concepts, Systems, and Practice*, Oxford: Oxford University Press.

Royal College of Psychiatrists (2002) *Suicide in Prisons*. Council Report CR99. February, London: Royal College of Psychiatrists.

Rudd, M. D., Joiner, T. and Rajab, M. H. (2001) *Treating Suicidal Behaviour: An Effective, Time-limited Approach*, New York: Guilford Press.

Runeson, B., Tidemalm, D., Dahlin, M., Lichtenstein, P. and Långström, N. (2010) 'Method of attempted suicide as predictor of subsequent successful suicide: National long-term cohort study', *British Medical Journal, 340*: c3222.

Saunders, K. E. A. and Hawton, K. (2006) 'Suicidal behaviour and the menstrual cycle', *Psychological Medicine, 36*: 901–12.

Shadigian, E. M. and Bauer, S. T. (2005) 'Pregnancy-associated death: A qualitative systematic review of homicide and suicide', *Obstetrical and Gynecological Survey, 60*: 183–90.

Sharkey, L. (2010) 'Does overcrowding in prisons exacerbate the risk of suicide among women prisoners?' *The Howard Journal of Criminal Justice, 49*: 111–24.

Shaw, J., Baker, D., Hunt, I. M., Moloney, A. and Appleby, L. (2004) 'Suicide by prisoners', *British Journal of Psychiatry, 184*: 263–67.

Singleton, N., Meltzer, H., Gatward, R., Coid, J. and Deasy, D. (1998) *Psychiatric Morbidity among Prisoners in England and Wales*, London: HMSO.

Speckens, A. E. M. and Hawton, K. (2005) 'Social problem solving in adolescents with suicidal behaviour: A systematic review', *Suicide and Life-Threatening Behavior, 35*: 365–87.

van Velsen, C. (2010) 'Psychotherapeutic understanding and approach to psychosis in mentally disordered offenders', in A. Bartlett and G. McGauley (eds) *Forensic Mental Health: Concepts, Systems, and Practice*, Oxford: Oxford University Press.

de Vogel, V., de Ruiter, C., Bouman, Y. and de Vries Robbé, M. (2009) *Structured Assessment of Protective Factors (SAPROF): Guidelines for the assessment of protective factors for violence risk*, English version, Utrecht, The Netherlands: Forum Educatief.

Völlm, B. and Dolan, M. (2009) 'Self-harm among UK female prisoners: A cross-sectional study', *Journal of Forensic Psychiatry and Psychology, 20*: 741–51.

Webster, C. D., Martin, M., Brink, J., Nicholls, T. L. and Middleton, C. (2004) *Short-term Assessment of Risk and Treatability (START): An Evaluation and Planning Guide*, Hamilton, Ontario: St. Joseph's Healthcare.

Whitlock, J., Eckenrode, J. and Silverman, D. (2006) 'Self-injurious behaviors in a college population', *Pediatrics, 117*: 1939–48.

Whittle, M. (1997) 'Malignant alienation', *Journal of Forensic Psychiatry and Psychology, 8*: 5–10.

Wilcox, H. C., Conner, K. R. and Caine, E. D. (2004) 'Association of alcohol and drug use disorders and completed suicide: An empirical review of cohort studies', *Drug and Alcohol Dependence, 76 (SUPPL.)*: S11–19.

Windfuhr, K. and Swinson, N. (2011) 'Suicide and homicide by people with mental illness: A national overview', in R. Whittington and C. Logan (eds) *Self-harm and Violence: Towards Best Practice in Managing Risk in Mental Health Services*, p. 55–78, Chichester: Wiley-Blackwell.

World Health Organization (2007) *Preventing Suicide in Jails and Prisons*, Geneva: WHO. Accessed at www.who.int/mental_health/prevention/suicide/resource_jails_prisons.pdf.

Wulsin, L. R., Vaillant, G. E. and Wells, V. E. (2005) 'A systematic review of the mortality of depression', *Psychosomatic Medicine, 6*: 6–17.

Zapf, P. A. (2006) *Suicide Assessment Manual for Inmates* (SAMI), Vancouver, Canada: Mental Health, Law and Policy Institute, Simon Fraser University.

6 Pathological firesetting by adults

Assessing and managing risk within a functional analytic framework

John L. Taylor and Ian Thorne

Introduction and definitions

Intentional firesetting has very significant consequences for individuals, communities, and the economy. There were 79,700 deliberate fires in the UK in 2005, resulting in 111 fatalities and 2,700 non-fatal injuries (Department of Communities and Local Government, 2007). In the US in the same year, deliberate fires caused 490 deaths and 9,100 non-fatal injuries (Hall, 2007). Government research estimates the direct costs of arson to the economy of England and Wales to be £2.2 billion per annum (Canter and Almond, 2002).

Despite the scale and impact of deliberate fires, very few arson offenders are apprehended and convicted. For example, in 2001, fire services in England and Wales attended 110,000 fires where deliberate ignition was suspected (Arson Control Forum, 2003). Of this total, 60,472 fires were classified by the police as arson offences (involving 'reckless' behaviour or an 'intention to damage property'). Just 8 per cent (4,817) of these recorded offences were 'detected' (that is, the suspect was cautioned or charged) and only 2.5 per cent (1,500) suspects were found guilty of arson in the courts. Of the 899 more serious arson offences dealt with by the Crown Court in 2001, 63 defendants (7 per cent) received Hospital Orders under section 37 of the *England and Wales Mental Health Act* 1983 (Arson Control Forum, 2003).

Most research on deliberate firesetting has involved children and juveniles (Palmer, Caufield and Hollin, 2005). However, adults were responsible for just over half of all intentional fires detected in the USA in 2005 (Hall, 2007). As those who set fires for financial or political gain do not generally come to the attention of forensic mental health practitioners, the focus of this chapter is on adults who deliberately set fires in the context of associated mental health or emotional problems. At the outset, we make the point that, in our view, there is an urgent need for further work on this important problem. However, acknowledging current clinical need, in this chapter we provide an overview of research on firesetter characteristics, classification systems and explanatory theories. Attention is then given to the assessment of firesetting behaviour, risk and associated clinical issues within a structured clinical judgement framework, before providing some guidance on psychological interventions for firesetting behaviour and related issues.

Pyromania is classified in the fourth edition of the *Diagnostic and Statistical Manual of Mental Disorders* (DSM-IV; American Psychiatric Association, 1994) as an impulse-control disorder. This is likely to remain the case in the forthcoming fifth edition (DSM-5). Confusingly, the defining features of the disorder include deliberate and purposeful setting of fires involving 'considerable advance preparation' (p. 614). The DSM-IV definition also includes fire fascination and pleasure and gratification associated with setting fires as diagnostic criteria. The effect of these criteria is to narrow the pyromania definition and make it unlikely to apply to all but a very few arsonists. The DSM-IV definition also specifically excludes firesetters with intellectual disabilities (ID) as a group whose firesetting is a result of impaired judgement.

A distinction has been made between *arsonists,* who are apprehended, charged, and convicted of starting deliberate fires, and *firesetters* who have committed acts of arson that have not have resulted in charges being brought or convictions (Swaffer, Haggett and Oxley, 2001). Health and other human services that work with people with mental health problems and offending histories frequently deal with offenders who have committed acts of arson that have not been processed through the criminal justice system. Therefore the term 'firesetters' is the most appropriate to describe the population discussed in this chapter.

Jackson (1994) distinguished between 'pathological' and other types of firesetters (p. 95). Five criteria were suggested by Jackson as indicating pathological firesetting: (i) recidivism; (ii) fire to property rather than fire against other people; (iii) firesetting alone or repetitively with a single identified accomplice; (iv) evidence of personality, psychiatric, or emotional problems; and (v) the absence of financial or political gain as a motive for setting fires. Jackson, Glass and Hope (1987) considered this to be a more clinically relevant and useful concept that takes into account the evidence available concerning the prevalence and development of firesetting behaviour in people with mental health and emotional problems.

Classification and theoretical perspectives on firesetting

There is a significant literature involving firesetters that has described their features in terms of socio-demographic, developmental, mental health and offending history characteristics. Gannon and Pina (2010) provide a helpful review of this literature. Whilst these descriptions of firesetter characteristics are of interest to researchers and clinicians, they do not offer a coherent account of the aetiology, development and maintenance of firesetting behaviour that provides the basis of a formulation to guide clinical intervention and management plans. This is a common problem in research on clinical risk. It is now recognized that we need to move beyond cumulative risk models to a better understanding of what, why, where and how risk factors function at the individual level (see Cooke and Michie, this volume; also Johnstone, this volume).

There have been many attempts to organize information about firesetters into different schemes to help our understanding, assessment and treatment of this phenomenon. Over the years, many authors have offered typologies of firesetters based on the personal characteristics of perpetrators, their motives for firesetting, and other features such as place of residence (e.g. Geller, 1992; Inciardi, 1970; Lewis and Yarnell, 1951; Prins, 1994; Prins, Tennant and Trick, 1985). Motives for firesetting have been the focus of some of the more extensive studies. Firesetters released on parole from a US prison over a five-year period were the subject of a file review study by Inciardi (1970). Those motivated by revenge comprised the largest group (58 per cent). More pertinent to the clinical context, Rix (1994) conducted clinical interviews with 153 firesetters referred to psychiatric services in the UK over a 10-year period. Similar to Inciardi's findings, Rix found revenge to be the most frequently cited motive for firesetting (33 per cent) in this study group. In a different clinical context, Murphy and Clare (1996) found that anger was the most frequently reported antecedent to firesetting in a group of 10 adults with intellectual disabilities (ID). This finding was replicated by Taylor, Thorne, Robertson and Avery (2002) in their assessment of 14 adults with ID detained in secure hospital settings following convictions for arson. Underlining the anger-revenge construct as an antecedent to firesetting, numerous other studies have also reported revenge as the most prevalent motive for firesetting amongst adult populations (see Gannon and Pina, 2010 for a review).

An important limitation of schemes that categorize firesetters or firesetting behaviour is that they don't account for the diversity or heterogeneity of firesetter characteristics or the complex interaction of dispositional, situational and environmental factors that can lead to firesetting behaviour. Historically, the concept of an irresistible impulse or drive to set fires, which underpins the DSM-IV definition of pyromania, has led to assumed associations between arson and fire fascination, sexual gratification, displaced aggression, and psychoses. Jackson (1994) explored the research literature supporting these associations and concluded that there is little evidence to support clear and straight-cut, linear relationships between firesetting and any of these factors.

In an attempt to better explain firesetting behaviour, Jackson, et al. (1987) described recidivistic arson within a 'functional analysis paradigm' (p. 175). Deliberate firesetters are viewed as a psychosocially disadvantaged group with associated mood and self-esteem problems, and impairments in their abilities to communicate effectively and to influence their environments. In this framework, arson is conceived as a maladaptive response influenced by antecedents, positive and negative reinforcing contingencies, and other social-learning processes, including individual and vicarious fire experiences. The triggering event is likely to be emotionally significant, for example disappointment or insult, leading to feelings of anger and negative affect (Bumpass, Brix and Preston, 1985). However, fire is likely to be selected as the response because it provides a non-confrontational form of communication for these often under-assertive individuals (Harris and Rice, 1984; Smith and Short, 1995). While there may not be a human target, the action elicits immediate and powerful reinforcing consequences in the form of avoidance, caregiving, revenge, or the amelioration of negative affective states.

Thus, in the short term at least, the ineffectual firesetter achieves a degree of control over their environment. This is what Jackson (1994) describes as the 'Only Viable Option Theory' (p. 107), which can have a powerful maintaining effect on firesetting behaviour.

The functional analysis paradigm (Jackson, 1994) provides a multi-factor explanation for the development of firesetting behaviour, from childhood curiosity and experimentation to pathological arson. This paradigm, well established in the behavioural literature, can be extremely useful in framing individual assessments. For example, many arsonists, due to their socially disadvantaged backgrounds and abusive early experiences, frequently have significant difficulties in interacting in a socially adaptive manner with family, peers and the school environment. This in turn reduces their opportunities for learning or engaging in pro-social means of emotional expression. This combination of factors leads to the expression of emotion, or attempts to resolve interpersonal problems, through the medium of fire. The choice of fire as the only viable option might be particularly relevant for people with mental health problems and developmental disabilities given the social and emotional problems often associated with such conditions.

Case example illustrating the functional analytic approach

Paul is a 34-year-old man with borderline intellectual functioning. He presents as an extremely passive and reticent individual. Paul was convicted of arson and detained under a *Mental Health Act* 1983 hospital order. He had a previous conviction for arson with intent to endanger life, and a history of childhood firesetting and hoax calls to the emergency services. Paul experienced a disturbed, deprived and abusive family history. He was taken into care as a child and moved into a supervised community home upon reaching adulthood. Previous firesetting behaviour was associated with relationship difficulties with his mother. Following his reception into care, visits to or from his mother tended to be eagerly anticipated, but intermittently received, resulting in feelings of rejection and resentment. Paul tended to suppress his feelings of frustration and express his anger and bitterness indirectly through the medium of fire.

Paul's index offence involved setting fire to a building whilst he was living in a residential community placement. In a functional analysis of the index offence, Paul indicated that he had been the victim of inappropriate sexual advances from another resident. He had attempted to bring this issue to the attention of support staff. However, he felt his concerns had not been taken seriously and that the alleged perpetrator had not been dealt with appropriately. Parallels can be drawn with Paul's previous firesetting behaviour, which was preceded by anger and strong feelings of rejection and injustice. As an anxious person with little self-confidence who often experiences low mood, Paul finds interpersonal problem-solving difficult. His firesetting behaviour is an effective means of communicating and ventilating negative emotional states, and of eliciting care-giving behaviour through a medium he has experience of being reinforcing.

Assessment of firesetting behaviour

The functional analytical paradigm enables practitioners to use clinical and file information, augmented by the results of formal assessments, to reach clinically defensible decisions concerning risks and factors influencing risks presented by particular patients (Taylor and Halstead, 2001). This is consistent with the structured professional judgement (SJP) approach to risk assessment described by Hart and Logan (2011).

In any forensic clinical context, it is important to collect and collate information systematically from a range of sources (self and informant reports, behavioural observations, file review, clinical assessment). The functional analytical paradigm provides a framework for this assessment that allows the clinician to formulate the patient's risk, needs and intervention plans.

In the following section an approach to assessing firesetting behaviour is described that involves the use of a guiding framework and a number of fire-specific file-review and clinical-assessment tools that can inform structured clinical judgements concerning firesetting risk and indicate areas requiring therapeutic and management interventions.

A guiding framework for firesetter assessment

Taylor, Thorne and Slavkin (2004) reported on the use of a newly designed *Pathological Fire-Setters Interview* (*PFSI*). This is a structured interview, augmented with collateral information from patients' records, staff observations and patient- and informant-completed clinical measures and risk assessments that enables practitioners to collect and organize information within a functional analytic framework (cf. Jackson, 1994). The PFSI comprises the following components that map onto this framework:

- personal details – demographic details and offending history;
- setting conditions (situational) – e.g., family background, experience of physical/sexual abuse, care and educational history;
- setting conditions (dispositional) – e.g., psychiatric, psychological, neurological, self-harm, and drug/alcohol history, physical disabilities, speech impediments and social skills problems;
- immediate antecedents to firesetting – e.g., major mental illness, depression, anxiety, anger, interpersonal/physical conflict, alcohol/drug misuse, suicidal ideation/gestures;
- offence-specific factors – e.g., acted alone/with others, motives (anger, revenge, tension relief, care-seeking, fire fascination/excitement), intention to do harm/damage, feelings during/after fire, consequences of firesetting, involvement in fire-fighting (calling/helping emergency services); and
- offending history – details of previous firesetting behaviour, previous sex/ violence/property offences, and physical assaults since admission.

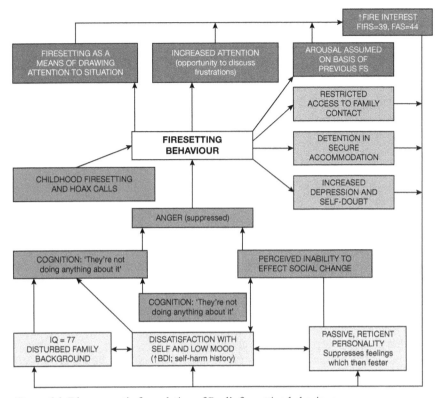

Figure 6.1 Diagrammatic formulation of Paul's firesetting behaviour

Elements of the PFSI can be populated using information concerning the index client drawn from a number of sources. In the following sections, a number of fire-specific, clinical and risk-factor assessment tools are described that can provide information that may be used to facilitate an analysis of a firesetter's behaviour using the PFSI as a framework. See Figure 6.1 for a diagrammatic representation of a formulation for Paul's firesetting informed by the PFSI and results of some of the assessment measures described below.

Fire-specific assessments

Murphy and Clare (1996) developed the *Fire Setting Assessment Schedule* (*FSAS*) for use with adult firesetters with ID. The construction of the FSAS was guided by the functional analytical approach to firesetting, which proposes that firesetting is associated with a number of psychological functions, including the need for peer approval, the need for excitement, a need to alleviate or express sadness, mental illness, a wish for retribution, and a need to reduce anxiety. The FSAS comprises 16 items concerning cognitions and feelings *prior to* setting fires, such as: 'I started fires to make people pay attention and listen to me'; 'I started fires to get out of going somewhere or doing something'; 'I started fires because I felt angry with people'; and a further 13 items pertaining to the individual's thoughts and feelings *after* setting fires, for example: 'After the fires began I felt calmer'; 'After the fires people took more notice of me'; and 'I felt happier after the fires'. All items are rated as true or false.

Murphy and Clare (1996) found in a small study involving adult firesetters with ID that the most frequently endorsed antecedent items on the FSAS were anger, followed by being ignored and then feelings of depression. Consistent with these findings, Taylor, et al. (2002) found that anger, being ignored, and depression (in rank order) were the most frequently endorsed items on the FSAS in terms of antecedents to and consequences of mild-borderline IQ firesetters' behaviour. In a further small study of women with mild ID who had set fires, Taylor, Robertson, Thorne, Belshaw and Watson (2006) also found that anger and depression were the most frequently endorsed items in participants prior to fire-raising incidents.

Murphy and Clare (1996) also developed the *Fire Interest Rating Scale (FIRS)* for use with clients with ID and histories of firesetting. The FIRS consists of 14 descriptions of fire-related situations, for example: 'Watching a bonfire out-doors, like on bonfire night'; 'Watching a fire engine come down the road'; 'Striking a match to set fire to a building'. Respondents are asked to rate how they would feel in each situation using a seven-point scale from 'most upsetting/absolutely horrible' to 'very exciting, lovely, nice'.

As part of a firesetters intervention manual used by UK Fire and Rescue Services, Muckley (1997) produced the *Fire Assessment Scale (FAS)*. This is a self-report measure completed by firesetters consisting of 20 statements concerning the respondent's attitudes, beliefs and behaviour such as: 'The best thing about fire is watching it spread'; 'People often set fires when they are angry'; 'Fires can easily get out of control'. Respondents rate the degree to which they agree with each statement using a five-point Likert scale from 'strongly agree' to 'strongly disagree'.

The FSAS, FIRS and FAS were all developed in routine clinical settings and have not been subject to rigorous reliability and validity evaluations. However, if used carefully by experienced clinicians as part of a comprehensive assessment they can be helpful in providing data to inform an analysis of firesetting using the PFSI.

Assessment of firesetter risk factors

As pointed out by Gannon and Pina (2010), there is little literature available to guide the assessment of firesetting risk factors. A number of the actuarial factors (e.g. early history of firesetting, number of fires set, and age at first fire) have been found to be predictive of recidivistic firesetting by mentally disordered offenders (Rice and Harris, 1996). In the same vein, Dickens, Sugarman, Edgar, Hofberg, Tewari and Ahmad (2009), in a study of UK arsonists, found that recidivism was associated with being young and single, an early age of onset for criminality, property offending, a history of violence, substance abuse and relationship problems.

The *Historical-Clinical-Risk Management-20* (HCR-20; Webster, Douglas, Eaves and Hart, 1997) is one of the most widely used and extensively evaluated structured clinical judgement tools in the forensic practice field. The HCR-20 manual defines violence as '. . . actual, attempted, or threatened harm to a person or persons' (p. 24). Thus, as suggested by Gannon and Pina (2010), and the HCR-20 manual, firesetting that is clearly aimed at causing others harm (actual or intended) can be considered a form of violence within this definition and thus assessed using the HCR-20.

However, as described above, the factors influencing firesetting behaviour can be complex and extend beyond historical and actuarial causes. In an attempt to capture information relating to a wider range of risk factors, including current clinical issues, Taylor and colleagues developed the *Northgate Firesetter Risk Assessment* (*NFRA*; Taylor and Thorne, 2005). This is a tool modelled on the HCR-20 format that incorporates a number of historical and clinical items empirically linked to firesetting behaviour. The NFRA was developed for use with adults with mild-borderline ID and histories of firesetting. It comprises five historical risk factors (child and adult firesetting histories, targeted firesetting, history of hoax calls, and history of self-harm/suicide attempts) and six clinical items (depression/stress, anger, conflict-resolution issues, impulsivity, major mental illness and low social attention) that are consistent with the literature concerning pathological firesetters characteristics and identified recidivism risks. The evidence associating these factors with firesetting behaviour is incorporated into the NFRA, which is described in detail in Appendix 1.

The clinical items of the NFRA can be used to monitor fluctuations in the presence and strength of risk factors for particular patients during their rehabilitation pathway and in response to any clinical and management interventions offered. NFRA historical items can inform the formulation of an individual's firesetting behaviour within the functional analytic framework. For example, items H1 to H4 will help to describe the patient's history of firesetting and level of fire interest. Item H5 is useful in looking at dispositional setting conditions.

Taylor, et al. (2002) developed a series of *Goal Attainment Scales* (*GAS;* Kiresuk and Sherman, 1968) to support the clinical evaluation of the responses of firesetters with mild-borderline ID to a group therapy intervention. Based on their answers in a semi-structured interview, a group therapist and an independent rater used GASs to score clients in relation to six offence-related treatment targets: (i) 'acceptance of guilt'; (ii) 'acknowledgement of responsibility'; (iii) 'understanding of victim issues'; (iv) 'understanding of high risk elements of offence cycle'; (v) 'appropriate expression of emotion'; and (vi) 'ability to form and maintain relationships'. Assessors used a five-point scale (from (0) 'much worse than expected', through (2) 'satisfactory', to (4) 'much better than expected') for each GAS using operationalized scoring criteria.[1] Patients' scores on the GASs can also indicate increased or lowered risk for firesetting if incorporated into the functional analytic approach using the FSAS assessment framework.

Clinical assessment

Research indicates that a range of mental health and emotional problems can be associated with firesetting behaviour. Reliable and valid clinical measures can thus augment any fire-specific and firesetter risk assessments administered (Jackson, 1994; Swaffer, et al., 2001).

In their work with firesetters with mild-borderline ID, Taylor, et al. (2002) assessed anger using the *Novaco Anger Scale* (*NAS*; Novaco, 2003). This is a 48-item self-report measure that yields a summary score for anger disposition and has good reliability and validity for a version of this scale modified especially for offenders with ID (Novaco and Taylor, 2004). For depression, a well-known 13-item brief self-report measure, the *Beck Depression Inventory-Short Form* was used (*BDI*; Beck and Beck, 1972). Each BDI item is rated on a four-point scale that relates to particular symptoms or signs associated with depression. In order to assess issues related to social effectiveness, Taylor and colleagues used the *Culture-Free Self-Esteem Inventory-2nd Edition, Form AD* (*CFSEI-2*; Battle, 1992). This is a widely used and reliable self-report measure of self-esteem. The inventory is made up of 40 'yes/no' items that are summed to give a *Total* index score.

Use of such clinical measures alongside relevant fire-specific measures will enable practitioners to provide evidence to support their ratings for particular risk assessment items (e.g., mental health problems – including depression and anxiety, anger, impulsivity) as well as formulate the treatment needs and consider *responsivity* issues linked to the patient's learning style, skills and abilities as suggested by Andrews and Bonta (2003).

Treatment of firesetting behaviour

With the exception of a small number of dated and arcane case-study reports in the behavioural literature (e.g. Lande, 1980; Royer, Flynn and Osadca, 1971), most of the literature concerning therapeutic interventions for firesetters has involved children and adolescents (see Barnett and Spitzer, 1994 and Palmer, Caulfield and Hollin, 2007 for reviews). Canter and Almond (2002), in a report for the UK Government, concluded that arson treatment programmes have not been evaluated in a consistent or objective manner. The dearth of research available to support interventions for adult perpetrators is surprising, taking into account the impact of firesetting behaviour at a number of levels. It has been suggested that this situation is related to the heterogeneity of the offence histories of many firesetters who receive treatment via exposure to generic offending behaviour programmes (Gannon and Pina, 2010), although there is no empirical data available to support this assertion. Given the concern that pathological firesetting in particular raises, with its historical associations with 'madness' and 'badness', it is perhaps less surprising that what sparse evidence is available emanates from the mental health treatment field.

Some early intervention work involved social skills training approaches that yielded positive results (e.g. Hurley and Monahan, 1969; Rice and Chaplin, 1979).

More recently cognitive behavioural approaches to working with firesetters have been developed, mainly in mental health and ID service settings (Palmer, Caulfield and Hollin, 2005). Swaffer, et al. (2001, p. 469) described a group treatment programme to 10 firesetter patients in a high-security hospital in the UK. The intervention, based on an approach suggested by Jackson, et al. (1987) involved four modules delivered sequentially: (i) education concerning fire and its risks (12 sessions); (ii) development of coping skills including problem-solving and assertiveness training (24 sessions); (iii) insight and self-awareness, including functional analyses of firesetting behaviour (12 sessions); and (iv) relapse prevention – developing strategies to break offending cycles (14 sessions). Unfortunately, as the authors were describing a programme that was still being delivered, they were unable to report any results concerning changes following the intervention on the range of assessments used in the programme.

In relative terms there has been a significant amount of interest in the treatment and management of firesetters with ID in the forensic clinical literature. This may be due to the historical association between firesetting and low intelligence (e.g. Walker and McCabe, 1973), although more recent research found that firesetting accounted for only a small proportion (4 per cent) of those referred to ID services due to offending and antisocial behaviour (O'Brien, et al., 2010). On the other hand, the proportion of people in secure ID services with histories of firesetting is significant. Hogue, et al. (2006) found that just over 21 per cent of those detained in low/medium secure services in a UK study sample had an index offence of arson. This might explain why clinicians working in these service settings have attempted to develop interventions to address firesetting behaviour, a number of which have been described in the literature.

In the UK, Clare, Murphy, Cox and Chaplin (1992) reported a case study involving a man with mild ID admitted to a high-secure hospital following convictions for two offences of arson. Significant clinical improvements were observed following a comprehensive treatment package. The client was discharged to a community setting and had not engaged in any fire-related offending behaviour at 30 months follow-up. Hall, Clayton and Johnson (2005) described the delivery of a 16-session group cognitive-behavioural approach to six male patients with ID and histories of firesetting detained in a UK specialist NHS medium secure unit. Unfortunately, outcome data were not provided, although most group participants were reported to have responded positively to the intervention in terms of their clinical presentations, and two patients were successfully transferred to less secure placements following completion of the programme.

Taylor, et al. (2002) reported a group study involving 14 men and women with ID and arson convictions who were assessed pre- and post-treatment on a number of fire-specific (FAS, FIRS and GAS), anger, self-esteem and depression measures. The intervention is a cognitive-behaviourally framed approach developed especially for this patient group. It is a multifaceted programme based on the approach outlined by Jackson (1994), which is underpinned by the 'functional analysis paradigm' (Jackson, et al., 1987, p. 175). It comprises seven modules delivered over approximately 45 sessions that involve work on offence cycles, education about the costs associated with setting fires, training of skills to enhance future coping with emotional problems associated with previous firesetting behaviour, and work on personalized plans to prevent relapse. A detailed description of the treatment modules and aims is given in Table 6.1. Given the demonstrated importance of anger/revenge as an antecedent to firesetting in this population (Murphy and Clare, 1996; Taylor, et al., 2002) up to 10 sessions are dedicated to

Table 6.1 Structure and aims of the Northgate Firesetters Treatment Programme

Sessions	Module	Aims
1–2	Establishing the group	• To break the ice and initiate group discussion and levels of rapport. • To give a general introduction to the programme and its aims. • To establish the rules of the group and agree a contract.
3–5	Group cohesion exercises – focus on *disclosure* and *self-esteem*	• To further establish group rapport. • To encourage group members to self-disclose information about themselves. • To introduce the concept that feelings can affect behaviour. • To demonstrate that in the short term self-esteem can rise and fall, but we need to feel good about ourselves in general. • For group members to discover and share positive things about themselves – strengths, achievements, successes, and personal qualities.
6–9	Family and related issues – focus on *Life Maps*	• Each group member to understand the concept of and produce a basic *Life Map*. • To allow group members to add interpretations of their major life events. • To enable fact-finding and the placement of the individual within various systems (e.g. familial, educational, institutional, friendship and support networks, offending history, conflict resolution). • To gain some basic insight into group members' schemas (e.g. worthlessness, self-blame, suspiciousness, rejection, entitlement, control).
10	Offence Analysis I – focus on *cognitive distortions*	• To help group members to understand the concept and purpose of excuse-making. • To encourage group members to display their characteristic cognitive distortions at this stage. • To prompt group participants to begin to recognize denial and minimization in relation to firesetting.
11–22	Offence Analysis II – focus on *individual offence accounts*	• To get each group member to give an active account of their offence. • To establish for each group member the factors that may have triggered their offending and the consequences that could also maintain it. • To identify and undermine any distortions that group members use to minimize the seriousness of their offending or their responsibility for it.

Sessions	Module	Aims
23–24	Offence Analysis III – focus on *preliminary formulation* and *identification of risk factors*	• To review participants' offence accounts, giving each the opportunity to make amendments as required. • To develop initial hypotheses, in collaboration with participants, about the function of their firesetting for the offence described. • To explain the concept of *risk factors*. • To identify preliminary *risk factors* for each group member.
25–26	Information and Education – including local *Fire and Rescue Service* presentation	• To help group members to begin to understand that firesetting is not a victimless offence. • To encourage participants to think about the real and potential consequences of their firesetting. • To leave clients with strong reminders of the potential costs (financial and human) of firesetting, which may act as a motivator not to reoffend and an intrusion into any fire-related fantasies.
27	Alternative Skills Training I – *Communication and its Purpose*	• To explore the purposes of communication. • To identify the ways in which we communicate with each other. • To recognize why communication is important. • To identify the skills necessary for effective communication.
28	Alternative Skills Training II – *Communicating Emotions*	• To familiarize participants with different emotional states. • To encourage group members to describe feelings that these states induce. • For group members to explore the ways that they communicate feelings, and decide which are helpful and which are unhelpful ways of expressing feelings.
29–40	Alternative Skills Training III – focus on *understanding and coping effectively with anger*	• To explain that anger is a normal emotion. • To identify the types of situation that provoke personal anger reactions. • To develop anger-reducing strategies including arousal-reduction techniques and cognitive reframing. • To practise skills in coping with provocation, especially assertive communication and strategic withdrawal.
41	Risk Management I – focus on *identifying risk factors*	• To reacquaint group members with the concept of risk factors. • To further develop preliminary lists of risk factors for each group member. • To facilitate a greater understanding of group members' own risk factors.
42–43	Risk Management II – focus on *developing risk coping strategies*	• To identify risk factors that apply to more than one group member. • To recognize the need for planning ways to deal with risk factors when they arise in the future. • To recap on some of the strategies that group members might use in order to deal with their risk factors.
44	Risk Management III – focus on *preparing for lapses*	• To understand the concept of a *lapse*. • To acknowledge that lapses will occur (i.e. they will encounter and, on occasions, fail to cope with a particular risk factor). • To develop a positive attitude to recovery from lapses.

developing anger coping strategies using an evidence-based intervention developed by Taylor and Novaco (2005).

The intervention described by Taylor, et al. (2002) successfully engaged these patients, all of whom completed the programme delivered over a period of four months. Despite their intellectual and cognitive limitations, all participants showed high levels of motivation and commitment. Following treatment, significant improvements were obtained on the fire-specific and anger and self-esteem scales.

In an extension of this work, Taylor, et al. (2004) described a case series of four detained men with ID and arson convictions and (2006) used the same methods in a further case series of six women with ID and convictions for arson. In these case series reports participants engaged well in treatment and all showed improved attitudes with regard to personal responsibility, victim issues and awareness of risk factors associated with their firesetting behaviour. All but one of the female participants had been discharged to community placements at two-year follow-up, and there had been no reports of participants setting any fires or engaging in fire risk-related behaviour.

Conclusions

Firesetting is a significant problem for the wider community and for forensic mental health practitioners considering risk and management issues. There has been a good deal of empirical research concerning the characteristics of firesetters, classification of firesetter types, and to a lesser extent explanatory theories. However, there is a dearth of evidence available to guide the professional in considering approaches to assessing clinical needs and risk, and in delivering effective therapeutic interventions to meet these needs and reduce risk.

Much of the literature that is available concerns children and younger firesetters, despite adults being responsible for more than half of all deliberate fires set. This chapter has focused on the assessment and treatment of pathological firesetters, who tend to be recidivists who set fires alone in the context of mental-health or emotional problems and in the absence of any financial or political gain. These are the types of deliberate firesetter most frequently encountered by professionals working in forensic mental health and correctional settings. We suggest that Jackson, et al.'s (1987) functional analytic framework is useful in helping to assess and formulate the needs of this heterogeneous group of firesetters, taking into account a range of explanatory factors including psychosocial disadvantage, impaired development of personality, cognitive and interpersonal functioning, individual and situational antecedents, proximal triggers, and maintaining positive and negative contingencies.

Assessment of firesetting behaviour can be described as more of an art than a science at this point as there are very few tools available that have been adequately evaluated in terms of their reliability and validity. However, it is recommended that the forensic mental health practitioner considers at least three areas of assessment in working with firesetter clients: fire-specific assessment; assessment of firesetter risk factors; and assessment of relevant clinical factors. There is a small amount of material in the literature available to guide practitioners with regard to fire-specific assessment, although this is limited and requires further research to establish normative data and reliability and validity. Firesetter risk assessment is at a very early stage of development, with no empirical research to support it. A prototype scheme developed for people with mild-borderline ID is offered in this chapter, taking into account some of the available evidence concerning firesetter characteristics and recidivism factors. Forensic practitioners are encouraged to develop and evaluate this and similar schemes with a range of client groups in the forensic mental health and offender-management systems. Clinical factors and conditions associated with firesetting behaviour (depression, anxiety, low self-esteem, psychotic symptomatology, and so on) should be assessed using established measures and techniques relevant to the population from which the individual client is drawn.

Treatment of adult firesetters is very poorly developed and there is a dearth of evidence to support those approaches that have been reported. It has been suggested that this is because firesetting is often seen as part of a general pattern of offending and can thus be addressed via general offender management programmes. This is unlikely to be the case for pathological firesetters and there have been few attempts at developing intervention programmes for those who find themselves in forensic mental health services as a result of firesetting behaviour.

Similar to other areas of offender treatment, cognitive behavioural approaches appear to offer some hope in addressing fire-related interests and attitudes, and associated clinical factors. An example of such a programme designed for firesetter patients with mild-borderline ID is detailed in this chapter, along with some preliminary evidence to support its effectiveness. However, the impact of these types of interventions on reducing the risks presented by firesetters and their recidivism rates over time has not been established. As suggested by others, there is an urgent need for adequately funded research programmes to address the gaps in the literature – primarily the development of reliable and valid risk assessment procedures and the robust and controlled evaluation of treatment effectiveness.

Note

1   Available on request from the authors.

Appendix 1
Northgate firesetter risk assessment

Historical items	Code 0 = No; 1 = Maybe; 2 = Yes
H1 Incidents of childhood (pre-16) firesetting	
H2 Previous incidents of firesetting as an adult	
H3 Previous incidents of targeted firesetting	
H4 Previous hoax calls to emergency services	
H5 Previous self-harm or suicidal gestures	

This assessment incorporates many risk factors associated with risk for firesetting. Each historical and clinical item should be scored and a final risk judgement made on the basis of these scores. *Please attempt to complete all items – even those that might not appear relevant to the client.*

Historical items

H1   Incidents of childhood (pre-16) firesetting

A number of studies have found that firesetters tend to have a previous history of firesetting/arson, for example, Koson and Dvoskin (1982) estimated that 38 per cent of their sample of firesetters had previous convictions for arson (see also Soothill and Pope, 1973; Hurley and Monahan, 1969). It is difficult to study reoffence rates for firesetting as there tends to be a very small reconviction rate for arsonists.

Look for evidence of previous firesetting incidents during childhood. This includes 'vandalistic' (adolescent) firesetting and experimental match play by children. It also includes firesetting committed for a variety of motives, e.g. financial reward, to cover up another crime, for political purposes, revenge, and firesetting due to the presence of a mental disorder or committed as an attention-seeking act.

No   No previous firesetting incidents in childhood.
Maybe   One possible/less serious previous incident of firesetting in childhood.
Yes   Any serious incident of firesetting in childhood or two or more less serious incidents of childhood firesetting.

H2 Previous incidents of firesetting as an adult

A number of studies have found that firesetters tend to have a previous history of firesetting/arson, for example, Koson and Dvoskin (1982) estimated that 38 per cent of their sample of firesetters had previous convictions for arson (see also Soothill and Pope, 1973; Hurley and Monahan, 1969). It is difficult to interpret reoffending rates for firesetting as there tends to be a very low conviction rate for arsonists.

Look for evidence of previous firesetting incidents as an adult. This includes firesetting committed for financial reward, to cover up another crime, for political purposes, and for mixed motives (e.g. during a phase of minor depression, as a cry for help, while under the influence of drugs or alcohol). It also includes firesetting due to the presence of a formal mental disorder (e.g. severe affective disorder, schizophrenic illness, organic mental disorder, and mental impairment), due to motives of revenge or committed as an attention-seeking act.

No   No previous incidents of firesetting as an adult.
Maybe   Possible/less serious previous incident of firesetting as an adult.
Yes   Definite serious previous incident(s) of firesetting.

H3 Previous incidents of targeted firesetting

Eighty per cent of arsonists set fire to property, usually of a residential nature (Bradford, 1982). There is a common bias amongst firesetters in their choice of targets (i.e. schools, official buildings, hospitals, care and custodial settings). Furthermore, in recidivistic firesetters, there is a tendency to choose the same type of target (e.g. warehouses, residential property, hospitals, and family homes). Look for evidence of previous targeting.

No   No previous incident of targeted firesetting.
Maybe   Possible/less serious previous incident of targeted firesetting.
Yes   Definite serious previous incident of targeted firesetting.

H4 Previous hoax calls to emergency services

Hoax calls have the potential to mobilize the emergency services and thereby permit the firesetter to exert a level of control over the environment which cannot be obtained in other ways (Vreeland and Levin, 1980). Many firesetters will call the emergency services themselves and remain at the scene of the fire, perhaps undertaking some role in evacuating the premises or extinguishing the fire, and therefore gain approval.

No   No previous hoax calls to emergency services.
Maybe   Possible/less serious (or one) previous hoax calls to emergency services.
Yes   Definite serious (two or more) previous hoax calls to emergency services.

H5   *Previous self-harm/suicidal gestures*

At one level self-harm can be associated with attention- or care-seeking. Several studies have noted a higher incidence of suicide attempts amongst firesetters (e.g. McKerracher and Dacre, 1966; Rice and Harris, 1991). Look for the presentation of previous deliberate self-harm committed by the client.

No   No previous deliberate self-harm/suicidal gestures.
Maybe   Possible/less serious deliberate self-harm/suicidal gestures.
Yes   Definite serious deliberate self-harm/suicidal gestures.

Clinical items

C1   *Recent build-up of depression and/or stress*

Studies undertaken with a forensic ID population indicate that self-reported feelings of depression can be a clear antecedent to firesetting behaviour in these clients. Feeling sad or depressed was found to be the third most identified antecedent emotion in a study evaluating treatment for firesetters by Taylor et al. (2002). Several other authors have also cited depression as a significant antecedent in their study groups – Vreeland and Levin (1980), Jackson et al. (1987), and Stewart (1993). Murphy and Clare (1996) found depression or sadness were the frequently reported antecedents in their study of people with ID who had set fires.

With regard to stress, Hurley and Monahan (1969) reported high levels of anxiety in 68 per cent of their sample, with 28 per cent reporting that they had set fires as a means of releasing 'tension'. More generally, Jackson et al. (1987) adopt the view that arson might have provided an effective means of changing or escaping from difficult circumstances. These may be internal, or external, such as a recent trauma, current life difficulties, exit events (bereavement, divorce, separation), financial worries, legal problems, social or medical strains or evidence of multiple problems, or a combination of both. Arson potentially serves multiple functions for the same individual.

Look for any visible or expressed signs of enduring depression/sadness or stress (or build-up) that the client has displayed within the last six months.

Recommendation: Use information from *Beck Depression Inventory* (BDI), *Zung Anxiety Scale* (ZAS), or other appropriate instruments.

No   No build-up of depression/stress.
Maybe   Possible/less serious build-up of depression/stress.
Yes   Definite serious build-up of depression/stress.

C2   *High levels of anger*

Treatment studies undertaken with a forensic ID population suggest that self-reported feelings of anger are the most frequent antecedent to firesetting behaviour in these clients (Taylor, et al., 2002, 2004, 2006). Hurley and Monahan (1969) reported that 26 per cent of their sample set fires as an act of revenge.

Look for evidence of anger, hatred (Virkkunen, 1974) and revenge directed at key others in client's residential setting.

Recommendation: Use information from *Novaco Anger Scale* (NAS), *State-Trait Anger Expression Inventory* (STAXI), *Provocation Inventory* (PI) and *Ward Anger Rating Scale* (WARS).

No   No evidence of high levels of anger.
Maybe   Possible/less serious evidence of high levels of anger.
Yes   Definite serious evidence of high levels of anger.

C3   Poor interpersonal conflict resolution skills

Factors such as borderline ID (Jackson et al., 1987), a high incidence of physical abnormality (Lewis and Yarnell, 1951), limited schooling (Bradford, 1982), a history of teasing, bullying and peer rejection (Jackson et al., 1987), lead to problems of social isolation. Hurley and Monahan (1969) reported problems such as shyness, fear of involvement and social distrust in 74 per cent of their sample of arsonists. Furthermore, harsh and punitive parenting (Siegelman and Folkman, 1971; Block et al., 1976) model poor problem-solving.

Due to skills deficits, confidence, or opportunity, firesetters can have impaired interpersonal conflict-resolution skills. Thus, they can lack assertiveness, avoid face-to-face confrontation due to fear of negative consequences, punishment or rejection, and are more likely to adopt socially inappropriate solutions.

No   No evidence of poor conflict-resolution skills.
Maybe   Possible/less serious evidence of poor conflict-resolution skills.
Yes   Definite serious evidence of poor conflict-resolution skills.

C4   Impulsivity

Impulsivity and sensation-seeking have often been linked to general offending behaviour (Barratt, 1994; Moeller, et al., 2001) and whilst these factors have not yet been thoroughly researched in offender populations with intellectual disabilities, the work of other authors (e.g. Glaser and Deane 1999) has suggested that offences carried out by these clients are related to impulsiveness, regardless of offence type.

Bourget and Bradford (1989) suggested the possibility of a general impulse-control problem in their study group of female firesetters and suggested that female firesetters tend to choose a target invested with emotional meaning, acting out of revenge and attention-seeking behaviour. They also concluded that firesetting is not an isolated abnormal behaviour and appears to be linked with other manifestations of deficient impulse control.

Recommendation: Use information from Eysenck *Impulsivity-Venturesomeness-Empathy Scale* (IVE), specifically the impulsivity score, PI total score and subscale scores, and NAS items 1, 33, 35, 12, 43.

No   No impulsivity.
Maybe   Possible/less serious impulsivity.
Yes   Definite/serious impulsivity.

C5   Current or recent signs of major mental illness (using DSM/ICD criteria)

Bradford and Dimock (1986) noted that their sample of firesetters frequently presented with a major psychiatric disorder. In particular, Virkkunen et al. (1974) found a substantial number of people with schizophrenia were represented in the population of firesetters they studied. Furthermore, the researchers noted that hallucinations and delusions were associated with arson in one third of the cases.

Novaco and Taylor (2004) found that over 50 per cent of detained male offenders had a dual diagnosis (intellectual disability plus psychiatric disorder) and Taylor et al. (2002) found that 10 out of 14 convicted arsonists in their treatment study had a dual diagnosis.

Recommendation: Use information from *Psychiatric Assessment Schedules for Adults with Developmental Disabilities* (PAS-ADD Checklist – if above threshold scores then full PAS-ADD should be carried out).

No   No active symptoms of major mental illness.
Maybe   Possible/less serious active symptoms of major mental illness.
Yes   Definite/serious active symptoms of major mental illness.

C6   Low social attention

Low social attention (i.e. feeling *not* listened to) was a frequently identified antecedent emotion in a study of males and females with intellectual disabilities and a history of firesetting – Taylor et al. (2002). Low social attention/feeling *not* listened to was also mentioned as something which was actually helped by firesetting (e.g. firesetting produced a positive response to the individual in terms of social interaction).

Murphy and Clare's (1996) study of a similar population sample identified low social attention as a frequently mentioned prior emotion. Similarly, an increase in social attention was the second most frequently mentioned consequence of firesetting in this client group of offenders with mild ID. Many other sources in the firesetting literature contain information that suggest similar findings (e.g. Vreeland and Levin, 1980, Bradford, 1982 and Bourget et al.,1989).

Look for evidence of the person:

- having generally poor communication skills with a generally diffident/ unassertive demeanour;
- the person having a limited pool of skills and behaviours with which to interact and draw people's attention to their worries and emotional distress, and;

- the lack of an identifiable person-target (the person is upset about something but cannot identify who/what is responsible, or who can help, or the target is not obtainable).

No   No issues regarding low social attention (not feeling listened to).
Maybe   Possible issues regarding low social attention.
Yes   Definite serious issues for the individual regarding low social attention.

References

American Psychiatric Association (1994) *Diagnostic and Statistical Manual of Mental Disorders (4th ed.)*, Washington: American Psychiatric Association.

Andrews, D. A. and Bonta, J. (2003) *The psychology of criminal conduct (3rd ed.)*, Cincinnati, OH: Anderson.

Arson Control Forum (2003, March) *Research bulletin no.1. Arson: From reporting to conviction*, London: The Office of the Deputy Prime Minister.

Barnett, W. and Spitzer, M. (1994) 'Pathological firesetting 1951–91: A review', *Medicine, Science and Law, 34*: 4–20.

Barratt, E. S. (1994) 'Impulsivity and aggression', in J. Monahan and H. J. Steadman (eds) *Violence and Mental Disorder: Developments in risk assessment*, Chicago: The University of Chicago Press.

Battle, J. (1992) *Culture-Free Self-Esteem Inventory*, Austin, TX: Pro-Ed.

Beck, A. T. and Beck, R. W. (1972) 'Screening depressed patients in family practice: A rapid technique', *Postgraduate Medicine, 52*: 81–85.

Block, J. H., Block, J. and Folkman, W. S. (1976) *Fire and Young Children: Learning survival skills*, USDA Forest Service Research Note, PSW-119.

Bourget, D. and Bradford, J. M. W. (1989) 'Female arsonists: A clinical study', *Bulletin of the American Academy of Psychiatry and Law, 17*: 293–300.

Bradford, J. and Dimock, J. (1986) 'A comparative study of adolescents and adults who wilfully set fires', *Psychiatric Journal of the University of Ottawa, 11*: 228–34.

Bradford, J. M. W. (1982) 'Arson: A clinical study', *Canadian Journal of Psychiatry, 27*: 188–92.

Bumpass, E. R., Brix, R. J. and Preston, D. (1985) 'A community-based program for juvenile firesetters', *Hospital and Community Psychiatry, 36*: 529–33.

Canter, D. and Almond, L. (2002) *The burning issue: Research strategies for reducing arson*, London: The Office of the Deputy Prime Minister.

Canter, D. and Fritzon, K. (1998) 'Differentiating arsonists: A model of firesetting actions and characteristics', *Legal and Criminological Psychology, 3*: 73–96.

Clare, I. C. H., Murphy, G. H., Cox, D. and Chaplin, E. H. (1992) 'Assessment and treatment of firesetting: A single-case investigation using a cognitive-behavioural model', *Criminal Behaviour and Mental Health, 2*: 253–68.

Department of Communities and Local Government (2007) *Fires statistics, United Kingdom, 2005*, London: Author.

Dickens, G., Sugarman, P., Edgar, S., Hofberg, K., Tewari, S. and Ahmad, F. (2009) 'Recidivism and dangerousness in arsonists', *Journal of Forensic Psychiatry and Psychology, 20*: 621–39.

Gannon, T. A. and Pina, A. (2010) 'Firesetting: Psychopathology, theory and treatment', *Aggression and Violent Behavior, 15*: 224–38.

Geller, J. (1992) 'Pathological firesetting in adults', *International Journal of Law and Psychiatry, 15*: 283–302.

Glaser, W. and Deane, K. (1999) 'Normalisation in an abnormal world: A study of prisoners with an intellectual disability', *International Journal of Offender Therapy and Comparative Criminology, 43*: 338–56.

Grant, J. E. and Kim, S. W. (2007) 'Clinical characteristics and psychiatric morbidity of pyromania', *Journal of Clinical Psychiatry, 68*: 1717–22.

Hall, J. R. (2007, November) *Intentional fires and arson*, Quinsey, MA: National Fire Protection Association.

Hall, I., Clayton, P. and Johnson, P. (2005) 'Arson and learning disability' in T. Riding, C. Swann, and B. Swann (eds) *The handbook of forensic learning disabilities* (pp. 51–72), Oxford: Radcliffe Publishing.

Harris, G. T. and Rice, M. E. (1984) 'Mentally disordered fire-setters: Psychodynamic versus empirical approaches', *International Journal of Law and Psychiatry, 7*: 19–43.

Hart, S. D. and Logan, C. (2011) 'Formulation of violence risk using evidence-based assessments: The structured professional judgment approach', in P. Sturmey and M. McMurran (eds) *Forensic case formulation*, Chichester: Wiley Blackwell.

Hogue, T. E., Steptoe, L., Taylor, J. L., Lindsay, W. R., Mooney, P., Pinkney, L., Johnston, S., Smith, A. H. W. and O'Brien, G. (2006) 'A comparison of offenders with intellectual disability across three levels of security', *Criminal Behaviour and Mental Health, 16*: 13–28.

Hurley, W. and Monahan, T. M. (1969) 'Arson: The criminal and the crime', *British Journal of Criminology, 9*: 4–21.

Inciardi, J. (1970) 'The adult firesetter', *Criminology, 8*: 145–55.

Jackson, H. F. (1994) 'Assessment of fire-setters', in M. McMurran and J. Hodge (eds) *The assessment of criminal behaviours in secure settings* (pp. 94–126), London: Jessica Kingsley.

Jackson, H. F., Glass, C. and Hope, S. (1987) 'A functional analysis of recidivistic arson', *British Journal of Clinical Psychology, 26*: 175–85.

Kiresuk, T. and Sherman, R. (1968) 'Goal attainment scaling: A general method of evaluating comprehensive mental health programmes', *Community Mental Health Journal, 4*: 443–53.

Kolko, D. J. and Kazdin, A. E. (1989) 'The Children's Firesetting Interview with psychiatrically referred and non-referred children', *Journal of Abnormal Child Psychology, 17*: 609–24.

Koson, D. F. and Dvoskin, J. (1982) 'Arson: A diagnostic study', *Bulletin of the American Academy of Psychiatry and the Law, 10*: 39–49.

Lande, S. D. (1980) 'A combination of orgasmic reconditioning and covert sensitisation in the treatment of a fire fetish', *Journal of Behaviour Therapy and Experimental Psychiatry, 11*: 291–96.

Lewis, N. D. C. and Yarnell, H. (1951) *Pathological firesetting (pyromania)*, New York: Nervous and Mental Disease Monographs, No 82.

McKerracher, D. W. and Dacre, J. I. (1966) 'A study of arsonists in a special security hospital', *British Journal of Psychiatry, 112*: 1151–54.

Moeller, F. G., Barratt, E. S., Dougherty, D. M., Schmitz, J. M. and Swann, A. C. (2001) 'Psychiatric aspects of impulsivity', *American Journal of Psychiatry, 158*: 1783–93.

Muckley, A. (1997) *Addressing firesetting behaviour with children, young people and adults: A resource and training manual*, Redcar and Cleveland Psychological Service.

Murphy, G. H. and Clare, I. C. H. (1996) 'Analysis of motivation in people with mild learning disabilities (mental handicap) who set fires', *Psychology, Crime and Law, 2*: 153–64.

Novaco, R. W. (2003) *The Novaco Anger Scale and Provocation Inventory (NAS-PI)*, Los Angeles: Western Psychological Services.

Novaco, R. W. and Taylor, J. L. (2004) 'Assessment of anger and aggression in male offenders with developmental disabilities', *Psychological Assessment, 16*: 42–50.

O'Brien, G., Taylor, J. L., Lindsay, W. R., Holland, A. J., Carson, D., Price, K., et al. (2010) 'A multi-centre study of adults with learning disabilities referred to services for antisocial or offending behaviour: Demographic, individual, offending and service characteristics', *Journal of Learning Disability and Offending Behaviour, 1*: 5–15.

O' Sullivan, G. H. and Kelleher, M. J. (1987) 'A study of fire-setters in the south-west of Ireland', *British Journal of Psychiatry, 151*: 818–23.

Palmer, E. J., Caulfield, L. S. and Hollin, C. R. (2005) *Evaluation of interventions with arsonists and young firesetters*, London: Office of the Deputy Prime Minister.

— (2007) 'Interventions with arsonists and young firesetters: A survey of the national picture in England and Wales', *Legal and Criminological Psychology, 12*: 101–16.

Prins, H. (1994) *Fire-raising: Its motivation and management*, London: Routledge.

Prins, H., Tennant, G. and Trick, K. (1985) 'Motives for arson (fireraising)', *Medicine, Science and the Law, 25*: 275–78.

Rice, M. E. and Chaplin, T. C. (1979) 'Social skills training for hospitalised male arsonists', *Journal of Behaviour Therapy and Experimental Psychiatry, 10*: 105–8.

Rice, M. E. and Harris, G. T. (1991) 'Firesetters admitted to a maximum security psychiatric institution,' *Journal of Interpersonal Violence*, 6: 461–75.

— (1996) 'Predicting the recidivism of mentally disordered firesetters', *Journal of Interpersonal Violence, 11*: 364–75.

— (2008) 'Arson', in V. N. Parillo (ed.) *The encyclopaedia of social problems,* California, USA: Thousand Oaks.

Richie, E. C. and Huff, T. G. (1999) 'Psychiatric aspects of arsonists', *Journal of Forensic Science, 44*: 733–40.

Rix, K. J. B. (1994) 'A psychiatric study of adult arsonists', *Medicine Science and Law, 34*: 21–34.

Royer, F. L., Flynn, W. F. and Osadca, B. S. (1971) 'Case history: Aversion therapy for firesetting by a deteriorated schizophrenic', *Behaviour Therapy, 2*: 229–32.

Ryle, A. (1993) *Cognitive analytic therapy: Active participation in change. A new integration in brief psychotherapy*, London: Churchill Livingstone.

Siegelman, E. Y. and Folkman, W. S. (1971) *Youthful Firesetters: An explanatory study in personality and background*, USDA Forest Service Research Note, PWS-230.

Smith, J. and Short, J. (1995) 'Mentally disordered firesetters', *British Journal of Hospital Medicine, 53*: 136–40.

Soothill, K. L. and Pope, P. J. (1973) 'Arson: A twenty-year cohort study', *Medicine, Science and the Law, 13*: 127–38.

Stewart, L. A. (1993) 'Profile of female fire-setters: Implications for treatment', *British Journal of Psychiatry, 163*: 248–56.

Swaffer, T. Haggett, M. and Oxley, T. (2001) 'Mentally disordered firesetters: A structured intervention programme', *Clinical Psychology and Psychotherapy, 8*: 468–75.

Taylor, J. L. and Halstead, S. (2001) 'Clinical risk assessment for people with learning disabilities who offend', *The British Journal of Forensic Practice, 3*: 22–32.

Taylor, J. L. and Novaco, R. W. (2005) *Anger treatment for people with developmental disabilities: A theory, evidence and manual based approach*, Chichester: Wiley.

Taylor, J. L., Robertson, A., Thorne, I., Belshaw, T. and Watson, A. (2006) 'Responses of female fire-setters with mild and borderline intellectual disabilities to a group-based intervention', *Journal of Applied Research in Intellectual Disabilities, 19*: 179–90.

Taylor, J. L. and Thorne, I. (2005) *Northgate Firesetter Risk Assessment*, Unpublished manual: Northgate and Prudhoe NHS Trust.

Taylor, J. L., Thorne, I., Robertson, A. and Avery, G. (2002) 'Evaluation of a group intervention for convicted arsonists with mild and borderline intellectual disabilities', *Criminal Behaviour and Mental Health, 12*: 282–93.

Taylor, J. L., Thorne, I. and Slavkin, M. L. (2004) 'Treatment of firesetting behaviour', in W. Lindsay, J. Taylor, and P. Sturmey (eds) *Offenders with developmental disabilities* (pp. 221–41), Chichester, UK: Wiley.

Tennent, T. J., McQuaid, A., Loughnane, T. and Hands, A. J. (1971) 'Female arsonists', *British Journal of Psychiatry, 119*: 497–502.

Virkkunen, M. (1974) 'On arson commited by schizophrenics'. *Acta Psychiatrica Scandinavica, 50*: 152–60.

Vreeland, R. and Levin, B. (1980) 'Psychological aspects of firesetting', in D. Canter (ed.) *Fires and human behaviour*, Chichester: Wiley.

Walker, N. and McCabe, S. (1973) *Crime and insanity in England volume 2 – New solutions and new problems*, Chicago: Adeline Pubishing Co.

Webster, C. D., Douglas, K. S., Eaves, D. and Hart, S. D. (1997) HCR-20: *Assessing risk for violence (version 2)*, Vancouver, British Columbia: Simon Fraser University.

7   Risk management

Beyond the individual

David J. Cooke and Lorraine Johnstone

'People are violent not only because of who they are but because of where they are.'
(Wortley, 2002, p. 3)

It is a truism that behaviour does not occur in a vacuum. As the economist Herbert Simon observed, rational behaviour is shaped by a pair of scissors, one blade of which is the characteristics of the actor, the other blade being the characteristics of the environment (Simon, 1990). This is equally true for violent behaviour. The past twenty years have seen growing confidence – at times misplaced confidence (Cooke and Michie, 2010; Cooke and Michie, this volume) – in our ability to evaluate risk of future violence. However, the primary focus of these efforts has been the characteristic of the actors, not the characteristics of their setting. The preoccupation with the individual is not surprising given that, for most psychologists, their expertise – and their predilection – is the evaluation of the individual; the individual's psychopathology, their motives, their personality, their functional deficits. These features are clearly important, but, as Simon noted, they are only one blade of the scissors that shape behaviour.

The focus of this chapter is an account of attempts to characterize the environment of prisons and forensic hospitals that act to enhance or mitigate violence risk; the overarching aim is to identify, manage, and understand the ways in which complex organizations can influence the violence within them.

The start of this long journey – at least for the first author – was a puzzle. Following conventional clinical psychology training, with its then heavy emphasis on the psychometric evaluation of the individual, I was confronted with the conundrum that Scotland's 'most violent men' were not being violent. The Barlinnie Special Unit was designed to hold difficult, disruptive and violent prisoners (Boyle, 1977; Cooke, 1989). All the prisoners had significant risk factors for violence. For example, they had lengthy histories of serious and persistent violence – both instrumental and reactive – major psychological disturbance including personality disorder, psychopathic traits, problems of addiction, and some episodic major mental illness. The majority had killed. They had sub-cultural values that celebrated violence. And those who considered the future, devalued it, expressing no interest in whether they remained in prison forever or not. In sum, they were risky. Yet curiously, over the 21-year life of the unit, only two assaults occurred

(Cooke, 1989; Cooke, 1997). As individuals, the prisoners remained challenging, hostile, impulsive, and angry but critically they were rarely violent; the most parsimonious account of the observed change was not that substantial changes had been wrought in the individuals – the changes were in their environment.

In the 1980s, Scottish prisons were subject to much prisoner unrest. At worst, this led to an epidemic of rooftop demonstrations where hostages were taken, abused, and humiliated. Direct observation gained through involvement with the incident management teams in four of these serious incidents – as well as professional commentaries (Coyle, 1987; Scratton, Sim, and Skidmore, 1991) – further highlighted the importance of context; specifically, ill-treatment by staff, inadequate regime quality, limited availability of privileges, and the inaccessibility of prisons for family visits, amongst other things. In the aftermath of these incidents, a conference was held in camera where senior civil servants, prison officials, outside experts and – critically – ten prisoners who had activity engaged in the riots, sat together for three days to debate the way forward. A dramatic volte-face took place in the official position, encapsulating a switch from explanations couched in terms of personality pathology to explanations couched in terms of environments (Cooke and Johnstone, 2010; Cooke, Wozniak and Johnstone, 2008). This analysis accepted the critical role of institutional factors, including the absence of sophisticated frontline custodial staff, deterrent sentences, shifts in parole policy, overcrowding, geographical remoteness, and impoverished regimes. The change in mindset was from doing things *to* prisoners to doing things *with* prisoners (Scottish Prison Service, 1990).

On reflection, the salience of situations should not have been a surprise. Famously, Mischel (1968; see also Mischel, 2004) challenged the field of personality psychology by showing the limited predictive power that personality variables have for observed behaviour; he argued that the characteristics of the situation in which an individual is placed has as much, if not more, influence on their behaviour. This is not just theory. Situational management of risk has a long and distinguished history in the area of crime prevention. Situational strategies include the use of anti-robbery screens in banks and off-licences, soothing lighting, reduced crowding, the provision of toughened beer glasses in public houses, and CCTV and neighbourhood watch schemes in areas of high crime (Clarke, 1985; Clarke, 1997). Striking confirmatory case examples exist within the violence literatures. In a famous prison laboratory study, Haney, Banks and Zimbardo (1973) found that young men who had been randomly assigned to either the role of prison guard or the role of prisoner rapidly adopted negative behaviour in the simulated prison: 'guards' became abusive and aggressive, 'prisoners' became so distressed that almost half had to be released because of their acute emotional responses. Haney (2006), commenting on the study years later, noted 'None of the personality or attitudinal measures used in the study explained the behavior of the participants, which seemed to occur entirely as a function of the extreme nature of the environment in which they had been placed' (p. 130).

In other domains, such as preventative medicine, the important distinction between the strategies that target high-risk individuals and those that target the whole population is well recognized (Rose, 1992). Population strategies are often situational in nature. Population strategies are particularly effective where, as is the case for violence, the known risk factors are relatively weak (see Cooke and Johnstone, 2010 for a fuller discussion).

Unfortunately, the influence of situational factors on violence risk has not been subject to rigorous research testing and the findings that do exist are inconsistent at times (see Byrne and Hummer, 2007; Gadon, et al., 2006; Wortley, 2002). Nonetheless, some key papers have suggested a link between the organizational, environmental, systemic, staff, and managerial levels of institutional functioning and violence in prisons (e.g., Bloom, Eisen, Pollock and Webster, 2000; Byrne and Hummer, 2007; Cooke, 1991; Cooke, 1997; Ditchfield, 1991; DiLulio, 1987; Gendreau, Coggins and Law, 1997; Rice, Harris, Varney and Quinsey, 1989; Silver, Mulvey and Monahan, 1999; Wortley, 2002) and mental health settings (Richter and Whittington, 2006).

Towards the systematic evaluation of situational risk factors for violence

The last twenty years has seen major strides in the professional study of violence risk in individuals. The seminal work of Hart, Kropp, Webster and others, in the development of the structured professional judgement approach (SPJ) to the evaluation of violence risk, has contributed substantially to the field. These SPJ approaches are evidence-based, they are comprehensive, flexible – designed to deal with the generalities, but also the idiosyncrasies of individual cases – they allow the application of professional judgement and discretion, and guide management strategies. We decided that the time was ripe to approach the problem of situational factors more systematically; we wanted to produce an evidence-based, but practical, procedure, for use by practitioners: we resolved that the SPJ provided the best fit for the purpose. *Promoting Risk Interventions by Situational Management* (PRISM) was the result (Johnstone and Cooke, 2008).

We developed PRISM using three steps. In order to capture the evidence base, we first carried out a systematic review of the literature on institutional violence in both forensic hospitals and prisons. Systematic reviews differ from traditional reviews (e.g. Cooke, 1991) because rigorous methods are employed for locating, appraising, and synthesizing evidence from the research literature. In order to make the study replicable, it is not only necessary to specify the criteria for the inclusion or exclusion of studies, but also the search strategy – including the databases that are to be reviewed – must be delineated before embarking on the review. Tellingly, while a very large number of studies were identified, only very few had direct relevance to the central purpose of the review – the understanding of situational risk factors for violence (Gadon, Johnstone, and Cooke, 2006). We formed the view that the restricted nature of the literature highlighted the lack of attention that has been given to this class of risk factors.

The second step in developing PRISM was the collection of qualitative information from prisoners and staff currently, or previously, employed in prison and/or health settings. This process clarified which situational variables were associated with institutional violence – compensating for the paucity of empirical studies – but it also provided a rich source of putative explanations concerning why these variables might increase the risk of violence (Gadon, Johnstone and Cooke, 2006). It informed our thinking not merely about 'what?' risk factors to consider but 'why?' these risk factors should be considered – understanding risk processes has implications both for the development of effective risk management strategies and also for providing a deeper understanding of the mechanism by which situational risk factors impact on individual patients or prisoners.

Having gathered this evidence from both research and practice, we moved to the third step in the development of PRISM: this was to distil that evidence – using rationale criteria – into a set of practice guidelines. These guidelines were designed to lead from assessment, through formulation and scenario planning, to effective risk interventions.

A brief description of PRISM

From the outset, the focus of PRISM was institutional violence. We used a broad definition, 'the actual, attempted, or threatened harm towards another person within the institutional setting. Institutional violence may be construed broadly to include acts such as verbal aggression (including threats of harm or behaviour which is intimidating), physical assault and sexual violence' (p. 16). We also used a broad definition of situational risk factors in order to capture the diversity and complexity of the organizations studied; and we thus refer to them as features of the context within which the violence takes place. Using a rationale approach, we derived five domains of risk factors (see Figure 7.1).

The first domain is concerned with the *History of Institutional Violence*. Violent behaviour in the two-year period prior to the PRISM evaluation is considered. To some degree, the decision to consider a two-year period is arbitrary but, based on experience, we considered that it was sufficiently long to provide a sample of violent incidents while sufficiently short that the situational risk factors are likely to have remained the same. We broke this domain into four risk factors. It includes: (1) *Previous institutional violence* (i.e., the level of violence within the last two years); (2) *Escalating institutional violence* (i.e., increase in violence in the last two years); (3) *Diversity of institutional violence* (i.e., occurrence of different types of violence – different perpetrators, victims, levels of seriousness, weapon use, and so on); and (4) *Change in number and/or type of complaints submitted* (i.e., any increase or decrease in number or types of complaints).

The second domain is concerned with *Physical and Security Factors*. We broke this domain into two risk factors: (1) *Supervision and control measures* (i.e., the extent to which the availability and implementation of supervision and control is carefully targeted and matched to the level of risk posed); and (2) *Physical layout and resources* (i.e., the extent to which the structural quality, level of cleanliness and hygiene, noise levels, temperature and space, and so on, are appropriate for

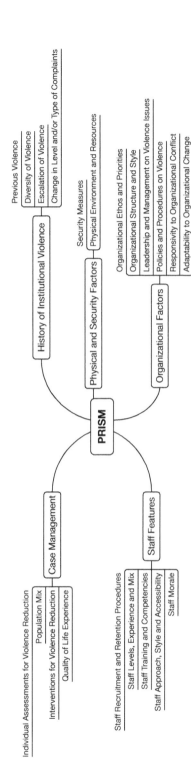

Figure 7.1 Domains of risk factors in the PRISM

the purposes of the institution and are compliant with health-and-safety and human-rights legislation).

The third domain is concerned with *Organizational Factors* and focuses on the strengths and weaknesses of the relevant organizational structures, not only within the institution per se, but the organization in which it is embedded. We broke down this domain into six risk factors: (1) *Organizational structure and style* (i.e., the extent to which the organization has a clear structure and style to its management); (2) *Organizational ethos towards violence* (i.e., the extent to which the organization fosters a zero-tolerance ethos on violence); (3) *Leadership and management on violence-related issues* (i.e., the extent to which the institution promotes a strategic approach to the implementation of violence risk assessment by having a dedicated lead); (4) *Effective policies and procedures on violence* (i.e., the extent to which the organization has a clear policy which explicitly states a pledge to promote a violence-free work environment); (5) *Responsivity to conflict* (i.e., the extent to which the organization responds to conflict either between staff groups, or prisoner groups, or between prisoners and staff, and so on); and (6) *Adaptability to change* (i.e., the extent to which the organization can adapt to change – positive or negative).

The fourth domain is concerned with *Staff Features* and is focused on determining the strengths and weaknesses of the staff compliment. We broke down this domain into five risk factors of concern: (1) *Recruitment procedures* (i.e., the extent to which there are appropriate recruitment and retention procedures for appropriately trained and skilled staff to ensure the effective day-to-day running of the institution); (2) *Staff numbers and mix* (i.e., the extent to which an appropriate number of staff are available to ensure the effective day-to-day running of the organization and the extent to which there are an appropriate number of staff to manage the needs of the prisoner group; included in this item is the extent to which staff are appropriately mixed in terms of their competencies and experience); (3) *Staff training* (i.e., the extent to which staff are given appropriate levels of training on issues regarding risk assessment and risk management and the extent to which this training matches their role); (4) *Staff morale* (i.e., the extent to which staff perceive appropriate working conditions, levels of support, both professional and personal, and how engaged they are with the institution); and (5) *Staff approach and style* (i.e., the extent to which staff foster and engage prisoners in communication and collaboration where possible).

The fifth and final domain is the *Case Management* domain. This domain is concerned with risk factors associated with the population residing in the institution and the matching of risk management interventions to their aggregate risk and needs. We broke this domain into four risk factors: (1) *Case formulation* (i.e., the extent to which prisoners are appropriately assessed for their violence risk and needs, the extent to which these assessments correspond with existing professional standards of risk assessment such as the HCR-20 (Webster, Douglas, Eaves, and Hart, 1997) and the extent to which staff monitor these risks on a day-to-day basis); (2) *Programmes/therapies for violent prisoners* (i.e., the extent to which the institution makes available and delivers effective programmes);

(3) *Population mix* (i.e., the extent to which the institution appropriately considers prisoner placement decisions); and (4) *Quality of life experiences* (i.e., the extent to which prisoners have access to positive experiences, such as recreation, education, contact with the outside world, and so on).

PRISM as an action-orientated process

As practitioners, from the outset we wanted to make PRISM action orientated. We were conscious that a PRISM evaluation could be construed as an 'inspection', something which would be inimical to effective change. It was important to ensure that the process was collaborative. One way to achieve this was to emphasize that all risk assessments require a multi-method and multi-source approach; the best way to achieve this in an institutional setting is to engage with a multidisciplinary team. A multidisciplinary approach not only facilitates the collection of a broad range of good-quality data but it also enhances 'buy-in' from staff; 'buy-in' is fundamental to the achievement of change.

The PRISM process is a seven-step process; the principles underpinning systematic case studies provided helpful guidance when developing this process (Yin, 2003). First, the team is selected and trained in the PRISM approach and they are then assigned tasks. Second, the team gathers information about the PRISM risk factors. A multi-method approach to data gathering is utilized, with the reliability and validity of the data being assessed. Third, the multi-disciplinary team, as a group, debates and evaluates the evidence concerning each risk factor and decides whether the risk factor is currently *problematic, needs improvement,* or is *satisfactory.* A *not known* option is used when there is inadequate information to rate the item: the use of this option is discouraged; essentially, it is used as a stimulus for more information gathering.

Fourth, future scenarios of violence, which might occur in that particular institution or section of the institution, are envisioned by the multi-disciplinary team using the techniques of scenario planning. Scenario planning has a long history and is applied in the management of uncertain and negative futures (Miller and Waller, 2003). A risk scenario can be considered to be a short narrative, or risk formulation, designed to capture the essence of a complex set of information and translate it into a meaningful account about what – and how – risk factors may be relevant for future violence. Scenarios are methods for thinking systematically about the future and they should guide decision-makers concerning interventions designed to obviate risk (see Hart and Logan, 2011; Hart, et al., 2003). Fifth, having identified key risk scenarios, the next step is to prioritize where to intervene in terms of urgency.

Sixth, the team and responsible managers consider each scenario and develop appropriate, and targeted, intervention strategies. It is vital, if these strategies are to be effective, that they are developed with cooperation amongst professionals working in different areas of the institution, with different skills, roles, responsibilities, and knowledge bases. Critically, risk interventions should be realistic and achievable; it is important to plan to fit with the short-, medium- and long-term capabilities and capacities of the institution. The seventh, final and perhaps the critical step, is the communication of risk. Communications need to be clear, concise, and simple, and expressed in a fashion that facilities appropriate action. Fundamentally, the PRISM entails a process that is designed to assist multidisciplinary teams to apply evidence-based practice to develop effective anti-violence interventions. But does it work?

PRISM in the real world: some institutional case studies

PRISM was developed to facilitate the understanding of institutional risk factors in real-world settings; it was designed to be sufficiently flexible to be useful for a range of tasks. Below we describe three case studies that demonstrate a variety of uses of PRISM – critical incident review, multiple case comparisons within a prison system, and cross-comparison of three segregation units within one prison in New Zealand.

Barbados prisons in transition

One of the first real-world uses of PRISM was in Barbados (Cooke and Wozniak, 2010). Barbados is a former British colony in the Eastern Caribbean with a population of just over a quarter of a million people. On 30 March 2005, a fight broke out among a small group of prisoners in Her Majesty's Prison Glendairy, a large Victorian prison built in 1855. The prison held all the prisoners on the island: a thousand prisoners; males and females, adults and young offenders, convicted and remand, and even a group of adult males on death row. Over three days, the single violent incident escalated to the point where a large number of prisoners rioted and took control of the prison and engaged in widespread destruction and arson. The prison was severely damaged and was no longer habitable – the only prison in Barbados was lost and a major logistical and political crisis ensued. To meet the challenge, the government required all metal fabrication facilities on the island to cease their normal activities and build temporary accommodation within the dormitories of a former US naval base, Harrison's Point. The majority of remand and low-security prisoners were housed in dormitories in 'cages' built from metal reinforcing rods; for higher-security prisoners the 'cages' contained one or two prisoners. The nature of the prison experience can be characterized in a number of ways: the principal remand units contained approximately 140 prisoners in four adjoining 'cages'; there was only one toilet and shower for each section of 35 prisoners. Triple bunks were provided but these were insufficient in number, with the result that some prisoners had to sleep on the floor. Exercise, work opportunities, and education were severely restricted for all but a small number of prisoners; most prisoners were forced to spend the vast majority of their day in their dormitory. Other essential services were restricted for many, water and toilet access being the major ones.

Shipping containers were used to segregate prisoners under punishment; these containers were hot during the day and cold at night. The perimeter security of

Harrison's Point was limited and any investment in improving the perimeter of the temporary facility was not cost-effective; therefore, control within the prison was rigorous. Movement for most prisoners was extremely limited and when it was permitted – or required – it generally entailed prisoners having to wear manacles and leg irons and being escorted by staff with dogs and 'supervised' by armed staff. Family members were denied the opportunity to visit or communicate with their relatives in prison other than via video or audio connection. By any objective standards, this was a regime based on limited prisoner movement and extreme personal control.

Inevitably, because the prison had been lost, there had been a loss of critical information. Our first task was to collect information from as many sources as possible, and this was achieved in a number of ways: through the first Barbados prisoner survey (response rate 93 per cent) and the first Barbados prison staff study, through individual interviews and focus groups with prisoners and prison staff, and by informal discussion with ex-prisoners (Cooke and Wozniak, 2010).

It is not surprising that we found many problematic areas in the functioning of the prison system in Barbados; the government and prison service are to be commended for allowing us to examine their system. Indeed, while the regime at Harrison's Point was impoverished and challenging, none of this should distract from the achievement of the Barbados authorities in creating a prison capable of housing over 1,000 prisoners in a matter of weeks.[1]

PRISM allowed us to systematically characterize the regime both in Glendairy prior to the riot and in Harrison's Point subsequent to the riot. We identified many and various areas of concerns in all the PRISM domains in regard to both Glendairy prison and Harrison's Point; however, our particular concern was to the future. During our second visit to Barbados, the new purpose-built prison was being constructed; our primary concern that the dysfunctional culture, attitudes, and practices that grew up in Glendairy, and which were hardened in the fire and conflicts of the riot and its aftermath, would be transferred to the new prison. We made a large number of recommendations regarding new approaches to prison management, procedures for improving staff morale, staff training, leadership and management, strategies for enhancing staff–prisoner relationships, methods for resolving problems of population mix and the benefits of a coherent information system. In couching our recommendations, we drew on best practice internationally but, critically, we tailored the recommendations to fit within the culture and resources of the Barbados Prison Service: recommendations must be realistic to be effective (Cooke and Wozniak, 2010).

High security facilities in New Zealand

The New Zealand Department of Corrections is a highly sophisticated corrections service. Two research psychologists, Nick Wilson and Armon Tamatea, carried out the first PRISM study in New Zealand (Wilson and Tamatea, 2010). A prior study had indicated that in New Zealand prisons gang members were over-represented in incidents of violence. The gangs were well recognized and included nationwide organized criminal groups such as Black Power and the Mongrel Mob. Perpetrators of prison violence were significantly younger (40 per cent under 25 years of age) and more likely to be of Maori descent. The majority of violent incidents occurred in remand (awaiting conviction or sentence) or maximum-security units. The focus of Wilson and Tametea's compelling study were New Zealand's only three dedicated maximum-security units, situated next to each other in a prison in Auckland; these units were selected for study in the wake of a number of serious, and high-profile, assaults – prisoner upon prisoner and prisoner on staff.

Following a careful and detailed PRISM assessment, the authors found that management and staff held distorted views of violence and safety. There were significant problems from a lack of leadership focused on violence management, and there was an absence of specific recruitment and training for the peculiar challenges of working under conditions of maximum security. They highlighted the very restricted unlock regime that operated, a regime with no treatment options and only limited recreational activities. The specific management challenges that they identified related to population mix, with gang issues at times preventing prisoner movement, and more broadly there was a problem of siltage, with other prisons reluctant to take transfers of prisoners from these high-security units. There was evidence of staff buy-in to the PRISM process. For example, Wilson and Tametea discovered that corrections staff found the use of risk scenarios a 'natural' move to a future focus; from a focus on blaming for past problems to more pragmatic interventions. It is heartening to note that they found the PRISM process to be an intervention in and of itself resulting in changes, including the paying of more attention to staff mix, the implementation of an active management approach, and the injection of some greater flexibility in regard to quality of life experiences.

Comparing prisons in Scotland

The PRISM was devised and grew up in Scotland, so it is appropriate that the largest study undertaken so far is a multiple case study of five Scottish prisons (Johnstone and Cooke, 2010). As noted above, in the 1980s, the Scottish Prison Service (SPS) was a failing organization (Cooke, Wozniak, and Johnstone, 2008). In an unprecedented U-turn, the new solution was not to isolate but to integrate the 'difficult' prisoners, to encourage them to participate actively in their sentence planning, and to provide opportunities for quality of life experiences, dignity, respect, and responsibility-taking (SPS, 1990). In addition, the role of the prison officer was redefined from a purely custodial function to a supporting function. Twenty years on, while it is by no means a violence-free organization, the SPS is in a position where, overall, it can boast reducing rates of violence. Notwithstanding, the picture is not uniform and despite these landslide changes in penal philosophy, there is a dearth of high-quality, robust, and replicable research specifically designed to identify 'what works' in terms of Scotland's approach to situational risk management. The organization supported the study of five prisons, which were selected because not only were they heterogeneous in purpose and design, but they also varied in level of perceived violence. The prisons were diverse, from Scotland's only prison for female offenders, through the main national facility for young offenders, to a high-security prison holding prisoners serving sentences of four years or more, a local prison for untried and convicted male prisoners (young offenders and adults), and, finally, a smaller local prison. We opted to use a multiple case study design as such a design is appropriate when the purpose of the research is to investigate 'a contemporary phenomenon within its real-life context especially when the boundaries between phenomenon and context are not clearly evident' (Yin, 2003, p. 13). Case study designs have the advantages that they tolerate differences across cases while, at the same time, they allow broad generalizations to be achieved.

At the conclusion of each evaluation, each site received a detailed and highly individualized report outlining the specific risk factors, scenarios and risk management interventions appropriate to their setting. For the purposes of illustrating the application of the tool, common themes to emerge are presented here. All sites were rated *problematic* or *needs improvement* on *Previous violence* and *Diversity of violence*. Tellingly, in most settings it was impossible to rate the *Complaints* item due to inadequate data. Three of the five sites were rated as *problematic* in terms of their supervision and control procedures, and three of the five prisons were rated as *problematic* on the *Policies and procedures on violence* factor. Three of the five sites were rated as *problematic* on *Leadership and management on violence issues* and four of the five sites were rated as *problematic* on *Effective policies and procedures*. All but one site received a *problematic* or *needs improvement* rating on *Staff levels, experience and mix*. None of the sites were viewed as having satisfactory *Staff morale*. Three of the sites had *problematic* ratings on *Population mix*, four were rated *problematic* in terms of *Case Management* and all sites were rated as having inadequate *Interventions for violence reduction*. The evaluations also revealed that policies and procedures with respect to identifying and managing risks in individual prisoners could be improved.

Across all settings, the most likely scenario was verbal and physical aggression between individual prisoners or between prisoners and staff. One setting identified a high risk of collective violence. All settings were rated as having a low likelihood of sexual violence.

A range of risk management interventions were proposed. These were matched to the risk-factor ratings and the scenarios to be managed. Examples included an improved and more sensitive violence-recording procedure, a review of the complaint procedure, staff training on the importance of attending to all forms of violence, including minor incidents, ongoing communication across the tiers of staff with regard to security and control, immediate intervention with regard to some of the physical environments rated 'not fit for purpose', improved policies and procedures on violence issues, having a competent leader on violence-related issues in post, a review of staffing issues – levels, mix and retention procedures, better individualized violence risk assessments, improved access to treatment programmes, and better processes to ensure acceptable population mix.

The fieldwork demonstrated the practical utility of PRISM in that it was found to facilitate comprehensive assessments of each setting and to achieve positive ratings on user-satisfaction. Feedback from participants indicated that the PRISM process encouraged collaboration and 'buy-in' from different staff, with different perspectives and priorities. Indeed, the assessment process itself appeared to have functioned as an intervention whereby team members had the opportunity to learn about the relevance of situational risk factors and how these factors might be tackled in creative ways.

The above are just three examples of PRISM case studies. We believe that they have demonstrated the content validity of the PRISM process, but also that they have demonstrated its utility. However, good evidence of the approach can only accrue through the application of the method in diverse settings, and specifically by its use by other practitioners. Other studies have been carried out; Cregg and Payne (2010) considered an institution for incarcerated youths (15–17 years) in England, Neil (2010) studied a unit within a Scottish high-security forensic hospital, and Johnstone, in collaboration with colleagues, is in the process of facilitating an evaluation of a continuing care inpatient ward in a Scottish psychiatric hospital.

The case studies we have featured highlight some applications of PRISM but we consider that there are others. First, colleagues in New Zealand have indicated that PRISM will provide a set of guiding principles when developing a new treatment regime for sexual and violent offenders. It will assist those tasked with planning and implementing the new regime to consider the situational factors that need to be taken into account from the very beginning. This promotes a proactive approach to violence prevention. Second, PRISM could play a part in the training of practitioners and other professionals working within institutions containing those with the potential for violence. Training may enhance awareness and lead to creative interventions.

Third, we believe that PRISM can be used to inform theory by helping to identify the latent – or unobservable – 'risk processes' that underpin the risk factors that we assess. The research strategy that led to the development of PRISM helped to answer the 'What?' question, that is, what institutional risk factors should we attend to when we are considering risk of future violence in prisons or forensic hospitals. However, to effect change, it is necessary to answer the 'Why?' question too; why, for example, might lack of staff training or lack of clear management or poor information systems lead to an increase risk of violence? It is as if the evaluator has to carry out a 'conceptual factor analysis' based upon their understanding of the processes that underpin violence (Cooke and Wozniak, 2010). Each risk factor needs to be considered and then deconstructed in order to identify the potent elements of it that contribute to future risk. The key elements of these risk factors are likely to be underpinned by a limited set of risk processes; for example, promotion of a sense of injustice, promotion of a sense of uncertainty, promotion of a loss of agency, promotion of cultural expectations to be violent (e.g. through gang membership). Consideration of 'why?' a risk factor may be relevant should assist our understanding of distinct but related risk processes that – individually and together – shape the topography of violence (see Cooke and Michie, 2010; Cooke and Wozniak, 2010).

PRISM: things we have learned so far

Underpinning the philosophy of all forms of SPJ approaches is the core principle that they should be evidence based. PRISM is still relatively new, the evidence base is just developing, but we believe that we are learning some key lessons from the case studies already carried out so far; these lessons relate both to practical issues to do with effective interventions and theoretical issues to do with the interplay between situational risk factors and violence.

We discovered that the PRISM process is, by its very nature, an intervention and it fosters an understanding and collaboration amongst members of staff in the institution who would ordinarily not have anything to do with each other, and who often would have little appreciation of the skills and commitments of others in the workplace. This can be energizing. From a practical perspective we have learned that the model is relatively complex and for optimal use the PRISM team needs to contain some members who are *au fait* with the SPJ approach to risk assessment and risk management. The organization needs to commit appropriate staff across a range of levels to achieve an effective assessment.

Looking to the future, we think that there are three key tasks. The first task is to carry out development work – reviews and interviews (expert and stakeholder) – to determine whether the approach can be generalized across types of settings. We see no immediately obvious reasons why the principles of effective organizational functioning should not generalize to other types of organizations: secure care settings for juveniles, community-based services for offenders or out-patient settings for forensic patients, residential settings for populations presenting with challenging behaviour (e.g., older adults care homes or inpatient wards, resources for patients with learning disabilities), and so on. But this assumption requires testing.

The second task is to carry out developmental work to determine whether these situational factors also influence markers of distress, disturbance and dysfunction in closed settings other than violence; these markers might include suicidal and parasuicidal behaviour, depression and anxiety, reluctance to engage with regime, or failure to benefit from treatment activities, absconding, and other risk-taking behaviours, perhaps even relapses in mental illness. The third task is to develop a taxonomy of strategies for risk management. One of the findings that struck us, looking at the available studies across settings, is the commonality of problems. We believe that while responses need to be tailored to the individual institution, there are common strategies that can be adapted to fit specific circumstances. The wheel does not need to be reinvented.

We conclude this brief chapter by arguing that the situational approach has a number of advantages and the application of PRISM might be viewed as a first step in unlocking these advantages in a systematic manner (Cooke and Johnstone, 2010; Johnstone and Cooke, 2008). What are these advantages? First, the interventions derived from a situational approach are applicable across a whole institution and can have a broad – and significant – impact in situations where there are insufficient resources to deliver individualized interventions. Second, situational interventions should influence the group of 'difficult' prisoners or patients who, almost by definition, are unlikely to engage with individualized approaches. Third, these interventions can be cost-effective, with current assets being brigaded more effectively.

We started this chapter by observing that behaviour can be thought of as being shaped by a pair of scissors, with one blade being the characteristics of the actor and the other blade being the characteristics of the environment. PRISM goes some way to providing the missing second blade.

Note

1   The three reports submitted by the authors to the Office of the Attorney General in Barbados are available online at www.icpa.ca.

References

Bloom, H., Eisen, R. S., Pollock, N. and Webster, C. D. (2000) *WRA-20: Workplace risk assessment*, Toronto: workplace.calm.inc.

Boyle, J. (1977) *A Sense of Freedom*, London: Handbooks.

Byrne, J. M. and Hummer, D. (2007) 'Myths and realities of prison violence', *Victims and Offenders*, 2: 77–90.

Clarke, R. B. G. (1985) 'Deliquency environment as a dimension', *Journal of Child Psychology and Psychiatry*, 262: 515–23.

Clarke, R. G. (1997) *Situational Crime Prevention: Successful case studies* (2nd edition), New York: Harrow and Heston.

Cooke, D. J. (1989) 'Containing violent prisoners: An analysis of the Barlinnie Special Unit', *British Journal of Criminology*, 29: 129–43.

— (1991) 'Violence in prisons: The influence of regime factors', *The Howard Journal of Criminal Justice*, 30: 95–109.

— (1997) 'The Barlinnie Special Unit: The rise and fall of a therapeutic experiment' in E. Cullen, L. Jones and R. Woodward (eds) *Therapeutic Communities for Offenders* (pp. 101–20), London: Wiley.

Cooke, D. J. and Johnstone, L. (2010) 'Somewhere over the rainbow: Improving violence risk management in institutional settings', *International Journal of Forensic Mental Health Services*, 9: 150–58.

Cooke, D. J. and Michie, C. (2010) 'Limitations of diagnostic precision and predictive utility in the individual case: A challenge for forensic practice', *Law and Human Behavior*, 34: 258–74.

Cooke, D. J. and Wozniak, E. (2010) 'PRISM applied to a critical incident review: A case study of the Glendairy prison riot', *International Journal of Forensic Mental Health Services*, 9: 159–72.

Cooke, D. J., Wozniak, E. and Johnstone, L. (2008) 'Casting light on prison violence: Evaluating the impact of situational risk factors', *Criminal Justice and Behavior*, 35: 1065–78.

Coyle, A. G. (1987) 'The Scottish experience of small units', in A. E. Bottoms and R. Light (eds) *Problems of Long-term Imprisonment*, Aldershot: Gower.

Cregg, M. and Payne, E. (2010) 'PRISM with incarcerated young people: Optical illusion or reflection of reality?', *International Journal of Forensic Mental Health Services*, 9: 173–79.

DiLulio, J. J. (1987) *Governing Prisons: A comparative study of correctional management* (1st edition), London: Collier Macmillan.

Ditchfield, J. (1991) *Control in Prison: A review of the literature*, London: HMSO.

Gadon, L., Johnstone, L. and Cooke, D. J. (2006) 'Situational variables and institutional violence: A systematic review of the literature', *Clinical Psychology Review*, 26: 534.

Gendreau, P., Coggins, C. and Law, M. A. (1997) 'Predicting prison misconducts', *Criminal Justice and Behavior*, 24: 414–31.

Haney, C. (2006) *Reforming Punishment: Psychological limits to the pains of confinement*, Washington DC: American Psychological Association.

Haney, C., Bank, C. and Zimbardo, P. (1973) 'Interpersonal dynamics in a simulated prison', *International Journal of Criminology and Penology*, 1: 69–97.

Hart, S. D. and Logan, C. (2011) 'Formulation of violence risk using evidence-based assessments: The structured professional judgment approach', in P. Sturmey and M. McMurran (eds) *Forensic Case Formulation*, Chichester: Wiley-Blackwell.

Hart, S. D., Kropp, P. R., Laws, R., Klaver, J., Logan, C. and Watt, K. A. (2003) *The Risk of Sexual Violence Protocol (RSVP)*, Burnaby: Mental Health, Law, and Policy Institute, Simon Fraser University.

Johnstone, L. and Cooke, D.J. (2008) *PRISM: Promoting Risk Intervention by Situational Management: Structured professional guidelines for assessing situational risk factors for violence in institutions* (1st edition), Burnaby, Canada: Mental Health, Law, and Policy Institute. Simon Fraser University.

— (2010) 'PRISM: A promising paradigm for assessing and managing institutional violence: Findings from a multiple case study analysis of five Scottish prisons', *International Journal of Forensic Mental Health Services*, 9: 180–91.

Miller, K. D. and Waller, G. H. (2003) 'Scenarios, real options and integrated risk management', *Long Range Planning*, 36: 93–107.

Mischel, W. (1968) *Personality and Assessment*, New York: Wiley.

— (2004) 'Towards an integrative science of the person', *Annual Review of Psychology*, 55: 22.

Neil, C. (2010) *The Presence and Relevance of Situational Risk Factors for Violence in the State Hospital: A case study*. Report prepared for the Risk Group, State Hospital, Scotland (unpublished).

Rice, M. E., Harris, G. T., Varney, G. W. and Quinsey, B. L. (1989) *Violence in Institutions: Understanding, prevention and control*, Toronto: Hans Huber.

Rose, G. (1992) *The Strategy of Preventative Medicine*, Oxford: Oxford Medical Publications.

Scottish Prison Service (1990) *Opportunity and Responsibility: Developing new approaches to the management of the long term prison system in Scotland*, Edinburgh: HMSO.

Scratton, P., Sim, J. and Skidmore, P. (1991) *Prisons Under Protest* (1st edition), Milton Keynes: Open University Press.

Silver, E., Mulvey, E. P. and Monahan, J. (1999) 'Assessing violence risk among discharged psychiatric patients: Towards an ecological approach', *Law and Human Behavior*, 23: 237–55.

Simon, H. A. (1990) 'Invariants of human behaviour', *Annual Review of Psychology*, 41: 1–19.

Webster, C. D., Douglas, K., Eaves, D. and Hart, S. D. (1997) *HCR-20: Assessing Risk for Violence* (2nd edition), Vancouver: Simon Fraser University.

Whittington, R. and Richter, D. (2006) 'From the individual to the interpersonal: Environment and interaction in the escalation of violence in mental health settings', in D. Richter (ed.) *Violence in Mental Health Settings* (pp. 47–65), UK: Springer.

Wilson, N. J. and Tamatea, A. (2010) 'Beyond punishment: Applying PRISM in a New Zealand maximum security prison', *International Journal of Forensic Mental Health Services*, 9: 192–204.

Wortley, R. (2002) *Situational Prison Control: Crime prevention in correctional institutions*, Cambridge: Cambridge University Press.

Yin, R. K. (2003) *Case Study Research: Design and methods* (3rd edition), Thousand Oaks: Sage.

Part III
Key client groups

8 Risk assessment and management with clients with cognitive impairment

Suzanne O'Rourke

Introduction

The influence of cognitive impairment is pervasive in all aspects of the care of mentally disordered offenders (MDOs). Substantial evidence now exists that the most common diagnoses among our clients, including schizophrenia, antisocial personality disorder (ASPD) and psychopathy, are associated with specific cognitive deficits (e.g., Blair, 2003; Dolan and Park, 2002; Nuechterlein, et al., 2004). These deficits are compounded by their increased risk of acquired brain injury as a result of violence and substance abuse. In a cohort study of 256 special hospital patients, 91 per cent had either a diagnosis of schizophrenia or learning disability, a neurological injury or illness, or a history of drug and alcohol abuse indicative of probable impairment (O'Rourke and Hartley, 2011). Amongst a group of 125 special hospital patients, 79 per cent had one or more *Wechsler Adult Intelligence Scale 3rd Edition* (WAIS-III) IQ or index scores in the borderline range or below (O'Rourke and Hartley, 2011).

The great majority of MDOs have a diagnosis of schizophrenia, an illness now firmly established as a neurodevelopmental disorder (Marcopulos, et al., 2008) amidst calls for cognitive impairment to become part of its diagnostic criteria in the *Diagnostic and Statistical Manual of Mental Disorders 5th Edition* (DSM-5, e.g., Keefe, 2008). The National Institute of Mental Health Initiative, Measurement and Treatment Research to Improve Cognition in Schizophrenia (MATRICS) identified seven core cognitive deficits in schizophrenia: processing speed, attention/vigilance, working memory, verbal and visual learning and memory, reasoning and problem solving, and verbal comprehension. MATRICS suggested that, while the evidence is still preliminary, an additional factor – social cognition – was also worthy of further investigation and measurement in outcome trials (Nuechterlein, et al., 2004). Meta-analytic reviews suggest an average deficit in people with schizophrenia of approximately one standard deviation below that of control populations (Dickinson, et al., 2007), accounting for between 20 and 60 per cent of variance in functional outcome (Green, et al., 2000). Although a quarter of clients with a diagnosis of schizophrenia may fall within the normal range on neuropsychological measures, they are likely to represent a subgroup whose initially higher levels of functioning have obscured similar deficits, meaning that all individuals with schizophrenia should be considered to have suffered cognitive impairment (Keefe, 2008).

The association between violence and neurological impairment has been illustrated using a range of methods and populations (Krakowski, 2005), and cognitive impairment should be integral to the risk assessment and management of MDOs. Indeed, cognitive impairment is being considered for incorporation into the 3rd edition of the *Historical-Clinical-Risk Management-20* (HCR-20), the widely recognized gold-standard risk assessment tool in the field (Douglas, 2008). The relevance of cognitive risk factors should be considered in all stages of the structured professional judgement approach to risk assessment. Their relevance as motivators or disinhibitors to violence should be considered along with their potential to impede rehabilitation efforts. Risk management plans should include programmes to address specific cognitive deficits or adaptations to reduce their negative impact. Risk formulations and scenario planning should take full account of their role in triggering violence, influencing its manifestation and the success of rehabilitation efforts.

Cognitive impairment is a heterogeneous term and is not per se associated with violence in MDOs. Rather it encompasses a range of deficits that are either directly linked to violent offending, perform a mediating role in possible offence pathways, or reduce the efficacy of rehabilitation. Despite this, cognitive impairment is an aspect of the client's functioning that is often ignored in forensic assessment. The core role that it plays in the aetiology of our clients' behaviours, prognosis, and ultimately risk, means that core competencies in neuropsychology are required if we are to fully address their risk assessment and management.

The purpose of this chapter is to describe the neuroanatomical correlates of violence and the areas of cognitive functioning that should be considered during the risk assessment and management of MDOs. The chapter will begin by describing the neuroanatomy of violence and aggression before considering in detail the cognitive deficits relevant to risk assessment and how they can be measured and addressed. While MDOs with schizophrenia will provide the focus for this chapter, those with other psychiatric diagnoses should also be considered at risk of cognitive impairment as specific deficits are associated with almost all major diagnostic categories (e.g., Bora, et al., 2009b; Bora, et al., 2010).

Neuro-anatomy of violence and aggression

A large body of evidence now suggests that the prefrontal cortex (PFC) is implicated in aggression (Hoptman, 2003; Morgan and Lilienfeld, 2000; Pietrini and Bambini, 2009). The prefrontal regions that have most often been implicated in antisocial behaviour are the orbitofrontal cortex (OFC), ventromedial prefrontal cortex (VMPFC), ventrolateral prefrontal cortex (VLPFC) and, more debatably, the dorsolateral prefrontal cortex (DLPFC) (Dolan and Park, 2002; Blair, 2005; Brower and Price, 2001).

The key to understanding aggression from a neuroscience perspective lies in both the amygdala and the prefrontal cortex (Pietrini and Bambini, 2009). The amygdala is thought to be responsible for the accurate identification of threats, the perception of other's emotions, and fear conditioning itself, all of which are implicated in the offending pathway (e.g. Adolphs, 2008). In turn, the OFC is considered to have a role in the inhibition of aggressive responses, and the VMPFC in deciding if a stimulus is considered to have positive or negative emotional content. Thus, the amygdala and VMPFC determine a person's emotional or instinctive response to a stimulus, while the OFC may have a role in inhibiting this response (Pietrini and Bambini, 2009).

Psychopathy, the personality disorder most associated with risk of violence, is primarily associated with the OFC and VMPFC areas, which control our ability to inhibit behaviour and respond to conflict (Blair, 2005). Blair's integrated emotions systems (IES) model suggests that when stimulus-response contingencies change, no longer producing the expected or desired outcome, deficits in the OFC reduce the individual's ability to reverse their responses, a situation where the expected outcome or reward fails to materialize and frustration and reactive aggression ensues (Blair, 2005). Psychopathy has also been associated with deficits in functions mediated by the amygdala, part of the limbic system responsible for the processing of emotions including identifying threats, fear conditioning, and the activation of empathic responses (Blair, 2003). The IES model suggests that a specific deficit in the amygdala prevents psychopaths from making stimulus–reinforcement associations; for example, the ability to learn appropriate behaviour from the aversive stimuli provided by the distress of others, leading to impaired socialization and moral referencing more generally (Blair, 2005). Particularly interesting is the recent study of Craig, et al. (2009), which identified significant abnormalities in the white matter tract linking the amygdala and OFC in psychopaths. Their findings may not simply elucidate the mechanisms underlying psychopathy but also those underlying antisocial behaviour more generally.

Clinical practice guidelines: cognitive functions that contribute to increased risk

In the absence of imaging technology in daily practice, it is to the cognitive, rather than anatomical, correlates of violence that we must turn to inform dynamic risk assessment and management, as these are both more easily assessed and amenable to amelioration. This section elaborates on the aspects of cognitive impairment that are essential to consider in any risk assessment and management plan for an MDO with cognitive impairment.

Executive functions

It should come as no surprise, given the association of the PFC with violence, that executive function deficits, which rely on this brain region, are also associated with violence (e.g., Brower and Price, 2001; Morgan and Lilienfeld, 2000). Broad deficits in executive function are correlated with treatment outcomes in prison populations (Fishbein, et al., 2006), but it is its specific subcomponents, impulsivity or disinhibition, insight and affect recognition, that may account for much of this relationship.

Impulsivity/inhibition

Impulsivity forms a key characteristic of a number of aggression typologies, most notably 'impulsive aggression' (Feshbach, 1964) and 'reactive aggression' (Raine, et al., 2006). Impulsivity is also a dynamic risk factor for violence (HCR-20) and a diagnostic criterion for psychopathy as measured by the *Psychopathy Checklist Revised* (PCL-R, Hare, 2003).

Dolan and Fullam (2004) identify a number of facets of the concept of impulsivity:

> the tendency to respond quickly and without reflection (Barrat and Patton, 1983), the inability to inhibit behaviour when inhibition is the appropriate response (Schachar and Logan, 1990) or the inability to delay gratification when tolerance of delays produces a less risky outcome (Rachlin, 1974).
>
> (Dolan and Fullam, 2004, p. 428)

In common with antisocial personality disorder (ASPD), psychopathy and violence generally, impulsivity has been associated with OFC abnormalities (Dolan and Fullam, 2004; Dolan, et al., 2001) and response inhibition with the right pre-frontal cortex (Aron and Poldrack, 2005). Impulsivity forms part of the DSM-IV diagnostic criteria for ASPD, borderline personality disorder and attention deficit hyperactivity disorder (ADHD) (American Psychiatric Association, 2000) and is integral to many other psychiatric disorders, including bipolar affective disorder and substance abuse (Moeller, et al., 2001). Further, impulsivity is considered the symptom of ADHD that most contributes to this group's increased risk of offend-ing (Babinski, et al., 1999; Willcutt, et al., 1999). Impulsivity facilitates aggressive acts by preventing their inhibition. Berkowitz (2008) suggests that a lack of serotonin weakens the amygdala's link with areas, including the OFC, which would normally have an inhibitory effect, resulting in 'a greater readiness to react violently to disturbing occurrences' and to 'not hold back when he or she is instigated to attack' (p. 120).

Impulsivity is a significant predictor of violence risk (Monahan, et al., 2001; Webster, et al., 1997) and it may be this failure to inhibit behavioural responses that acts as the key mediator between impairment in the frontal lobes and aggression (Blair, 2005). Higher levels of impulsivity or poor inhibition have been associated with reactive violence in personality disordered inpatients (Dolan and Fullam, 2004) and outpatients (Doyle and Dolan, 2006), and with recidivism in sexual offenders (Prentky, et al., 1995).

A further relationship between impulsivity and violence may be mediated by the former's association with substance abuse (Henderson, et al., 1998), which is reliably associated with violence in both MDOs and offenders (e.g., Bonta, et al., 1998). While both impulsiveness and disinhibition can contribute to the decision to abuse substances, substance abuse itself can cause cognitive damage that may contribute further to violent offending. Substance abuse is associated with impaired executive functioning (e.g., Rogers and Robbins, 2001) leading to a spiralling relationship with aggression and possibly further deterioration in impulse control and affect regulation (London, 2000; Nestor, 2002). Impulsivity may further contribute to the exhibiting of violence by mediating the success of treatment interventions, predicting treatment responsivity in prisoners (Fishbein, et al., 2006).

Ideally, the assessment of impulsivity in clinical forensic practice should use behavioural measures, rather than self-report, as only these can truly reflect an individual's difficulty in inhibiting their responses. The availability of neuropsychological tools measuring this domain is, however, limited. The ability to inhibit verbal responses can be measured using the *Hayling Sentence Completion Test* (Burgess and Shallice, 1997), the ability to inhibit semantic processing using the *Stroop Test* (Trenerry, et al., 1989) and motor responding by *GoNoGo* or *StopSignal* tasks (e.g., Dolan and Park, 2002; Simmonds, et al., 2008). These latter tests appear particularly promising, being software-based and therefore both highly standardized and sensitive, but their commercial availability appears to be limited to the more comprehensive computer test batteries (e.g. *Cambridge Automated Neuropsychological Test Battery*, CANTAB) and appropriate norms may be limited. Typically, patients with high levels of behavioural impulsivity will initially respond quickly, impulsively and incorrectly on these measures, becoming almost immobilized and complaining that they do not understand or are unable to complete the task. Self-report measures have disadvantages, in that they can be transparent and easily manipulated, but benefit from considerable ease and speed of use. The *Barratt Impulsiveness Scale* is widely used (Barratt, 1994, cited in Douglas and Skeem, 2005) and may have some clinical utility (Doyle and Dolan, 2006). The *Impulsivity Checklist* is suggested by the HCR-20 (Webster and Jackson, 1997).

Cognitive-behavioural therapies, particularly dialectical behaviour therapy, appear promising in the treatment of impulsivity, including impulsive aggression in forensic settings (e.g. Shelton, et al., 2009), as do some pharmacological interventions (Chamberlain and Sahakian, 2007).

Insight

Insight is a multi-dimensional construct that comprises an awareness of symptoms, treatment need, and the consequences of illness (Amador, 1993). Debate remains about whether it reflects broader executive functioning deficits or cognitive flexibility specifically. Others have argued that, while cognitive impairment contributes to lack of insight in some cases, for many it reflects the use of denial as a coping style (e.g. Lysaker, et al., 2003), the latter differentiated by the absence of executive or right hemisphere deficits (Marcopulos, et al., 2008). Amongst patients with a diagnosis of schizophrenia, about half will have moderate to extreme impairments in their awareness of their symptoms, their need for treatment, and the consequences of their illness (Lincoln and Hodgins, 2008).

Insight is a dynamic risk criterion in the HCR-20 and correlates with violence and recidivism in schizophrenia (e.g., Soyka, et al., 2007), although further research is required (Bjørkly, 2006). DSM-IV considers insight to be one of the best predictors of poor outcome in patients with a diagnosis of schizophrenia, an association that could form the mechanism that leads to its increased association with risk (American Psychiatric Association, 2000). This may result from its association with poor treatment compliance (e.g., Smith, et al., 1999), an unawareness of their risk cycle and true consequences of offending, or the inability to benefit fully from therapeutic interventions.

Most professionals seeking to identify the presence of insight do so using the HCR-20 criterion (Webster, et al., 1997) or the insight and judgement item from the *Positive and Negative Syndrome Scale* (PANSS, Kay, et al., 1987), whilst the *Scale to Assess Unawareness of Mental Disorder* (SUMD, Amador, et al., 1993) is popular in the research literature. Insight warrants specific assessment in every violence risk assessment but its absence is easily observed at interview when patients assert that they require neither admission nor psychiatric intervention, denying any symptoms of mental ill health. There should be targeted interventions (Buckley, et al., 2004) to address both lack of insight as a coping style or to retrain those patients whose deficit stems from cognitive impairment (Lysaker, et al., 2003). Such efforts may be rewarded with increased motivation and understanding of the treatment process (Schwartz, et al., 1997).

Social cognition

The capacity to identify another's emotions is mediated by the ability, first, to accurately identify facial expressions, and second, to represent their mental state or make inferences regarding their intentions (Premack and Woodruff, 1978, cited in Rocca and Castagna, 2007), an ability termed Theory of Mind (TOM). Both attributes are considered necessary for genuine empathy to exist (Marshall, et al., 1995). Social cognition, of which these form part, was considered worthy of inclusion in the list of cognitive factors to be measured in the MATRICS initiative (Nuechterlein, et al., 2004).

Accurate recognition of facial affect is thought to be based in the amygdala (e.g., Adolphs, et al., 1999), but the neural networks involved differ for each emotion, making them dissociable; a patient can be impaired on one but not on others (Marsh, et al., 2007). Both psychopathy (Blair, et al., 2004) and ASPD are reliably associated with an inability to recognize fearful facial expressions (Marsh and Blair, 2008). Amongst subjects with a diagnosis of schizophrenia, a relative impairment in the recognition of negative emotions is evident throughout their illness, albeit less so during periods of remission (Rocca and Castagna, 2007). This is associated with poorer community (Kee, et al., 2009) and social functioning (Hooker and Park, 2002). Social cognition more broadly may be a better predictor of functional outcome than other cognitive deficits (Niendam, et al., 2009). Amongst prisoners, accurate identification of facial affect predicted treatment readiness, treatment gains, and alteration in behaviour (Fishbein, et al., 2006).

There are a number of mechanisms by which a deficit in affect recognition may contribute to violence. Marshall et al.'s (1995) multi-component model of empathy considers the accurate identification of the emotions of others the first stage necessary for an empathic response. Blair's (2005) violence-inhibition mechanism and IES models suggest the recognition of distress cues in others forms an aversive stimulus necessary for moral referencing and reducing the likelihood of aggression. Indeed, affective empathy has been correlated with affect recognition (Decety and Lamm, 2006) and evidence suggests that the same neural networks are activated during both the experiencing of, and the perception of, emotions (Decety and Lamm, 2006). The misinterpretation of affective cues may also facilitate retaliatory aggression, particularly when coupled with a hostile attributional bias.

Most assessments of affect recognition are based on the 'Pictures of Facial Affect Series' compiled by Ekman and Friesen (1976). In clinical practice, the *Facial Expressions of Emotion Stimuli and Tests* (FEEST), a computerized adaptation of this series, with the *Emotion Hexagon Test* when further detail is required, is easy to use and interpret (Young, et al., 2002). Deficits in affect recognition tend not to be apparent during client interviews as they are unaware of their difficulty but suspicion should be raised by multiple accounts of 'unexplained' reactive aggression during social interactions. Feedback and explanation of assessment results do tend to prompt surprise and puzzlement, often followed by a 'lightbulb' onset of insight when formulations of their offending behaviour are discussed. Care should, however, be taken that clients do not interpret this aspect of their formulation as a complete explanation for past behaviour that absolves them of responsibility for their actions.

The association between impaired affect recognition and relevant psychiatric diagnoses and violence, coupled with its correlation with functional outcome and treatment responsivity, means that great consideration should be given to its inclusion in assessments of risk and its management. This is particularly so given that there are now therapeutic interventions that may begin to address this aspect of risk (e.g., Frommann, et al., 2003).

Cognitive deficits that mediate risk

In addition to those cognitive impairments directly associated with violence risk, there are a number that may impact on risk by mediating treatment responsivity. Therapeutic interventions depend on the ability to attend to, manipulate, and recall large quantities of verbal material while devising alternative strategies, all qualities often compromised in the cognitively impaired.

Fishbein, et al. (2006), in a rare attempt to determine the effects of such deficits on treatment outcome in a correctional setting, sought to relate the cognitive impairments of 224 prisoners to their ability to benefit from a cognitive-behavioural intervention. Specific cognitive impairments were found to predict treatment readiness, gain, responsivity, and completion, in addition to a reduction in institutional infractions and segregations during treatment. Evidence from non-forensic programmes suggests that cognitive impairment can predict improvement in interventions targeting psychosocial (Green, et al., 2000) and daily-life skills (Kurtz, et al., 2008). In addition to mediating the efficacy of psychological interventions, cognitive impairments – including those associated with the OFC, a deficit more common in forensic populations – may also reduce the efficacy of antipsychotic medications (Molina, et al., 2004).

A number of specific cognitive deficits are also likely to mediate the efficacy of therapeutic interventions. Meta-analysis suggests there is now 'substantial' evidence for TOM impairment in schizophrenia that remains, albeit in a milder form, during remission (Bora, et al., 2009a). The ability to infer the mental states of others is pivotal to offender treatment programmes and impairments are likely to be negatively correlated with treatment success. TOM may also mediate the relationship between fear perception and violence by contributing to the second stage of Marshall, et al.'s (1995) model of empathy, namely perspective-taking. Although TOM tests are not commonly administered to MDOs, measures used in the research literature tend to follow those of Stone et al. (1998), comprising first- and second-order false-belief tasks and a *Faux Pas Test* (e.g., Dolan and Fullam, 2004). Tests of first-order beliefs require the ability to grasp that another person holds a mistaken belief even though you know the truth. Second-order tasks require a subject to appreciate what person A thinks about what person B thinks, while the *Faux Pas Test* assesses a subject's ability to understand that a faux pas has occurred, that is, to understand the perspectives of both the speaker and the hearer of the faux pas. Given the obvious relevance of TOM to the understanding of offence cycles and subsequent risk, it is perhaps surprising that such tasks are not routinely used, although their use has been recommended previously by Murphy (2005). At the very least, the utility of these tests for risk assessments warrants further examination.

Verbal learning and memory is a core cognitive deficit in schizophrenia and significantly related to functional recovery (e.g., Tabares-Seisdedos, et al., 2008). The ability to learn and recall verbal material is a core element of most offender treatment programmes and is likely to be strongly related to treatment outcome. The MATRICS review identified the *Hopkins Verbal Learning Test* (Brandt and Benedict, 2001) as the optimal assessment in populations with a diagnosis of schizophrenia due to its multiple versions but considered the *Neuropsychological Assessment Battery Daily Living Memory Subtest* (White and Stern, 2003) psychometrically comparable (Nuechterlein, et al., 2008).

Although low intelligence is no longer considered a direct risk factor for violence, a higher level of intelligence is regarded as a protective factor and is included in the *Structured Assessment of Protective Factors* for violence risk (SAFROF, De Vries and De Vogel, 2009, this volume). In psychopathy, the relationship appears more complex, with higher IQ being correlated with an earlier onset of violent crime and release or detention failure (Johansson and Kerr, 2005). Vitacco, et al. (2005, 2008), using a four-factor model of psychopathy, found both the antisocial and interpersonal factors, including superficiality, grandiosity, and deceitfulness, positively correlated with intelligence. Attention deficits do not appear to be causally related to an increased risk of violence; however, the resulting inability to concentrate for prolonged periods is likely to mediate an individual's ability to benefit from treatment interventions. MATRICS identified the *Continuous Performance Test-Identical Pairs* version (Cornblatt, et al., 1988) as the optimum assessment in patients with a diagnosis of schizophrenia (Nuechterlein, et al., 2008).

In addition to influencing treatment efficacy, cognitive impairment is implicated in other factors considered predictive of violence risk. It is central to treatment compliance, having been found the strongest predictor of patients' ability to manage medication, even controlling for symptom severity and attitude towards medication (Jeste, et al., 2003). Cognitive impairment also predicts current and future employment problems (Mueser, et al., 2001), and substance abuse through increased impulsivity (Henderson, et al., 1998).

Neuropsychological deficits may also influence violence risk more vicariously by contributing to functional outcome in schizophrenia. Cognitive impairment predicts 'recovery', functional outcome, social functioning, performance-based everyday life skills, and quality of life in schizophrenia (Fujii and Wylie, 2002; Fujii, et al., 2004; Kopelowicz, et al., 2005; Kurtz, et al., 2008; Rocca and Castagna, 2007), which may in turn affect patient ratings on risk factors, including exposure to destabilizers, relationship instability, lack of personal support, and stress (e.g. in the HCR-20). During a 19-year follow up period, verbal memory was found to predict community functioning and, independently, executive function to predict total duration of inpatient admissions (Fuji and Wylie, 2002), the former association likely reflecting the importance of learning potential.

Cognitive measures for risk assessment

For the assessment of violence risk, the contribution of cognitive assessment should be to focus on those elements of impairment that the evidence suggests directly impact on violence potential, namely impulsivity, insight and affect recognition, plus those that most directly mediate the success of efforts to manage risk, namely theory of mind, verbal learning, and memory.

For the clinician working with individuals with a diagnosis of schizophrenia or a related disorder, the question of the most appropriate assessments for identifying cognitive strengths and weaknesses has already been answered by the recent compilation of the MATRICS *Consensus Cognitive Battery* (MCCB) by the MATRICS group (Nuechterlein, et al., 2008). The MCCB comprises 10 tests, taking 60 to 90 minutes, measuring the core deficits identified in schizophrenia (Nuechterlein, et al., 2008). This battery provides an excellent tool for the identification of strengths and weaknesses in relation to normative data, their treatment and monitoring.

All assessors of cognition should be aware of the dependence of these tests on patient effort for their efficacy. Although not as common in forensic settings as one might suppose, there are many situations where respondents may either lack the motivation to perform optimally or be motivated to perform sub-optimally. Two helpful reviews of the literature in this area are provided by the British Psychological Society (2009) and Heilbronner, et al. (2009).

Cognitive remediation for risk management

Evidence suggests that cognitive impairment is relevant to the assessment of risk of violence in MDOs but a dynamic risk factor must also be amenable to change if it is to be useful for risk management. Although cognitive risk factors can be considered relatively time invariant, there is increasing evidence that they are amenable to treatment. Cognitive remediation refers to attempts to help those with cognitive deficits 'develop the underlying cognitive skills that will make them better able to function in daily tasks, including school, work, social interactions and independent living' (Medalia and Choi, 2009, p. 354). They suggest that it is useful to 'conceptualise cognitive remediation as a learning activity where people learn to pay attention, to problem solve, to process information quickly and to remember it better' (p. 355). It is in effect a series of learning activities that allow patients to practise skills such as concentrating, problem solving and information processing. These may be administered individually or in a group, using paper and pencil or computer software programmes.

Despite, or perhaps spurred on by, the inconclusive Cochrane review of cognitive remediation for schizophrenia (Hayes and McGrath, 2000), studies have continued throughout the intervening decade such that very different conclusions can now be reached. In their review of the literature, Medalia and Choi (2009) found that five of the six meta-analyses conducted in the interim had found moderate to large effect sizes of cognitive remediation on cognitive test performance and daily functioning.

Evidence suggests that cognitive remediation benefits both inpatients and outpatients (Bellucci, et al., 2003; Sartory, et al., 2005), and can contribute to improved problem solving (Medalia, et al., 2002) and social functioning (Wykes, et al., 2003), in addition to a reduction in relapse rates (Velligan, et al., 2000). Medalia and Choi (2009) provide an excellent review of the area. Perhaps most exciting in this literature is an increasing number of computerized interventions that adjust automatically to the patients' abilities and increase in difficulty as they progress while requiring minimal staff input and expertise (e.g., Cogniplus, COGPAK, Rehacom).

Conclusion

Existing research has highlighted the relevance and importance of this field. That our clients have cognitive impairments is not in question, but the mechanisms involved and relative importance of these for risk assessment and management, and ultimately their amelioration, warrants further investigation.

It is now clear that cognitive impairments are pervasive amongst our clients, a contributing factor to their past offences, the success of their therapies, and their risk of further offending. There is little excuse for failing to address them. Formulation of risk and its management should routinely be informed by the assessment of impulsivity, insight, and affect recognition. Pre-treatment screening for deficits in TOM, verbal learning, and memory should be accompanied by adaptations to treatment programmes to enhance the efficacy of interventions, ultimately reducing risk. Such an approach will require core clinical skills and access to neurological consultancy on occasion but the benefits of including these skills in both training and continuing professional development will do much to further enhance our ability to accurately assess and manage our clients' risk.

References

Adolphs, R. (1999) 'Recognition of facial emotion in nine individuals with bilateral amygdala damage', *Neuropsychologia*, 37: 1111–17.

Adolphs, R. (2008) 'Fear, faces and the human amygdala', *Current Opinion in Neurobiology*, 18: 166–72.

American Psychiatric Association (2000) *Diagnostic and Statistical Manual of Mental Disorders: DSM-IV-TR* 4th ed. Text revision, Washington DS: Author.

Aron, A. R. and Poldrack, R. A. (2005) 'The cognitive neuroscience of response inhibition: Relevance for genetic research in attention-deficit/hyperactivity disorder', *Biological Psychiatry*, 57: 1285–92.

Babinski, L. M., Hartsough, C. S. and Lambert, N. M. (1999) 'Childhood conduct problems, hyperactivity-impulsivity, and inattention as predictors of adult criminal activity', *Journal of Child Psychology and Psychiatry and Allied Disciplines*, 40: 347–55.

Barratt, E. (1994) 'Impulsiveness and aggression', in J. Monahan and H. J. Steadman (eds) *Violence and Mental Disorder: Developments in Risk Assessment* (pp. 61–79), Chicago: University of Chicago Press.

Barratt, E. S. and Patton, J. (1983) 'Impulsivity: Cognitive, behavioural and psychophysiological correlates', in M. Zuckerman (ed) *Biological Bases of Sensation Seeking, Impulsivity and Anxiety*, Hillsdale, NJ: Lawrence Erlbaum Associates, pp. 77–122.

Bellucci, D. M., Glaberman, K. and Haslam, N. (2002) 'Computer-assisted cognitive rehabilitation reduces negative symptoms in the severely mentally ill', *Schizophrenia Research*, 59: 225–32.

Berkowitz, L. (2008) 'On the consideration of automatic as well as controlled psychological processes in aggression', *Aggressive Behaviour*, 34: 117–29.

Bjørkly, S. (2006) 'Empirical evidence of a relationship between insight and risk of violence in the mentally ill: A review of the literature', *Aggression and Violent Behavior*, 11: 414–23.

Blair, R. J. R. (2003) 'Neurobiological basis of psychopathy', *British Journal of Psychiatry*, 182: 5–7.

— (2005) 'Applying a cognitive neuroscience perspective to the disorder of psychopathy', *Development and Psychopathology*, 17: 865–91.

Blair, R. J. R., Mitchell, D. G. V., Peschardt, K. S., Colledge, E., Leonard, R. A., Shine, J. H., Murray, L. K. and Perrett, D. I. (2004) 'Reduced sensitivity to others' fearful expression in psychopathic individuals', *Personality and Individual Differences*, 37: 1111–22.

Bonta, J., Law, M. and Hanson, K. (1998) 'The prediction of criminal and violent recidivism among mentally disordered offenders: A meta-analysis', *Psychological Bulletin*, 123: 123–42.

Bora, E., Yucel, M. and Pantelis, C. (2009a) 'Theory of mind impairment in schizophrenia: Meta-analysis', *Schizophrenia Research*, 109: 1–9.

Bora, E., Yücel, M. and Pantellis, C. (2009b) 'Cognitive endophenotypes of bipolar disorder: A meta-analysis of neuropsychological deficits in euthymic patients and their first-degree relatives', *Journal of Affective Disorders*, 113: 1–20.

— (2010) 'Cognitive impairment in affective psychoses: A meta-analysis', *Schizophrenia Bulletin*, 36: 112–25.

British Psychological Society (2009) 'Assessment of effort in clinical testing of cognitive functioning for adults: Report of a working party of the Professional Practice Board', Leicester: McMillan, BPS.

Brower, M. C. and Price, B. H. (2001) 'Neuropsychiatry of frontal lobe dysfunction in violent and criminal behaviour: A critical review', *Journal of Neurology, Neurosurgery, and Psychiatry*, 71: 720–26.

Buckley, P. F., Hrouda, D. R., Friedman, L., Noffsinger, S. G., Resnick, P. J. and Camlin-Shingler, K. (2004) 'Insight and its relationship to violent behavior in patients with schizophrenia', *American Journal of Psychiatry*, 161: 1712–14.

Chamberlain, S. and Sahakian, B. (2007) 'The neuropsychiatry of impulsivity', *Current Opinion in Psychiatry*, 20: 255–61.

Craig, M. C., Catani, M., Deeley, Q., Latham, R., Daly, E., Kanaan, R., Picchioni, M., McGuire, P. K., Fahy, T. and Murphy, D. G. (2009) 'Altered connections on the road to psychopathy', *Molecular Psychiatry*, 14: 946–53.

Decety, J. and Lamm, C. (2006) 'Human empathy through the lens of social neuroscience', *Scientific World Journal*, 6: 1146–63.

Dickinson, D., Ramsey, M. E. and Gold, J. M. (2007) 'Overlooking the obvious: A meta-analytic comparison of digit symbol coding tasks and other cognitive measures in schizophrenia', *Archives of General Psychiatry*, 64: 532–42.

Dolan, M. and Fullam, R. (2004) 'Behavioural and psychometric measures of impulsivity in a personality disordered population', *Journal of Forensic Psychiatry and Psychology*, 15: 426–50.

Dolan, M. and Park, I. (2002) 'The neuropsychology of antisocial personality disorder', *Psychological Medicine*, 32: 417–27.

Dolan, M., Anderson, I. M. and Deakin, J. F. W. (2001) 'Relationship between 5-HT function and impulsivity and aggression in male offenders with personality disorder', *British Journal of Psychiatry*, 178: 352–59.

Douglas, K. and Skeem, J. (2005) 'Violence risk assessment: Getting specific about being dynamic', *Psychology, Public Policy, and Law*, 11: 347–83.

Douglas, K. S. (2008) *Drawing upon contemporary risk assessment and management principles in the revision of the HCR-20 Violence Risk Assessment Scheme.* Accessed at http://www.ohrn.nhs.uk/conferences/past/25Nov08Douglas.ppt, on 18/02/2010.

Doyle, M. and Dolan, M. (2006) 'Predicting community violence from patients discharged from mental health services', *British Journal of Psychiatry*, 189: 520–26.

Feshbach, S (1964) 'The function of aggression and the regulation of the aggressive drive', *Psychological Review*, 71: 257–72.

Fishbein, D., Scott, M., Hyde, C., Newlin, D., Hubal, R., Serin, R. et al. (2006) 'Neuropsychological and emotional deficits predict correctional treatment response', Final Report to the National Institute of Justice.

Frommann, N., Streit, M. and Wölwer, W. (2003) 'Remediation of facial affect recognition impairments in patients with schizophrenia: A new training program', *Psychiatry Research*, 117: 281–84.

Fujii, D. E. and Wylie, A. M. (2002) 'Neurocognition and community outcome in schizophrenia: Long-term predictive validity', *Schizophrenia Research*, 59: 219–23.

Fujii, D. E., Wylie, A. M. and Nathan, J. H. (2004) 'Neurocognition and long-term prediction of quality of life in outpatients with severe and persistent mental illness', *Schizophrenia Research*, 69: 67–73.

Green, M. F., Kern, R. S., Braff, D. L. and Mintz, J. (2000) 'Neurocognitive deficits and functional outcome in schizophrenia: Are we measuring the "right stuff"?', *Schizophrenia Bulletin*, 26: 119–36.

Hare, R. D. (2003) *Pschopathy Checklist – Revised Technical Manual* (2nd ed), Toronto: Multihealth Systems, Inc.

Hayes, R. L. and McGrath, J. J. (2000) 'Cognitive rehabilitation for people with schizophrenia and related conditions', Cochrane Database of Systematic Reviews, Issue 3. Art. No.: CD000968. DOI:10.1002/14651858. CD000968.

Heilbronner, R. L., Sweet, J. J., Morgan, J. E., Larrabee, G. J., Millis, S. R. et al. (2009) 'American Academy of Clinical Neuropsychology Consensus Conference Statement on the Neuropsychological Assessment of Effort, Response Bias, and Malingering', *The Clinical Neuropsychologist*, 23: 1093–1129.

Henderson, M. J., Galen, L. W. and DeLuca, J. W. (1998) 'Temperament style and substance abuse characteristics', *Substance Abuse*, 19: 61–70.

Hert, M. de, Dekker, J. M., Wood, D., Kahl, K. G., Holt, R. I. G. and Moller, H. J. (2009) 'Cardiovascular disease and diabetes in people with severe mental illness: Position statement from the European Psychiatric Association (EPA), supported by the European Association for the Study of Diabetes (EASD) and the European Society of Cardiology (ESC)', *European Psychiatry*, 24: 412–24.

Hooker, C. and Park, S. (2002) 'Emotion processing and its relationship to social functioning in schizophrenia patients', *Psychiatry Research*, 112: 41–50.

Hoptman, M. J. (2003) 'Neuroimaging studies of violence and antisocial behaviour', *Journal of Psychiatric Practice*, 9: 265–78.

Jeste, S. D., Patterson, T. L., Palmer, B. W., Dolder, C. R., Goldman, S. and Jeste, D. V. (2003) 'Cognitive predictors of medication adherence among middle-aged and older outpatients with schizophrenia', *Schizophrenia Research*, 63: 49–58.

Johansson, P. and Kerr, M. (2005) 'Psychopathy and intelligence: A second look', *Journal of Personality Disorders*, 19: 357–69.

Kee, K. S., Horan, W. P., Salovey, P., Kern, R. S., Sergi, M. J., Fiske, A. P. et al. (2009) 'Emotional intelligence in schizophrenia', *Schizophrenia Research*, 107: 61–68.

Keefe, R. S. E. (2008) 'Should cognitive impairment be included in the diagnostic criteria for schizophrenia?', *World Psychiatry*, 7: 22–28.

Kopelowicz, A., Liberman, R. P., Ventura, J., Zarate, R. and Mintz, J. (2005) 'Neurocognitive correlates of recovery from schizophrenia', *Psychological Medicine*, 35: 1165–73.

Krakowski, M. (2005) 'Schizophrenia with aggressive and violent behaviours', *Psychiatric Annals*, 35: 45–49.

Kurtz, M., Wexler, B. E., Fujimoto, M., Shagan, D. S. and Seltzer, J. C. (2008) 'Symptoms versus neurocognition as predictors of change in life skills in schizophrenia after outpatient rehabilitation', *Schizophrenia Research*, 102: 303–11.

Lincoln, T. M. and Hodgins, S. (2008) 'Is lack of insight associated with physically aggressive behaviour among people with schizophrenia living in the community?', *Journal of Nervous and Mental Disease*, 196: 62–66.

London, E. (2000) 'Orbitofrontal cortex and human drug abuse: Functional imaging', *Cerebral Cortex*, 10: 334–42.

Lysaker, P. H., Bryson, G. J., Lancaster, R. S., Evans, J. D. and Bell, M. D. (2003) 'Patterns of neurocognitive deficits and unawareness of illness in schizophrenia', *Journal of Nervous and Mental Diseases*, 191: 38–44.

Marcopulos, B. A., Fujii, D., O'Grady, J., Shaver, G., Manley, J. and Aucone, E. (2008) 'Providing neuropsychological services for persons with schizophrenia: A review of the literature and prescription for practice', in J. E. Morgan and J. H. Ricker (eds) *Textbook of Clinical Neuropsychology*, New York: Taylor and Francis.

Marsh, A. A. and Blair, R. J. R. (2008) 'Deficits in facial affect recognition among antisocial populations: A meta-analysis', *Neuroscience and Biobehavioural Reviews*, 32: 454–65.

Marsh, A. A., Kozak, M. N. and Ambady, N. (2007) 'Accurate identification of fear facial expressions predicts prosocial behavior', *Emotion*, 7: 239–51.

Marshall, W. L., Hudson, S. M., Jones, R. and Fernandez, Y. L. (1995) 'Empathy in sex offenders', *Clinical Psychology Review*, 15: 99–113.

Medalia, A. and Choi, J. (2009) 'Cognitive remediation in schizophrenia', *Neuropsychology Review*, 19: 353–64.

Medalia, A., Revheim, N. and Casey, M. (2002) 'Remediation of problem-solving skills in schizophrenia: Evidence of a persistent effect', *Schizophrenia Research*, 57: 165–71.

Moeller, F. G., Barratt, E. S., Dougherty, D. M., Schmitz, J. M. and Swann, A. C. (2001) 'Psychiatric aspects of impulsivity', *American Journal of Psychiatry*, 158: 1783–93.

Molina, V., Sanz, J., Benito, C. and Palomo, T. (2004) 'Direct association between orbitofrontal atrophy and the response of psychotic symptoms to olanzapine in schizophrenia', *Journal of Psychopharmacology*, 19: 221–28.

Monahan, J., Steadman, H. J., Silver, E., Appelbaum, P. S., Robbins, P. C., Mulvey, E. P., et al. (2001) *Rethinking Risk Assessment: The MacArthur study of Mental Disorder and Violence*, New York: Oxford University Press.

Morgan, A. B. and Lilienfeld, S. O. (2000) 'A meta-analytic review of the relation between antisocial behaviour and neuropsychological measures of executive function', *Clinical Psychology Review*, 20: 113–36.

Mueser, K. T., Salyers, M. P. and Mueser, P. R. (2001) 'A prospective analysis of work in schizophrenia', *Schizophrenia Bulletin*, 27: 281–95.

Murphy, D. (2005) 'Mind-blindness in mentally disordered offenders', *Forensic Update*, 83: 17–23.

Nestor, P. G. (2002) 'Mental disorder and violence: Personality dimensions and clinical features', *American Journal of Psychiatry*, 159: 1973–77.

Niendam, T. A., Jalbrzikowski, M. and Bearden, C. E. (2009) 'Exploring predictors of outcome in the psychosis prodrome: Implications for early identification and intervention', *Neuropsychological Review*, 19: 280–93.

Nuechterlein, K., Barc, D. M., Gold, J. M., Goldberg, T. E., Green, M. F. and Heaton, R. K. (2004) 'Identification of separable cognitive factors in schizophrenia', *Schizophrenia Research*, 72: 29–39.

Nuechterlein, K. H., Green, M. F., Kern, R. S., Baade, L. E., Barch, D. L., Cohen, J., Essock, S., Fenton, W. S., Frese, F. J., Gold, J. M., Goldberg, T., Heaton, R. K., Keefe, R. S. E., Kraemer, H., Mesholam-Gately, R., Seidman, L. J., Stover, E., Weinberger, D. R., Young, A. S., Zalcman, S., Marder, S. R., (2008) 'The MATRICS consensus battery, part 1: Test selection, reliability, and validity', *American Journal of Psychiatry*, 165: 203–13.

O'Rourke, S. and Hartley, J. B. (2011) 'The State Hospital', Unpublished.

Pietrini, P. and Bambini, V. (2009) '*Homo ferox*: The contribution of functional brain studies to understanding the neural bases of aggressive and criminal behaviour', *International Journal of Law and Psychiatry*, 32: 259–65.

Premack, D. and Woodruff, G. (1978) 'Does the chimpanzee have a theory of mind?' *Behavioural and Brain Sciences*, 4: 515–26. Cited in Rocca, P. and Castagna, F. (2007) 'Social cognition in schizophrenia', *Clinical Neuropsychiatry*, 4: 185–90.

Prentky, R. A., Knight, R. A., Lee, A. F. S. and Cerce, D. D. (1995) 'Predictive validity of lifestyle impulsivity for rapists', *Criminal Justice and Behavior*, 22: 106–28.

Rachlin, H. (1974) 'Self-control', *Behaviorism*, 2: 94–107.

Raine, A., Dodge, K., Loeber, R., Gatzke-Kopp, L., Lynam, D., Reynolds, C. et al. (2006) 'The reactive–proactive aggression questionnaire: Differential correlates of reactive and proactive aggression in adolescent boys', *Aggressive Behavior*, 32: 159–71.

Rocca, P. and Castagna, F. (2007) 'Social cognition in schizophrenia', *Clinical Neuropsychiatry*, 4(5–6): 185–90.

Rogers, R.D. and Robbins, T.W. (2001) 'Investigating the neurocognitive deficits associated with chronic drug misuse, *Current Opinion in Neurobiology*, 11: 250–57.

Sartory, G., Zorn, C., Groetzinger, G. and Windgassen, K. (2005) 'Computerized cognitive remediation improves verbal learning and processing speed in schizophrenia', *Schizophrenia Research*, 75: 219–23.

Schachar, R. and Logan, G. (1990) 'Impulsivity and inhibitory control in normal development and childhood psychopathology', *Developmental Psychology*, 26: 710–20.

Schwartz, R.C., Cohen, B.N. and Grubaugh, A. (1997) 'Does insight affect long-term inpatient treatment outcome in chronic schizophrenia?', *Comprehensive Psychiatry*, 38: 283–88.

Shelton, D., Sampl, S., Kesten, K.L., Zhang, W. and Trestman, R.L. (2009) 'Treatment of impulsive aggression in correctional settings', *Behavioural Sciences and the Law*, 27: 787–800.

Smith, T., Hull, J.W., Goodman, M., Hedayat-Harris, A., Willson, D.F., Israel, L.M. et al. (1999) 'The relative influences of symptoms, insight, and neurocognition on social adjustment in schizophrenia and schizoaffective disorder', *Journal of Nervous and Mental Disease*, 187: 102–8.

Soyka, M., Graz, C., Bottlender, R., Dirschedl, P., and Schoech, H. (2007) 'Clinical correlates of later violence and criminal offences in schizophrenia', *Schizophrenia Research*, 94: 89–98.

Stone, V.E., Baron-Cohen, S. and Knight, R.T. (1998) 'Frontal lobe contributions to theory of mind', *Journal of Cognitive Neuroscience*, 10: 640–56.

Tabares-Seisdedos, R., Balanzá-Martinez, V., Sánchez-Moreno, J., Martinez-Aran, A., Salazar-Fraile, J., Selva-Vera, G. et al. (2008) 'Neurocognitive and clinical predictors of functional outcome in patients with schizophrenia and bipolar I disorder at one-year follow-up', *Journal of Affective Disorders*, 109: 286–99.

Velligan, D., Bow-Thomas, C., Mahurin, R. K., Miller, A.L. and Halgunseth, L. C. (2000) 'Randomized controlled trial of the use of compensatory strategies to enhance adaptive functioning in outpatients with schizophrenia', *American Journal of Psychiatry*, 157: 1317–23.

Vitacco M.J., Neumann, C. S. and Jackson, R. L. (2005) 'Testing a four-factor model of psychopathy and its association with ethnicity, gender, intelligence, and violence', *Journal of Consulting and Clinical Psychology*, 73: 466–76.

Vitacco, M. J., Neuman, C. S. and Wodushek, T. (2008) 'Differential relationships between the dimensions of psychopathy and intelligence: Replication with adult jail inmates', *Criminal Justice and Behaviour*, 35: 48–55.

Vries Robbé, M. de, and Vogel, V. de (2009). 'Assessing protective factors for (sexual) violence: Research results with the SAPROF', paper presented at the 9th Conference of the International Association of Forensic Mental Health Services, Edinburgh, Scotland.

Webster, C. D. and Jackson, M. (1997) 'A clinical perspective on impulsivity', in C. D. Webster and M. A. Jackson (eds) *Impulsivity: Theory, Assessment, and Treatment*, New York: Guilford.

Webster, C. D., Douglas, K. S., Eaves, D. and Hart, S. D. (1997) *HCR-20: Assessing Risk for Violence, Version 2*, Vancouver: Mental Health, Law and Policy Institute, British Columbia.

Willcutt, E. G., Pennington, B. F., Chhabildas, N. A., Friedman, M. C., and Alexander, J. (1999) 'Psychiatric comorbidity associated with DSM-IV ADHD in a non-referred sample of twins', *Journal of the American Academy of Child and Adolescent Psychiatry*, 38: 1355–62.

Wykes, T., Reeder, C., Williams, C., Corner, J., Rice, C. and Everitt, B. (2003) 'Are the effects of cognitive remediation therapy (CRT) durable? Results from an exploratory trial in schizophrenia', *Schizophrenia Research*, 61: 163–74.

Bibliography of test and rehabiliation batteries

CANTAB: Cambridge Cognition Ltd. Cambridge Ltd.

CogniPlus: http://www.schuhfried.at/index.php?id=259.

COGPAK: http://www.cogpack.com/USA/frames.htm.

CPT-IP: Cornblatt, B. A., Rish, N. J., Faris, G., Friedman, D. and Erlenmeyer-Kimling, L. (1988) 'The Continuous Performance Test, Identical Pairs Version (CPT-IP):1. New findings about sustained attention in normal families', *Psychiatric Research*, 26: 223–38.

Go No-Go: Simmonds, D. J., Pekar, J. J. and Mostofsky, S. H. (2008) 'Meta-analysis of Go/No-Go Tasks demonstrating that fMRI activation associated with response inhibition is task dependent', *Neuropsychologica*, 46: 224–32.

Hayling and Brixton: Burgess, P. and Shallice, T. (1997) *The Hayling and Brixton Tests. Test Manual,* Bury St Edmunds, UK: Thames Valley Test Company.

HVLT: Brand, J. and Benedict, R. H. B. (2001) *The Hopkins Verbal Learning Test-Revised*, Odessa, Fl: Psychological Assessment Resources, Inc.

NAB: White, T. and Stern, R. A. (2003) *Neuropsychological Assessment Battery: Psychometric and Technical Manual,* Lutz, Fl: Psychological Assessment Resources, Inc.

PANNS: Kay, S. R., Fiszbein, A. and Opler, L. A. (1987) 'The Positive and Negative Syndrome Scale (PANSS) for schizophrenia', *Schizophrenia Bulletin*, 13: 261–76.

PCL-R: Hare, R. D. (2003) *The Hare Psychopathy Checklist–Revised manual,* North Tonawanda, NY: Multi-Health Systems.

Pictures of Facial Affect: Ekman, P. and Friesen, W. V. (1976) *Pictures of Facial Affect,* Palo Alto, California: Consulting Psychologists Press.

Rehacom: http://rehacom.co.uk.

SUMD: Amador, X. F., Strauss, D. H., Yale, S. A., Flaum, M. M., Endicott, J. and Gorman, J. M. (1993) 'Assessment of insight in psychosis', *American Journal of Psychiatry.* 150: 873–79.

Stroop Test: Stroop neuropsychological screening test (SNST) (1989) Trenerry, M. R., Crosson, B. Deboe, J. and Leber, W. R., Psychological Assessment Resources, Inc.

FEEST: Young, A., Perrett, D., Calder, A. Sprengelmeyer, R. and Ekman, P (2002) *Facial Expressions of Emotion: Stimuli and Test (FEEST),* Bury St Edmunds, Suffolk: Thames Valley Test Company.

9 Making delinquency prevention work with children and adolescents

From risk assessment to effective interventions

Corine de Ruiter and Leena K. Augimeri

Introduction

Studies have shown that individuals with an early onset of delinquency, prior to the age of 12, are more at risk of later serious violent and chronic offending by three times, as compared to those individuals who begin their delinquent careers in adolescence (Loeber and Farrington, 2001; Moffitt, 1993). This particular group of serious and persistent juvenile offenders accounts for 50 per cent of all juvenile offending (Loeber and Farrington, 1998). The economic cost of serious antisocial behavior in children and adolescents is substantial and the implications for society can be enormous (Loeber, Slot, van der Laan, and Hoeve, 2008). Such antisocial behaviors typically start before the age of 14 (Loeber, et al., 2008) and include costs that may relate to accessing health, mental health, child welfare, and special education. For example, Romeo, Knapp and Scott (2006) reported an annual cost of approximately GB £6,000 per year for children between the ages of three and eight years demonstrating antisocial behavior. Koegl (2011) conducted a longitudinal analysis on a clinical sample of Canadian children with conduct problems and found, for those who entered the juvenile justice system, the costs per case averaged approximately US $100K per year over a nine-year period. When looking at high-risk offenders, cost per case increased to upwards of US $1.4 million, and Koegl (2011) commented that although crime prevention programs may reach and benefit a small fraction of children, they can still produce enormous savings to society. Foster, Jones, and the Conduct Problems Prevention Research Group (2005) also concluded that '. . . public expenditures may be reduced if resources are moved from coping with problem behaviors to preventing them' (p. 1771). A similar recommendation was formulated by Romeo, et al. (2006): 'Wider uptake of evidence-based interventions is likely to lead to considerable economic benefits in the short term, and probably even more in the long term' (p. 547).

Child and adolescent offenders are a heterogeneous group in terms of risk status and the factors that contribute to antisocial behavior. Over the past few decades, epidemiological and longitudinal research has been successful in identifying individual and contextual risk factors for young people engaging in future delinquency (Howell, 2003, 2009; Lahey, Moffitt, and Caspi, 2003; Loeber, Farrington, and Petechuk, 2003). Some of these factors are: lack of empathy or callous-unemotional traits[1] (White and Frick, 2010), Attention Deficit Hyperactivity Disorder (ADHD; Biederman, Mick, Faraone, and Burback, 2001; Fazel, Doll, and Långström, 2008), poor parenting styles (Snyder and Stoolmiller, 2002), and negative peer influences (Dishion, Spracklen, Andrews, and Patterson, 1996; Snyder, 2002). Furthermore, as much as possible, preventive interventions should target those risk factors that are causally linked to the antisocial behavior in each individual case. In order to facilitate such a tailor-made preventive strategy, a comprehensive psychosocial risk assessment framework is required (Augimeri, Enebrink, Walsh, and Jiang, 2010). Such a framework should include promotive and protective factors as well as risk factors, as the failure to consider both may lead to unbalanced and biased assessments (Rogers, 2000), particularly with regard to children and adolescents who are still developing. Some researchers (Farrington, Loeber, Jolliffe, and Pardini, 2008; Loeber, Slot, and Stouthamer-Loeber, 2008; Stouthamer-Loeber, Loeber, Wei, Farrington, and Wikström, 2002) conceptualize promotive factors as factors that lower the probability of problem behavior, regardless of risk level. Similarly, protective factors are factors that moderate the effects of risk on problem behavior (Fergusson and Lynskey, 1996; Pollard, Hawkins, and Arthur, 1999; Rutter, 2003). Protective factors are thus a subcategory of promotive factors that reduce the effects of risk factors on problem behavior (Farrington, et al., 2008). Research has shown that protective factors can act as buffers against risk factors and predict desistance from reoffending in children and adolescents (Lodewijks, de Ruiter, and Doreleijers, 2010; Stouthamer-Loeber, Wei, Masten, and Loeber, 2004).

The increase in our theoretical and empirical understanding of antisocial behavior in youth has resulted in great advances in evidence-based assessment and interventions. This chapter will provide an overview of validated structured risk assessment tools available for child and adolescent offenders as well as those at high risk of becoming so. Subsequently, we will review the scientific evidence base on multimodal risk management interventions for children and adolescents. The manner in which structured risk assessment and risk management are connected in everyday clinical practice will be illustrated with a case example from Toronto's Center for Children Committing Offences at the Child Develop-ment Institute (CDI). We will also provide a brief note on the implementation of evidence-based risk prevention at the community level. Finally, suggestions for future research into the further refinement of our structured risk assessment and clinical risk management strategies are presented.

Structured professional risk assessment for future offending and violence in children and adolescents

Factors that are empirically associated with increased risk of antisocial behavior in children and adolescents have been incorporated into instruments for structured risk assessment during the last decades. Furthermore, structured risk assessment tools typically contain static and dynamic items. In this context, the term 'static' implies that these items are not subject to change, as opposed to the dynamic items, which may vary. So-called structured professional judgment (SPJ) risk assessment tools contain a fixed set of empirically based risk factors (and sometimes also protective factors), which are weighed and integrated into a final risk estimate by an experienced forensic mental health professional (Douglas and Otto, 2010). However, the goal of the SPJ tools is risk prevention, not risk prediction; therefore, SPJ tools are not reliant on the total score, nor do they encourage the use of cutoff scores to predict varying levels of risk. The focus of SPJ tools is intervention planning with a goal to reduce and manage risk. By doing so, the SPJ tools encourage the assessors to draw on the strengths of both the clinical and actuarial approaches to clinical risk management decision-making (Borum and Douglas, 2003).

EARL-20 B and EARL-21G

Since their development over a decade ago, research on the *Early Assessment Risk Lists* for boys (EARL-20B) and girls (EARL-21G) has flourished (Augimeri, Enebrink, Walsh, and Jiang, 2010; Augimeri, Walsh, Liddon, and Dassinger, 2011). Previous EARL-20B studies have included findings on the tools' reliability and validity. Total EARL-20B score values showed acceptable mean inter-rater reliability (e.g., Mean = .92; Enebrink, Långström, and Gumpert, 2006), which is comparable to other structured professional judgment tools, such as the *Structured Assessment of Violence Risk in Youth* (SAVRY) (.81; Catchpole and Gretton, 2003) and *Short Term Assessment of Risk and Treatability* (START) (.87; Nicholls, Brink, Desmarais, Webster, and Martin, 2006). To date, a number of studies have been completed on the EARL-21G, all of which have produced similar positive findings to the EARL-20B in terms of the clinical utility, reliability and validity of the tool (Levene, Walsh, Augimeri, and Pepler, 2004). The predictive validity of the EARLs was examined in several studies and has been shown to be good for parent and teacher ratings of aggression and criminal outcomes (Augimeri, Desmarais, Koegl, Jiang, and Webster, 2009; Enebrink, et al., 2006). For example, Enebrink and colleagues (2006) found, for a sample of 76 clinic-referred children, that the EARL-20B summary risk rating (low, moderate, high) showed good predictive validity for parent and teacher ratings of reactive and proactive aggression at six months (rs = .47-.58) and 30 months (rs = .31-.50) follow-up. For a comprehensive review, see Augimeri, et al. (2010).

To further the ecological validity of the research on the EARLs, a cross-sector collaboration between researchers and practitioners was undertaken to examine their predictive quality and content validity (Augimeri, Pepler, Walsh, Jiang and Dassinger, 2010). The investigators found that the *Family* subscale significantly predicts future criminal offences for both the EARL-20B and EARL-21G, with the EARL Total score and *Responsivity* subscale score predicting for boys only. Several individual EARL risk items were also found to predict for boys: *Caregiver Continuity, Parenting Style, Onset of Behavioural Difficulties, Likeability, Peer*

Socialization, Authority Contact, Antisocial Attitudes, Antisocial Behaviour, and *Family Responsivity.* For girls, however, the one *Family* item, *Antisocial Values and Conduct,* was a strong predictor of criminal outcome.

This investigation generated a similar three-factor model structure for the EARL-20B, as previously reported in Augimeri (2005). The three factors are labeled *Child, Family,* and *Biological.* For girls, the findings did not replicate previous observations from a retrospective sample (i.e., *Family, Child* and *Amenability*; Augimeri, et al., 2011). A new three-factor model was produced, with a *Relational Disturbance* factor. It is comprised of the following items: *Caregiver Continuity, Abuse/Neglect/Trauma, Antisocial Values and Conduct* and *Sexual Development.* The newly generated three-factor model for the EARL-20B, with the *Family, Child* and *Biological* factors, accurately predicted entry into the criminal justice system for boys. Out of the three-factor model generated for the EARL-21G, consisting of *Family, Child* and *Relational Disturbance,* only the latter predicted increased risk of future criminal offences for girls. Overall, these findings indicate that some of the risk factors for aggression and delinquency are to a certain degree gender specific.[2] The practical utility of the distinction between these three factors, or domains, lies in their value in intervention planning. Depending on the weight of the different domains, different intervention priorities and strategies should be implemented.

SAVRY. The SAVRY (Borum, Bartel, and Forth, 2006) is a structured professional judgment guide devised for the assessment of youths aged between 12 and 18 who have been detained or referred for assessment of violence risk (Borum, Lodewijks, Bartel, and Forth, 2010). The SAVRY protocol consists of 24 risk items and six protective items. Risk items are categorized into three subsets: *Historical, Individual,* and *Social/Contextual,* with one risk factor that directly relates to deficiencies in empathy. The SAVRY also addresses additional factors or situational variables that may be person-specific, but their influence is crucial in comprehending the propensity for future violence. This approach is an inherent component to many structured professional judgment guides, allowing the qualified clinician to take into account issues not included in the 24 risk factors listed in the SAVRY. The SAVRY draws on the structured professional judgment approach in that the items are not summed to arrive at a risk rating but are used to inform clinical risk management plans. Clinicians weigh and evaluate the collection and pattern of risk factors to arrive at a global risk rating of low, moderate, or high, versus being reliant on cutoff scores to determine level of risk, as in non-SPJ tools. A unique feature of the SAVRY is its inclusion of six protective factors that might mitigate the youth's risk.

The psychometric properties of the SAVRY are promising. Using trained student raters, the single-rater intraclass correlation coefficient (ICC) was .81 for the SAVRY Risk Total score and .77 for the Summary Risk Rating (Catchpole and Gretton, 2003). Comparably, McEachran (2001) found relatively high inter-rater reliability (.83) for the SAVRY Risk Total and moderate coefficients (.72) for the Summary Risk Rating. In several Dutch studies of adolescent offenders from successive phases in the legal process (pre-trial, during residential stay and after release from a juvenile justice facility), the SAVRY showed good to excellent inter-rater reliability (Lodewijks, Doreleijers, de Ruiter, and Borum, 2008a; Lodewijks, Doreleijers, and de Ruiter, 2008b; Lodewijks, de Ruiter, and Doreleijers, 2009). For instance, in Lodewijks, et al. (2008a), the inter-rater reliability of the SAVRY domains and SAVRY Risk Total ranged from good to excellent (single measure ICC: Risk Total = .74, *Historical* = .74, *Social/Contextual* = .61, *Individual* = .82 and *Protective* = .86). The inter-rater reliability of the Summary Risk Rating was also excellent (ICC = .85).

As for predictive accuracy, in the initial validation sample (Bartel, et al., 2000), SAVRY Risk Total scores[3] were significantly related to measures of institutional aggressive behavior (r = .40) and aggressive conduct disorder symptoms (r = .52). SAVRY Summary Risk Ratings have also been found to correlate significantly with outcome measures of community violence (Gretton and Abramowitz, 2002; McEachran, 2001). Using the Receiver Operating Characteristic (ROC) analysis, Areas under the Curve (AUCs) for the SAVRY Risk Total averaged between .74 and .80 across these North-American studies. Interestingly, the overall risk judgment (Summary Risk Rating) consistently performed as well as, and often better than, the actuarial summation of the scores. For example, using the ROC analysis, McEachran (2001) found an AUC for the SAVRY Risk Total of .70, though the AUC for the SAVRY Summary Risk Rating was .89. SAVRY Risk Total scores also demonstrated high predictive validity in five samples of Dutch juvenile offenders (Lodewijks, et al. 2008a, 2008b, 2010). For instance, the AUC for the Summary Risk Rating was .86 for physical violence against persons within a secure residential institution (Lodewijks, et al. 2008a), and .71 for violent reoffending in the community after three years follow-up (Lodewijks, et al. 2008b). Significant associations were also found in all five samples between the *Individual* subscale and violent outcomes, and in four out of five samples between the *Social/Contextual* subscale and violent outcomes. Lodewijks, et al. did not find any association between the *Historical* scale and violent outcomes in any sample in their studies. The SAVRY was also significantly more accurate in predicting violent recidivism than unstructured clinical judgment (Lodewijks, et al., 2008b). A qualifying comment as to the clinical relevance of predictive validity studies is in order here: SPJ risk assessment tools are designed for risk management and risk prevention purposes (Douglas and Kropp, 2002). Thus, the ultimate test of these instruments lies in their ability to inform effective interventions to reduce future risk, though such research has not been conducted yet.

The practice of structured risk assessment with young offenders

Having available reliable and valid risk assessment tools such as those noted (i.e., EARLs, SAVRY) increases the chance that risk assessments will be evidence-based and accurate. Nevertheless, the quality of risk assessment is only partially determined by the quality of the device itself; the expertise of the professional that uses the tool is equally important. Through providing training workshops on the proper use of tools like the EARLs and the SAVRY, we have noticed that the added value of using structured risk assessment versus unstructured clinical judgment only becomes apparent when professionals are rigorous in the following ways. Their approach to the collection of information relating to the different risk factors must be thorough. In some cases, this includes a comprehensive assessment of intelligence, personality features, and psychopathology of the child/adolescent. Data must be collected from a variety of agents in addition to the child, such as his/her caretakers, teachers, health-care professionals, using a variety of sources of information such as their respective records (e.g., school records, police records and standardized measures) as it is important to corroborate such findings to arrive at a clear understanding of the child in question. Professionals who use risk=assessment tools for children and juveniles should be trained in child development and developmental psychopathology as the individuals in question are still developing. The issue of whether certain behaviors or personality traits are 'non-normative' or part of a developmental process often arises (Johnstone and Cooke, 2004). Lastly, it cannot be emphasized enough that users should always have the corresponding risk assessment guide at hand when assessing a case, to prevent definition drift, which seriously reduces the fidelity of the tools. These are the minimum standards for use mentioned in SPJ manuals but also in the major textbooks on forensic mental health assessment (e.g., Heilbrun, Grisso, and Goldstein, 2008). Hart (2001) stated that the 'ultimate goal' of risk assessment should be violence prevention, and that a 'good risk assessment should: (1) yield consistent or replicable results; (2) be prescriptive, and (3) transparent' (p. 15). The following clinical case and completed EARL-20B Summary Sheet provides an example of these important principles in practice.

Clinical case example: Mason Edwards

Mason is a nine-year old boy. He is articulate, bright and likeable, even though adults find his behavior challenging at times. He enjoys swimming, skating and playing with his toys. He says he wants to be a firefighter or police officer when he grows up. Reports indicate he is barely passing his class subjects; the most recent academic report card indicated the majority of his marks were in the 50–69 per cent range. The teacher reported that he is not performing to his ability, as his reading skills are above grade level. Currently, he is in a specialized class with nine other children who are also experiencing serious behavioral issues – the teacher feels his conduct is impeding his ability to focus, which is the cause of his poor academic performance. Socially, the teacher reports he has positive social skills and is able to make friends; however, he has difficulty keeping them. He has also been known to associate with other children who get into trouble.

   Mason and his older sister (aged 12) recently rejoined their family after being in foster care for the past four years. Crystal (Mason's mother) could not manage her children and they were placed in care. At the time, she was experiencing severe depression and other psychiatric problems. She frequently used punitive discipline and had difficulty supervising and monitoring her children. (This is still apparent today.) In addition, the children witnessed extreme violence from various partners towards their mother. During the time that Mason and his sister were away from their mother, she had two more children (a boy aged four and a girl aged one). The family is currently receiving government assistance (financial help) and living in subsidized housing. The house is large enough for the family but poorly maintained. It is in a very 'tough' neighbourhood; however, the area has access to community resources (e.g., children's mental health center, recreation activities), which Crystal has been able to access for some help. They are hoping to stay in this home for a few years as the family has moved five times in the past five years. Besides these supports and a few close friends that Crystal relies on, the family is quite isolated.

In addition to the multiple moves and issues presented above, this family is experiencing other stressors. Crystal reports that her children constantly argue and fight and that Mason's behavior is problematic. She feels he is manipulative, withdrawn, depressed, can be physically aggressive (he has punched holes in the wall and broken windows), and often lies. He has also been stealing from the local store since he was seven years old, which has resulted in police contact. She attributes his behavior to being angry and/or having been in care. Crystal reports that to help her cope she occasionally drinks alcohol and there is a suspicion that she also uses illegal drugs. Mason has also admitted on a self-report delinquency measure that he destroys property at home, has shoplifted, has been in physical fights with his older sister, which often resulted in her being bruised and at times caused her to bleed, fights with peers and has been sent home from school for 'bad behavior'. He also indicated that he does not like going home and prefers to hang out on the streets with older kids he knows (many of whom get into trouble with the law). He reports feeling as though he is treated the worst in his family and that his mother resents him because she compares him to his father whom she greatly dislikes. He indicates feeling hopeless and angry towards his mother as he feels she will not change and treats him unfairly compared to the rest of his siblings. Reports from other sources also indicate that Mason has experienced both excessive physical and emotional abuse by his mother and her previous partners. Mason understands the concept of right from wrong but feels that being physical is the only way to get what he wants. He has a hard time feeling empathic towards others because he feels 'no one loves or cares about him'. He indicates that this makes him feel sad and that, on occasion, he has thought about suicide. He has indicated he wants to get help to control his anger but is not sure it will help. Crystal, on the other hand, feels that she has attended a number of parenting courses and believes that it is Mason who needs the help and not her.

As noted above, one of the goals of risk assessment is to summarize all available and relevant information in a structured and transparent manner so that the clinician assessing the case can formulate an effective clinical risk management plan based on the child's level of risk and need. Figure 9.1 presents a sample of a completed EARL-20B Summary Sheet for Mason. The information is organized under three main risk categories: *Family, Child* and *Responsivity*. The information becomes 'transparent' as the corresponding information is noted beside each item (see italics). Each item is scored on a three-point scale (0 = not present, 1 = possibly present, 2 = definitely present). The *Critical Risk* section helps clinicians to 'red flag' areas of particular concern that require immediate attention. This is why it is important, as noted above, to use multiple sources of information (e.g., school reports, standardized measures) from a variety of respondents (e.g., parent/caregiver, teacher, child) to ascertain the level of risk and need. At the bottom of the form is a section entitled *Overall Clinical Judgment*. This allows the clinician the 'clinical freedom' to denote level of risk (low, moderate or high) independent of the Total Score. As noted previously, the EARLs are part of the SPJ family of risk assessment tools and do not rely on cutoff scores to denote level of risk. Typically, there will be correspondence between Total Score and final risk estimate; that is, the higher the score the greater the risk. The *Overall Judgment* also allows for additional information that may not get captured in the tool and/or protective information that may buffer the risk scores rendered. In addition, to further help clinicians formulate an effective clinical risk management plan based on the EARL assessment, an EARL Case Planning Form was developed (see the section below and Figure 9.2) that corresponds with the EARL Summary Sheet (see Figure 9.1).

Effective preventive and risk management interventions

Risk management in practice

A key aspect of good clinical risk assessment is the ability to then use the information to formulate an effective clinical risk management plan ('prescription for intervention'). This involves the completion of a structured professional judgment risk/need assessment tool such as the EARL-20B (for boys) or the EARL-21G (for girls), followed by a thorough eco-systemic assessment. It has been noted in the scientific literature that this process from risk assessment to management seems to be missing a key ingredient when it comes to designing effective crime-prevention programs for children and youth (Jones and Wyant, 2007). In 2001, Andrews introduced the principles of risk-need-responsivity for effective correctional programs. This highlighted the need to match level of risk and need with the appropriate treatment interventions to ensure successful treatment response.

Since the creation of the EARL-20B (1998; 2001) and the EARL-21G (2001), one of the authors developed the EARL Case Planning Form that corresponds with the EARL Summary Sheet (see Figure 9.1). This form evolved out of a need to assist clinicians in linking the information from the EARL risk assessment to clinical risk management strategies (pinpointing areas for immediate intervention).

Figure 9.2 provides a sample for the case of Mason Edwards. One begins by examining the *Overall Clinical Judgment* and the *Critical Risk Items*. Part of that examination involves exploring possible protective factors that may diminish the risk level in the identified critical risk items. Based on the information noted, the clinician decides the services that are available within the community to best meet the needs of the particular client system.

The EARL-20B Version 2 Summary Sheet
(To be used in association with the EARL-20B, Version 2 Manual)

Child's Name or ID#: __Mason Edwards__   Date: __2010–03–01__
(First name SURNAME)   (YYYY–MM–DD)

Assessor: __L.K.A__   Child's DOB: __2001–02–15__   Age: __9__
(YYYY–MM–DD)

Family Items		Rating (0-1-2)	Critical Risk
F1	Household Circumstances *government assistance, subsidized housing, poorly maintained*	2	
F2	Caregiver Continuity *single led family (mother), children in care/foster home (4 years)*	2	
F3	Supports *few close friends, community social service agency*	1	✓
F4	Stressors *parenting distress, high family mobility – 5 moves in 5 yrs, sibling rivalry, maternal depression*	2	
F5	Parenting Style *inconsistent, spanking/hitting (puncture), lack of supervision/monitoring*	2	✓
F6	Antisocial Values and Conduct *domestic violence (between Mom and partners), suspected alcohol/drug abuse*	2	

Child Items		Rating (0-1-2)	Critical Risk
C1	Developmental Problem *no identified concerns*	0	
C2	Onset of Behavioral Difficulties *7 years of age (started stealing)*	1	
C3	Abuse/Neglect/Trauma *witnessed extreme family violence, neglect, spanking*	2	✓
C4	HIA (Hyperactivity/Impulsivity/Attention Deficits) *impulsive, concentration problems*	1	✓
C5	Likeability *likeable (teacher/clinician), pleasant demeanor, attractive, articulate/bright*	0	✓
C6	Peer Socialization *history of problems with peers, able to make friends, difficulty keeping them*	1	✓
C7	Academic Performance *specialized beh class – beh. vs academics, at grade level (4) – reading above, marks poor*	2	✓
C8	Neighborhood *a tough area, resources available (mental health, recreation)*	1	
C9	Authority Contact *principal, teachers, police*	2	
C10	Antisocial Attitudes *antisocial thinking, weak in areas of cooperation and empathy, manipulative*	2	✓
C11	Antisocial Behaviour *stealing, aggression (physical/verbal), lying, oppositional, delinquent behavior*	2	
C12	Coping Ability *withdrawn, depressive symptoms (feels unloved, sad), suicide ideation*	2	✓

Responsivity Items		Rating (0-1-2)	Critical Risk
R1	Family Responsivity *did not follow through in past, feels it is her child's issue not hers*	2	✓
R2	Child Responsivity *guarded, would like to deal with his anger*	1	✓

Overall Clinical Judgment	LOW	MOD	HIGH		TOTAL SCORE	30
	LOW	MOD	✓			

Notes: *Mason has some very positive attributes – he is likeable, bright and articulate. He is a bit guarded in getting help but is interested in learning how to control his anger. He is in a grade 4 behavioral class functioning at grade level (his marks are low; his reading skills are above grade level). Teachers report that his behavior impedes his ability to stay focused. The goal – build on his strengths. Based on the above risk summary, the following clinical risk management strategies are recommended: (1) connect Mother to a children's mental health center where she can access a Parent Group – to learn effective parenting strategies; (2) build a support system for this family – ensure continued monitoring by child protection; (3) promote family responsivity by helping Mother with instrumental challenges (e.g., transportation, child care); (4) help Mom find a service to deal with her depression/anger; (5) enroll Mason in anger management program (e.g., SNAP®); (6) connect him to a structured community activity (e.g., swimming, skating) – build on his social skills and encourage him to make some new friends; (7) academic tutoring; (8) assess items C4 and C12 – HIA versus anxiety/depression (assess suicide ideation immediately) – it is suspected that the impulsivity and concentration problems may be tied into C3 (Abuse/Neglect/Trauma); and (9) promote child responsivity (e.g., weekly telephone reminder calls to get to group, individual befriending/mentoring at home and school to explore identified issues/ensure engagement).*

Figure 9.1 The EARL-20B Version 2 Summary Sheet

EARL CASE PLANNING ECO-SYSTEMIC ASSESSMENT FORM

NAME: *Mason Edwards*	ID # *01216*
BIRTHDATE: February *15, 2001*	ASSESSOR: *Helena Hrynkiw*
SCREENING DATE(S): *March 3, 2010*	SERVICE COORDINATOR: *Nicola Perring*
TOTAL EARL SCORE: *30*	OVERALL CLINICAL JUDGMENT: ☐ LOW ☐ MOD ☑ HIGH

CRITICAL RISK ITEM(S)		REASON
F3	Supports	Family has few identified supports in place; multiple stressors. Focus – strengthen the support system to diminish/buffer the stressors.
F5	Parenting Style	Parent is inconsistent, does not adequately monitor child and uses punitive discipline methods – could be contributing to the child's problematic behavior (e.g., not coming home after school, staying out late at night and 'hanging out' on the streets with older delinquent peers).
C3	Abuse/Neglect/Trauma	Child has experienced physical and emotional abuse and been exposed to extreme violence by mother's partners.
C4	HIA (Hyperactivity/Impulsivity/ Attention Deficits)	Issues noted in regards to impulsivity and concentration problems. No formal testing/assessment has been conducted. Not sure if this is in relation to HIA or possible anxiety or depression.
C5	Likeability	Adults see this boy as likeable. This is in fact an important positive attribute for this child. Need to build on this strength.
C6	Peer Socialization	History of strained peer relationships. Determine what the issues are and how to build on his positive qualities so that he can form and keep positive relationships/ friendships.
C7	Academic Performance	This child is not performing to his ability (teacher indicates he is above grade level in reading but functioning at 50-60%). Strengthen academic performance (in school supports and incentives) to ensure school success.
C10	Antisocial Attitudes	Concerns that this child lacks empathy. He can also be manipulative. Important for treatment to challenge cognitive distortions/thinking errors without making him feel alienated or interfere with therapeutic alliance.
C12	Coping Ability	This boy is displaying depressive symptoms. He is withdrawn, sad and feels unloved. He sometimes also talks about killing himself. Assess this right away to determine suicidal tendencies.
R1	Family Responsivity	Mother does not seem interested in service. She feels she is not in need of assistance ('It is my son's problem, not mine.'). Focus on engagement issues.
R2	Child Responsivity	Child is interested in getting help but guarded. Focus on engaging this child in a therapeutic relationship.

SUGGESTED CLINICAL RISK MANAGEMENT STRATEGIES – BASED ON EARL ASSESSMENT

CHILD:

☑ ANGER/IMPULSE CONTROL AND SOCIAL PROBLEM SOLVING SKILLS TRAINING

☑ STRUCTURED MENTORING PROGRAM

☑ SUPERVISED RECREATION WITH PEERS

☑ SCHOOL CONSULTATION – CLASSROOM BEHAVIOURAL MANAGEMENT

☑ SCHOOL ADVOCACY

☑ ACADEMIC TUTORING

☐ STIMULANT MEDICATION

☑ SPECIALIZED MENTAL HEALTH SERVICES (e.g. for psychoses, major affective disorder, trauma, substance abuse)

Figure 9.2 EARL Case Planning Eco-Systemic Assessment Form

TYPE OF SERVICE RECOMMENDED BASED ON OVERALL CLINICAL JUDGMENT LEVEL

☑ HIGH INTENSITY ☐ MODERATE INTENSITY ☐ LOW INTENSITY

RECOMMENDED SERVCE:

Based on the information above and corresponding EARL-20B risk assessment it is suggested that this child and his family be referred to a children's mental health center specializing in latency-aged children with disruptive behavior problems. A multi-modal cognitive behavioral service is highly recommended for Mason and his family (e.g., SNAP® Under 12 Outreach Project for Boys at the Child Development Institute). This program offers the following recommended service components that meet the suggested needs (SNAP® Boys Group, a self-control and problem solving group; SNAP® Parent Group that focuses on effective parent management strategies; Individual Counseling/Mentoring and connections to structured community recreation activities; SNAP Parenting, Individual family counselling; School Support/Advocacy to assist the child in school; and Academic Tutoring to booster the child's academics through a tutoring club). A psychiatric assessment is critical to address the identified depression and suicide ideation risk. As Mason's mother seems to be guarded as noted in the Family Responsivity (R1) risk item, all attempts need to be made to engage this family in service. To further ensure treatment success, establishing a strong therapeutic alliance/connection with both Mason and his mother is important. Ongoing treatment reviews (every six months) to ensure treatment compliance and outcome monitoring need to be conducted.

PLANNING

NEAREST INTERSECTION TO CHILD'S HOME: *Rogers Road and Black Creek*

CLOSEST APPROPRIATE SERVICE PROVIDER(S): *Child Development Institute*

AGENCY REFERRED TO: *Child Development Institute*	**DATE:** *August 5, 2010*

DESIGNATED PROGRAM: *SNAP® Under 12 Outreach Program for Boys*

CONTACT PERSON: *Karen Sewell*	**TITLE:** *Program Manager/Intake*
PHONE NUMBER: *416–654–8989*	**EMAIL ADDRESS:** *not applicable*

AGENCY ADDRESS: *46 St. Clair Gardens, Toronto, Ontario, M6E 3V4*

FOLLOW-UP PLAN: *Ensure family is actively participating in treatment; suggested recommendations have been implemented; ongoing treatment reviews; and monitoring of treatment outcomes.*

EARL ASSESSOR SIGNATURE: Helena Hrynkiw

Figure 9.2 (continued)

During the past few decades, the knowledge base on what is effective in the prevention and treatment of child and adolescent offending has increased tremendously. This knowledge base has been summarized in a number of excellent publications on the subject (e.g., Farrington and Welsh, 2007; Howell, 2003, 2009; Loeber, et al., 2008), and is now also available from websites of accredited rating bodies, such as the US Office of Juvenile Justice and Delinquency Prevention (http://www2.dsgonline.com/mpg/), the US White House initiative, Model Program Guides (http://www.findyouthinfo.gov) and the Canadian National Crime Prevention Centre (http://www.publicsafety.gc.ca/res/cp/res/2008-pcpp-eng.aspx). To a similar extent, our knowledge of what is *in*effective in reducing juvenile delinquency has accumulated. For example, correctional boot camps using the traditional military-style model of discipline are ineffective in reducing recidivism

(Aos, Phipps, Barnoski, and Lieb, 2001), and the potential for psychological and physical abuse of youngsters in these settings is substantial (MacKenzie, Wilson, Armstrong, and Gover, 2001). Examples of other ineffective approaches are 'Scared Straight', that is, bringing youth into prison and subjecting them to threats, bullying and intimidation (Lipsey and Wilson, 1998) and 'punishing smarter' techniques, such as home confinement, increased surveillance, and shock incarceration (Gendreau and Goggin, 1996). Some of these 'get tough' approaches even seem to result in slight increases in recidivism (Howell, 2003, p. 132). Nevertheless, many of these punitive approaches continue to be popular among policymakers, politicians and the general public, as they seem to fulfil a wish to confer a penalty on those who have caused harm to society.

A complete review of all evidence-based interventions available to reduce the risk of future antisocial behavior in children and adolescents is beyond the scope of this chapter. Instead, we will focus on two multimodal evidence-based interventions designed specifically for children and youth in conflict with the law that have received top effectiveness designations from the above-noted accredited rating bodies. These models include involvement with parents, youth, and other systems (e.g., schools) and they are the SNAP® (Stop Now And Plan) model for young children between 6 and 12 years of age and multisystemic therapy (MST) for youths between 12 and 17 years of age. These two interventions were selected because they coincide with the ecological, systems framework that is a central aspect of risk-prevention tools such as the EARLs and SAVRY.

SNAP® (Stop Now And Plan)

Twenty-five years ago, a small community-based organization (Earlscourt Child and Family Centre, now called Child Development Institute) in Toronto in Canada, which specialized in working with children with disruptive behavior problems, created an innovative model for young children in conflict with the law. The program, called SNAP® (for more details see www.stopnowandplan.com), evolved from the best possible treatment ingredients identified in the scientific literature on 'what worked' with children and youth with conduct problems. It resulted in gender-specific cognitive-behavioral multi-component models based in a scientist-practitioner framework. The programs are fully manualized, and use an *adaptive* intervention structure; treatment dosage is dependent on level of risk and need (Collins, Murphy and Bierman, 2004). To ensure treatment adherence and compliance, a *SNAP® Fidelity and Integrity Rating Index* is used to monitor SNAP® replications (see Augimeri, Walsh and Slater, 2011). The model has been subjected to ongoing rigorous evaluation research (e.g., randomized controlled trials, replications and third-party evaluations), all of which have consistently demonstrated positive treatment changes from pre- to post-treatment and sustained treatment gains at follow-up. This has resulted in the model achieving the highest effectiveness rating from accredited bodies (for details, see Augimeri, et al., 2011; Koegl, Augimeri, Ferrante, Walsh, and Slater, 2008).

The first SNAP® program (SNAP® Under 12 Outreach Project; SNAP® ORP) was initiated in 1985 as a result of changes in Canadian federal law in 1984 pertaining to the decriminalization of children under the age of 12 with the implementation of the *Young Offenders Act* (YOA). At the time of the introduction of the YOA, the Canadian federal government put the onus on the provinces and territories to come up with effective crime-prevention and intervention programs to meet the needs of young children under the age of 12 engaging in antisocial activities.

The SNAP® ORP consists of five key components: (1) a SNAP® Children's Club – a structured group that teaches boys impulse control and problem-solving skills using SNAP® strategies; (2) a concurrent SNAP® Parenting Group that teaches parents effective child-management strategies; (3) one-on-one family counseling based on 'Stop Now and Plan Parenting' or SNAPP; (4) individual child counseling/ mentoring for boys who are not connected with positive structured activities in their community and require extra support; and (5) academic tutoring to assist boys who are not performing at their age-appropriate grade level at school. Other components of the program that are deployed where appropriate include school advocacy and teacher consultation, victim restitution, and a Monday Night Club for high-risk boys who have completed the SNAP® Boys Group but still require support. In addition, a Leaders-In-Training (LIT) program is available to boys over 12 years of age who still require support as they enter into their teenage years. This component also provides the boys with job skills development by giving them opportunities to assist with therapeutic summer day camp and weekly activity groups at the Centre. Based on an assessment of their unique treatment needs, SNAP® ORP children and families access a range of these components; however, the two core components, the 12-week child-and-parent SNAP® groups, are offered to all children and their families.

The sister program of the SNAP® ORP, the SNAP® Girls Connection (SNAP® GC), began in 1996 when preliminary assessments of the then mixed-gender SNAP®ORP groups revealed that the program was not producing the same positive outcomes for girls as it was for boys. Over its 15-year history, the SNAP® GC has been established as the most advanced gender-specific intervention for girls under the age of 12 in conflict with the law (Pepler, Walsh, and Levene, 2004; Pepler, et al., 2010). Like the SNAP® ORP, two core components of the SNAP® GC are the SNAP® Girls' Club and a concurrent SNAP® Parenting Group. Upon completion of these components, however, girls over 8 years of age and their mothers may also participate in a third core component, Girls Growing up Healthy (GGUH) – a group for mothers and daughters that focuses on relationship building and includes such topics as physical and sexual health, puberty, female role models and girls in the media, and intimate relationships. Individual child counseling/mentoring, academic tutoring, one-on-one family counseling based on SNAPP and the LIT program are also made available, as needed.

Research on the SNAP® Under 12 Outreach Project (SNAP® ORP)

A number of randomized controlled trials (RCTs) of the SNAP® ORP program were conducted, and showed that treated children improved significantly more than children receiving an attention-only group or delayed treatment; effect sizes were large, exceeding 1.1 (Koegl, Farrington, Augimeri, and Day, 2008). The program lowers aggression and delinquent behaviors in the short term, with good evidence that these effects can be sustained over the intermediate future. There is also some indication that the program may produce long-term changes, such as preventing involvement in criminal activities in adolescence and adulthood. A closer look at program effects showed that the amount of treatment received influences treatment effectiveness in terms of immediate decreases in delinquency and aggression, and longer-term outcomes such as involvement in criminal activities (Augimeri, et al., 2007; Koegl, et al., 2008).

Research on the SNAP® Girls Connection (SNAP® GC)

The first quantitative evaluation of the SNAP® GC program was conducted during the first four years of the program's operation (Walsh, Pepler and Levene, 2002). The analysis examined behavioral change, comparing externalizing behavior scores upon admission, as well as at six- (N = 72) and twelve- (N = 58) month intervals using the Standardized Client Information System, a measure based on the *Child Behavior Checklist* (CBCL, Offord and Boyle, 1996). At both follow-up periods, girls showed significant improvements in externalizing behaviors, which is an aggregation of conduct and oppositional problem behaviors. The girls also displayed an increase in social skills – statistically significant improvements from admission to the six-month follow-up were found, and these improvements were maintained at twelve months. Effect sizes for the change in externalizing behaviors were in the small to medium range ($d = 0.42$ to 0.49), whereas improvement in social skills emerged as a large effect ($d = 0.72$).

The most recent evaluation of the SNAP® GC was a prospective study of girls referred to the program between 2002 and 2004 (Pepler, et al., 2010). A quasi-experimental design was used to randomly assign referred girls either to immediate treatment in the program (N = 45) or to a waiting-list control group (N = 35). Both groups were stratified in terms of the severity of girls' behavior problems at intake. Externalizing behaviors were assessed at admission, post-treatment, and at six-, twelve-, and eigtheen-month follow-up intervals using the CBCL. Results indicated a significant treatment effect of the program. In comparing the treatment group to the control group, behavior problems (e.g., aggression, rule-breaking, conduct disorder, oppositional defiant disorder, and social problems) decreased significantly more for girls who received the SNAP® GC intervention. There was also a significant decrease in parental reports of girls' externalizing behaviors from pre-to post-program ($d = .51$), and significantly more of the treatment girls (38 percent) moved into the non-clinical range on externalizing behaviors post-treatment compared to controls (10 percent). Also, treatment girls significantly improved in terms of their self-control and cooperation skills.

Recent SNAP® longitudinal research looking at levels of risk as assessed using the EARLs and long-term outcome, showed that 91.8 percent of the boys and

96.9 percent of the girls who participated in the SNAP® ORP and SNAP® GC had no history of criminal offences at follow-up (14 years was the average age at follow-up; Augimeri, et al., 2010). In the last few years, CDI has engaged in two studies with the Hospital for Sick Children and the University of Toronto. The first study focused on neuro-cognitive processes in relation to impulse control in SNAP®-treated children. It used dense-array EEG sensor nets to record children's brain activity before and after SNAP® treatment. Results of this study showed that, after the SNAP® treatment, there were significant improvements in children's externalizing behavior associated with changes in brain activity as evidenced by more dorsally mediated executive regulation and less ventrally mediated reactive regulation (Lewis, et al., 2008). Thus, SNAP® increases children's ability to inhibit aggressive impulses, shown at both the behavioral and the brain level. The second study by Granic, O'Hara, Pepler and Lewis (2007) focused on parent-child interactions and found that SNAP® children who showed significant improvement in their externalizing behavior from pre-to post-treatment also showed improved parent-child communication; they were able to 'repair' more easily after engaging in a difficult parent–child interaction.

Multisystemic therapy (MST)

Scott Henggeler and colleagues at the Medical University of South Carolina developed MST in the late 1970s to address several limitations of existing mental health services for serious juvenile offenders (i.e., ineffectiveness, lack of a systems focus). MST fits closely with findings from multidimensional causal models of delinquent behavior (Howell, 2009). Using interventions that are present-focused and action-oriented, MST directly addresses intrapersonal (e.g., cognitive) and systemic (i.e., family, peer, school) factors that are known to be associated with adolescent antisocial behavior. Moreover, because different combinations of these factors are relevant for different adolescents, MST interventions are individualized and highly flexible. This provides a good fit with individualized risk assessment.

MST typically uses a home-based model of service delivery to reduce barriers that keep families from accessing services (Henggeler, Schoenwald, Borduin, Rowland, and Cunningham, 2009). Therapists have small caseloads of four to six families, work as a team, are available twenty-four hours a day, seven days a week, and provide services at times convenient to the family. The average treatment occurs over approximately four months, with multiple therapist–family contacts occurring each week. MST therapists concentrate on empowering parents and improving their effectiveness by identifying strengths and developing natural support systems (e.g., extended family, neighbors, friends, church members) and removing barriers (e.g., poor parenting skills, high stress, poor relationships between partners). Specific treatment techniques used to facilitate these gains are integrated from those therapies that have the most empirical support, including behavioral, cognitive-behavioral, and the pragmatic family therapies.

Research on MST

The first controlled study of MST with juvenile offenders (Henggeler, et al., 1986) evaluated its effectiveness compared with usual community treatment for inner-city juvenile offenders and their families. The study's success led to several randomized controlled trials and quasi-experimental studies, examining the effectiveness of MST in other populations of youths who presented serious clinical problems. Henggeler and colleagues (1992, 1993) examined MST as an alternative to incarceration. The study included 84 violent and chronic juvenile offenders, of whom 54 percent had been arrested for violent crimes. Their mean number of arrests was 3.5, and they averaged 9.5 weeks of prior placement in correctional facilities. The average age of the youths was 15.2 years, and 77 percent were male. Youths were assigned randomly to receive MST (n = 43) or usual services provided by the South Carolina Department of Juvenile Justice (n = 41). The average duration of treatment was 13 weeks. Assessment batteries, consisting of stand-ardized measurement instruments, were administered pre- and post-treatment. The results of the study showed that MST was effective at reducing rates of criminal activity and institutionalization. At the 59-week post-referral follow-up, youths receiving MST had significantly fewer re-arrests and weeks incarcerated than did youths receiving usual services. Families receiving MST reported more cohesion, whereas reported family cohesion decreased in the usual services condition. Significantly, the relative effectiveness of MST was not moderated by demographic characteristics (e.g., race, age, social class, gender, and arrest and incarceration history). Similarly, pre-existing problems in family relations, peer relations, social competence, behavior problems, and parental symptomatology were not differentially predictive of outcomes. Moreover, a 2.4-year follow-up (Henggeler, et al., 1993) showed that MST doubled the percentage of youths who did not recidivate in comparison with usual services.

MST started to be transferred to community settings and to countries outside the United States in the mid 1990s and this provided an opportunity for independent evaluations of its effectiveness. For instance, Ogden and Halliday-Boykins (2004) directed a four-site randomized trial in which participants were 100 seriously antisocial adolescents in Norway. The Norwegian study's short-term outcomes at six months post-recruitment showed that MST was significantly more effective at reducing youth internalizing and externalizing symptoms and out-of-home placement as well as increasing youth social competence and family satisfaction with treatment (Ogden and Halliday-Boykins, 2004). Significantly, analyses demonstrated differential site effects – the one site with problematic adherence to the MST intervention protocols had the worst outcome. In addition, a two-year follow-up has shown that MST's effects on out-of-home placements and youth internalizing and externalizing problems were maintained (Ogden and Hagen, 2006).

In 2004, a meta-analysis of seven primary outcome studies and four secondary studies involving a total of 708 participants was published (Curtis, Ronan, and Borduin, 2004). Results indicated that across different presenting problems and samples, the average effect size of MST was d = .55 following treatment. Youths and their families treated with MST were functioning better than 70 per cent of youths and families treated alternatively. Results also showed that the average effect of MST was larger in studies involving graduate-student therapists (i.e., efficacy studies; d = .81) than in studies with therapists from the community (i.e., effectiveness studies; d = .26). Thus, ongoing quality assurance to monitor treatment fidelity seems to be important to optimize treatment effectiveness. A more recent and more stringent meta-analysis by the Cochrane Collaboration using eight RCTs indicated no significant differences between MST and usual services in terms of out-of-home-placements and arrests/convictions (Littell, Campbell, Green, and Toews, 2009). However, the sample size for this meta-analysis was small and effects were not consistent across studies.

Using data from three effect studies of MST on criminal outcomes, Aos and colleagues (Aos, et al., 2001) reported that, compared to alternative interventions (usual services, community services, or individual therapy), MST reduced the proportion of youth who committed criminal offenses (Standardized Mean Difference = -.31, SD = .10). They estimated that the net direct cost of the program per participant was US \$4,743. When they compared this cost with estimated economic benefits of anticipated reductions in crime, the estimated net benefits of MST range from US \$31,661 (for taxpayers only) to US \$131,918 (for taxpayers and crime victims) per MST program participant.

Implementing risk prevention at the community level

Bringing evidence-based intervention programs such as SNAP® and MST to communities requires more than just the training of therapists in the new treatment method. Dodge (2009) summarized the most important pitfalls in this process. The first is that evidence-based interventions are difficult to implement with high fidelity at full scale in entire communities (see the example of MST above; Curtis, et al., 2004). Treatment fidelity should be monitored continuously to prevent drift. Second, community-level improvements in the resources, financing, and access to individual-level interventions are often needed. Official government policies may or may not be in line with these needs. Finally, the third possible reason that interventions delivered to children and their families are not as effective as expected is that the antisocial behavior problems themselves are partially caused by community-level factors, such as neighborhood violence, cultural endorsement of aggression, and peer deviance and discrimination against specific groups, which can be changed only by community-level intervention. Clinicians 'work around' or 'work with' community risk factors mostly indirectly (Dodge, 2009).

To provide an illustration – the Centre for Children Committing Offences at the Child Development Institute (CDI) developed a comprehensive crime-prevention model for young children in conflict with the law that includes a three-pronged approach: police-community referral protocol, structured professional risk assessment (i.e., EARLs), and gender-sensitive evidence-based interventions (i.e., SNAP® Models) (Augimeri, et al. 2011). The Police-Community Referral Protocol (briefly summarized here, including some of the dos and don'ts) is an example of how community partners such as the Toronto Police and Fire Services, child-welfare organizations, school boards, children's mental health and other children's service agencies can work together to establish a single-entry access point through a Central Intake Line housed at CDI. Signed on February 1, 1999, this Protocol mandates the 15 participating organizations to make referrals to CDI within 48 hours, which, if the family agrees to participate (families who refuse are referred to child welfare), triggers a more in-depth clinical assessment within five working days (for details, see Koegl, et al., 2008).

In order to assess the Protocol's effectiveness and maintain a steady flow of referrals, there must be constant communication and coordination among Protocol stakeholders. In the 12 years that the Protocol has been in place, CDI has been able to identify four key ingredients and challenges associated with such an endeavor (the ingredients were also described in Koegl, et al., 2008). Specifically, lessons learned included the need to have the following:

1. *Protocol champion* – a person within a lead organization who is in regular contact with partnering agencies to: (a) assess and monitor the volume of referrals, (b) check whether children are being admitted into services, (c) inform referral sources about the status of referrals (e.g., whether families followed through with treatment), (d) monitor whether partnering organizations are actively participating in the referral process, and (e) ensure that staff are adequately trained to provide services. The Protocol champion should also mobilize local stakeholders and resources, and/or secure external funding when needed to support its continued development.

2. *Protocol marketing strategy* – so that frontline personnel within participating organizations (i.e., those most likely to encounter at-risk children) are aware of the Protocol and know how to make a referral through the Central Intake Line. For example, in Toronto, a Protocol poster was widely distributed to elementary schools, community centers, police and fire stations, child welfare offices, and children's mental health centers. We learned, however, that many of these posters were either never displayed or were removed over time. This led us to extend our marketing efforts beyond the poster itself to key personnel within our community who occupied positions of influence, and who could ensure that staff were aware of the Central Intake Line.

3. *Ongoing protocol training* – so that professionals (e.g., police, clinicians) understand the needs of high-risk children and their families so that they are able to engage and encourage them to participate in treatment. This is important at the point of referral but also during the provision of clinical services. For example, we know that families are more likely to consent to treatment if referring police officers assume a compassionate rather than authoritative stance when making a referral through the Central Intake Line (Coombs, 2005).

4. *A process for ongoing dialogue between the referral source and service provider* – our practice with the Toronto Police Service is to inform referring

officers about the status of their referral. In the absence of information, we have found that there is a tendency for officers – especially in cases where the family does not pursue treatment – to become cynical about the efficacy of the Protocol, which has historically led to a reduction in referrals. Two evaluations indicate that the Protocol has helped to seal a significant crack in the system by bringing organizations together to serve this specific population of youth. From these positive evaluations, and the fact that Protocol implementation costs relatively little in terms of financial resources, the Protocol model has been subsequently replicated in eight other communities across Canada (see Koegl, et al., 2008, p. 287–88).

Future directions in research and practice

The 'nothing works' era in juvenile-offender rehabilitation, which started with Martinson's (1974) analysis of 231 program studies and his conclusion that a 'radical flaw [exists] in our present strategies [such] that [rehabilitation] at its best, cannot overcome, or even appreciably reduce, the powerful tendency for offenders to continue in criminal behaviors' (p. 49), seems finally to have ended and turned into an era of 'evidence-based practice'. This is largely the result of numerous well-designed studies that identify the effectiveness of specific intervention programs and their critical components. However, the size of treatment effects reported in recent meta-analyses still leaves room for improvement. Further refinement of individual clinical risk management may be possible if we take recent research that is showing important interaction effects into account. For instance, Hawes and Dadds (2005) examined the impact of callous-unemotional (CU) traits on treatment outcomes in a 10-week behavioral parent-training inter-vention with young boys referred for conduct problems (N = 56; mean age 6.29 years). CU traits were associated with greater conduct problems at pretreatment and with poor outcomes at six-month follow-up. Boys with high CU traits were less responsive to discipline with time-out than boys without CU traits and reacted to this discipline with less affect. Recently, Hawes, Brennan and Dadds (2009) examined evidence that the role of the hypothalamic-pituitary-adrenal (HPA) axis in the development of antisocial behavior may differ across subgroups of children. A meta-analysis (Alink, van IJzendoorn, Bakermans-Kranenburg, et al., 2008) has supported the prediction that low levels of cortisol are associated with risk for childhood antisocial behavior, but the relationship is weaker than previously assumed. Recent studies suggest the association between cortisol levels and antisocial behavior may vary depending on type of antisocial behavior, patterns of internalizing comorbidity, and early environmental adversity. The findings are consistent with evidence that two early-onset pathways to antisocial behavior can be distinguished based on the presence or absence of callous-unemotional traits. Obviously, these ideas need further research, but improved insights into the role of interactions between different risk factors in the etiology of antisocial behavior seem essential to still further increase the effectiveness of present risk management strategies.

Lastly, the promise of risk assessment tools as *risk prevention* tools is still largely unfulfilled, since studies designed to demonstrate the preventive effects of these tools to formulate risk management and prevention plans still lie ahead. However, as noted in this chapter, there are promising new tools and interventions to help present-day practitioners develop effective intervention plans and community initiatives to help this group of children at risk.

Notes

1   Some scholars use the term psychopathy to refer to these types of traits in children and adolescents (Salekin and Lynam, 2010). This is still highly controversial, because of the great number of negative connotations (e.g., high risk, untreatable) professionals and laypeople alike associate with this term (Johnstone and Cooke, 2004), and because children and adolescents are still in development in terms of personality.
2   It is beyond the scope of this chapter to discuss in detail the relationship between gender and aggression. Although most research on juvenile offenders has been conducted on boys, there are some excellent resources that summarize what is known about aggression and antisocial behavior in girls: Moretti, Odgers, and Jackson, 2004; Pepler, Madsen, Webster, and Levene, 2005.
3   Although all SPJ guidelines advise against the simple summation of the individual risk factors in clinical practice, researchers have tended to ignore this and have examined the predictive value of these instruments' total (added) scores in comparison to the final risk judgement performed by the professional.

References

Alink, L. R. A., van IJzendoorn, M. H., Bakermans-Kranenburg, M. J., Mesman, J., Juffer, F. and Koot, H.M. (2008) 'Cortisol and externalizing behavior in children and adolescents: Mixed meta-analytic evidence for the inverse relation of basal cortisol and cortisol reactivity with externalizing behavior', *Developmental Psychobiolology*, 50: 427–50.

Andrews, D. A. (2001) 'Principles of effective correctional programs', in L. L. Motiuk and R. C. Serin (eds) *Compendium 2000 on Effective Correctional Programming*, Ottawa, Canada: Correctional Services of Canada.

Aos, S., Phipps, P., Barnoski, R. and Lieb, R. (2001) *The Comparative Costs and Benefits of Programs to Reduce Crime*, Olympia, WA: Washington State Institute for Public Policy. Retrieved from www.wsipp.wa.gov/crime/costben.html.

Augimeri, L. K. (2005) *Aggressive and Antisocial Young Children: Risk assessment and management utilizing the Early Assessment Risk List for Boys (EARL-20B)*, Doctoral dissertation, Ontario Institute of Studies in Education of the Toronto University, Toronto, ON, Canada.

Augimeri, L. K., Walsh, M. and Slater, N. (2011) 'Rolling out SNAP® an evidence-based intervention: A summary of implementation, evaluation and research', *International Journal of Child, Youth and Family Studies*, 2: 162–84.

Augimeri, L. K., Webster, C. D., Koegl, C. J. and Levene, K. (1998) *Early assessment risk list for boys: EARL-20B, Version 1, Consultation Edition*. Toronto, ON: Earlscourt Child and Family Centre.

Augimeri, L. K., Koegl, C. J., Webster, C. D. and Levene, K. (2001) *Early assessment risk list for boys: EARL-20B, Version 2*. Toronto, ON: Earlscourt Child and Family Centre.

Augimeri, L. K., Koegl, C. J., Levene, K. S. and Webster, C. D. (2005) 'Early Assessment Risk Lists for Boys and Girls', in T. Grisso, G. Vincent and D. Seagrave (eds) *Mental Health Screening and Assessment in Juvenile Justice*, New York: Guilford Press.

Augimeri, L. K., Farrington, D. P., Koegl, C. J. and Day, D. M. (2007) 'The Under 12 Outreach Project: Effects of a community based program for children with conduct problems', *Journal of Child and Family Studies*, 16: 799–807. Published online, January 10, 2007. DOI:10.1007/s10826-006-9126-x.

Augimeri, L. K., Enebrink, P., Walsh, M. and Jiang, D. (2010) 'Gender-specific childhood risk assessment tools: Early Assessment Risk Lists for Boys (EARL-20B) and Girls (EARL-21G)', in R. K. Otto and K. S. Douglas (eds) *Handbook of Violence Risk Assessment*, Oxford: Routledge.

Augimeri, L. K., Walsh, M. M., Liddon, A. D. and Dassinger, C. R. (2011) 'From risk identification to risk management: A comprehensive strategy for young children engaged in antisocial behavior', in A. Roberts and D. Springer (eds) *Juvenile Justice and Delinquency*, p.117–40, Sudbury, United States: Jones and Bartlett.

Augimeri, L. K., Desmarais, S. L., Koegl, C. J., Jiang, D. and Webster, C. D. (2009) *Assessing Risk for Antisocial Conduct Among Young Children: Psychometric properties of the Early Assessment Risk List for Boys (EARL-20B)*, Unpublished manuscript.

Augimeri, L. K., Pepler, D. P., Walsh, M. M., Jiang, D. and Dassinger, C. R. (2010) *Aggressive and Antisocial Young Children: Risk prediction, assessment and clinical risk management* (Program Evaluation Grant #RG-976 – The Provincial Centre of Excellence for Child and Youth Mental Health at CHEO), Toronto, ON: Child Development Institute.

Bartel, P., Borum, R. and Forth, A. (2000) *Structured Assessment for Violence Risk in Youth (SAVRY), Consultation Edition*, Tampa, FL: University of South Florida.

Biederman, J., Mick, E., Faraone, S. V. and Burback, M. (2001) 'Patterns of remission and symptom decline in Conduct Disorder: A four-year prospective study of an ADHD sample', *Journal of the American Academy of Child and Adolescent Psychiatry*, 40: 290–98.

Borum, R. and Douglas, K. (2003) 'New directions in violence risk assessment', *Psychiatric Times*, 20: 102–3.

Borum, R., Bartel, P. and Forth, A. (2005) 'Structured Assessment of Violence Risk in Youth (SAVRY)', in T. Grisso, G. Vincent and D. Seagrave (eds) *Mental Health Screening and Assessment in Juvenile Justice*, p. 311–23, New York: Guilford Press.

— (2006) *Manual for the Structured Assessment of Violence Risk in Youth (SAVRY)*, Odessa, FL: Psychological Assessment Resources.

Borum, R., Lodewijks, H., Bartel, P. A. and Forth, A. (2010) 'Structured Assessment of Violence in Youth (SAVRY)', in R. K. Otto and K. S. Douglas (eds) *Handbook of Violence Risk Assessment*, p.63–80, New York: Taylor and Francis.

Catchpole, R. and Gretton, H. (2003) 'The predictive validity of risk assessment with violent young offenders: A 1-year examination of criminal outcome', *Criminal Justice and Behavior*, 30: 688–708.

Collins, L. M., Murphy, S. A. and Bierman, K. L. (2004) 'A conceptual framework for adaptive preventive interventions', *Prevention Science*, 5: 185–96.

Coombs, J. (2005) *Engaging Families in Contact with the Toronto Police Protocol for Under-12 Children in Conflict with the Law: Qualitative observations and policy recommendations*, Ministry of Children and Youth Services: Mental Health Innovation Fund.

Curtis, N. M., Ronan, K. R. and Borduin, C. M. (2004) 'Multisystemic treatment: A meta analysis of outcome studies', *Journal of Family Psychology*, 18: 411–19.

Dishion, T. J., Spracklen, K. M., Andrews, D. W. and Patterson, G. R. (1996) 'Deviancy training in male adolescent friendships', *Behavior Therapy*, 27: 373–90.

Dodge, K. A. (2009) 'Community intervention and public policy in the prevention of antisocial behavior', *Journal of Child Psychology and Psychiatry*, 50: 194–200.

Douglas, K. S. and Kropp, P. R. (2002) 'A prevention-based paradigm for violence risk assessment: Clinical and research applications', *Criminal Justice and Behavior*, 29: 617–58.

Enebrink, P., Långström, N. and Gumpert, C. H. (2006) 'Predicting aggressive and disruptive behavior in referred 6- to 12-year-old boys: Prospective validation of the EARL-20B Risk/Needs Checklist', *Assessment*, 13: 356–67.

Enebrink, P., Långström, N., Hultén, A. and Gumpert, C. H. (2006) 'Swedish validation of the Early Assessment Risk List for Boys (EARL-20B), a decision-aid for use with children presenting with conduct-disordered behavior', *Nordic Journal of Psychiatry*, 60: 468–446.

Farrington, D. P. and Welsh, B. C. (2007) *Saving Children from a Life of Crime: Early risk factors and effective interventions*, New York: Oxford University Press.

Farrington, D. P., Loeber, R., Jolliffe, D. and Pardini, D. A. (2008) 'Promotive and risk processes at different life stages', in R. Loeber, D. P. Farrington, M. Stouthamer-Loeber and H. Raskin White (eds) *Violence and Serious Theft: Development and prediction from childhood to adulthood*, pp. 169–230, New York: Routledge.

Fazel, S., Doll, H. and Långström, N. (2008) 'Mental disorders among adolescents in juvenile detention and correctional facilities: A systematic review and meta-regression analysis of 25 surveys', *Journal of the American Academy of Child and Adolescent Psychiatry*, 47: 1010–19.

Fergusson, D. M. and Lynskey, M. T. (1996) 'Adolescent resiliency to family adversity', *Journal of Child Psychology and Psychiatry*, 37: 281–92.

Foster, E. M., Jones, D. E. and The Conduct Problems Research Prevention Group (2005) 'The high costs of aggression: Public expenditures resulting from Conduct Disorder', *American Journal of Public Health*, 95: 1767–72.

Gendreau, P. and Goggin, C. (1996) 'Principles of effective correctional programming', *Forum on Corrections Research*, 8: 38–41.

Granic, I., O'Hara, A., Pepler, D. and Lewis, M. (2007) 'A dynamic system analysis of parent-child changes associated with successful "real-world" interventions for aggressive children', *Journal of Abnormal Child Psychology*, 35: 845–57. Printed online: DOI 10.1007/s10802-007-9133-4.

Gretton, H. and Abramowitz, C. (2002) 'SAVRY: Contribution of items and scales to clinical risk judgments and criminal outcomes', Paper presented at the American Psychology and Law Society, Biennial Conference, Austin, Texas. Available from http://www.fmhi.usf.edu/mhlp/savry/SAVRY_Research.htm.

Hart, S. D. (2001) 'Assessing and managing violence risk', in K. S. Douglas, C. D. Webster, S. H. Hart, D. Eaves and J. R. P. Ogloff (eds) *HCR-20 Violence Risk Management Companion Guide*, pp. 13–26, Burnaby, British Columbia: Mental Health Law, and Policy Institute, Simon Fraser University.

Hawes, D. J. and Dadds, M. R. (2005) 'The treatment of conduct problems in children with callous-unemotional traits', *Journal of Consulting and Clinical Psychology*, 73: 737–41.

Hawes, D. J., Brennan, J. and Dadds, M. R. (2009) 'Cortisol, callous-unemotional traits, and pathways to antisocial behavior', *Current Opinion in Psychiatry*, 22: 357–62.

Heilbrun, K., Grisso, T. and Goldstein, A. (2008) *Foundations of Forensic Mental Health Assessment*, New York: Oxford University Press.

Henggeler, S. W., Melton, G. B. and Smith, L. A. (1992) 'Family preservation using multi-systemic therapy: An effective alternative to incarcerating serious juvenile offenders', *Journal of Consulting and Clinical Psychology*, 60: 953–61.

Henggeler, S. W., Melton, G. B., Smith, L. A., Schoenwald, S. K. and Hanley, J. H. (1993) 'Family preservation using multisystemic treatment: Long-term follow-up to a clinical trial with serious juvenile offenders', *Journal of Child and Family Studies*, 2: 283–93.

Henggeler, S. W., Rodick, J. D., Borduin, C. M., Hanson, C. L., Watson, S. M. and Urey, J. R. (1986) 'Multisystemic treatment of juvenile offenders: Effects on adolescent behavior and family interactions', *Developmental Psychology*, 22: 132–41.

Henggeler, S. W., Schoenwald, S. K., Borduin, C. M., Rowland, M. D. and Cunningham, P. B. (2009) *Multisystemic Therapy for Antisocial Behavior in Children and Adolescents, 2nd edition*, New York: Guilford Press.

Howell, J. C. (2003) *Preventing and Reducing Juvenile Delinquency: A comprehensive framework*, Thousand Oaks, CA: Sage.

— (2009) *Preventing and Reducing Juvenile Delinquency: A comprehensive framework, 2nd edition*, Thousand Oaks, CA: Sage.

Johnstone, L. and Cooke, D. J. (2004) 'Psychopathic-like traits in childhood: Conceptual and measurement concerns', *Behavioral Sciences and the Law*, 22: 103–22.

Jones, P. R. and Wyant, B. R. (2007) 'Target juvenile needs to reduce delinquency', *Criminology and Public Policy*, 6: 763–72.

Koegl, C. J. (2011) *High-risk antisocial children: Predicting future criminal and health outcomes*, Unpublished doctoral dissertation, University of Cambridge.

Koegl, C. J., Augimeri, L. K., Ferrante, P., Walsh, M. and Slater, N. (2008) 'A Canadian programme for child delinquents', in R. Loeber, N. W. Slot, P. van der Laan and M. Hoeve (eds) *Tomorrow's Criminals: The development of child delinquency and effective interventions*, pp. 285–300, Aldershot: Ashgate.

Koegl, C. J., Farrington, D. P., Augimeri, L. K. and Day, D. M. (2008) 'Evaluation of a targeted cognitive-behavioural programme for children with conduct problems: The SNAP® Under 12 Outreach Project: Service intensity, age and gender effects on short- and long-term outcomes', *Clinical Child Psychology and Psychiatry*, 13: 419–34.

Lahey, B. B., Moffitt, T. E. and Caspi, A. (2003) *Causes of Conduct Disorder and Juvenile Delinquency*, New York: Guilford.

Levene, K. S., Walsh, M. M., Augimeri, L. K. and Pepler, D. (2004) 'Linking identification and treatment of early risk factors for female delinquency', in M. Moretti, C. Odgers and M. Jackson (eds) *Girls and Aggression: Contributing factors and intervention principles: Perspectives in law and psychology (Vol. 19)*, pp. 147–64, New York: Kluwer Academic/ Plenum Publishers.

Lewis, M. D., Granic, I., Lamm, C., Zelazo, P. D., Stieben, J. Todd, R. M., Moadab, I. and Pepler, D. (2008) 'Changes in the neural bases of emotion regulation associate with clinical improvement in children with behaviour problems', *Development and Psychopathology*, 20: 913–39.

Lipsey, M. W. and Wilson, D. B. (1998) 'Effective interventions with serious juvenile offenders: A synthesis of research', in R. Loeber and D. P. Farrington (eds) *Serious and Violent Juvenile Offenders: Risk factors and successful interventions*, pp. 313–45, Thousand Oaks, CA: Sage.

Littell, J. H., Campbell, M., Green, S. and Toews, B. (2009) 'Multisystemic Therapy for social, emotional, and behavioral problems in youth aged 10–17', *Cochrane Database of Systematic Reviews* 2005, Issue 4. Art. No.: CD004797. DOI: 10.1002/14651858. CD004797.pub4.

Lodewijks, H. P. B., Doreleijers, T. A. H., de Ruiter, C. and Borum, R. (2008a) 'Predictive validity of the Structured Assessment of Violence Risk in Youth (SAVRY) during residential treatment', *International Journal of Law and Psychiatry*, 31: 263–71.

Lodewijks, H. P. B., Doreleijers, T. A. H. and de Ruiter, C. (2008b) 'SAVRY risk assessment in relation to sentencing and subsequent recidivism in a Dutch sample of violent juvenile offenders', *Criminal Justice and Behavior*, 35: 696–709.

Lodewijks, H. P. B., de Ruiter, C. and Doreleijers, T. A. H. (2009) 'Gender differences in violent outcome and risk assessment in adolescent offenders after residential treatment', *International Journal of Forensic Mental Health*, 7: 133–46.

— (2010) 'The impact of protective factors in desistance from violent reoffending: A study in three samples of adolescent violent offenders', *Journal of Interpersonal Violence*, 25: 568–87.

Loeber, R. and Farrington, D. P. (eds) (2001) *Child Delinquents: Development, intervention and service needs*, Thousand Oaks, CA: Sage.

Loeber, R. and Farrington, D. P. (2001) 'The significance of child delinquency', in R. Loeber and D. P. Farrington (eds) *Child Delinquents: Development, intervention and service needs*, pp. 1–24, Thousand Oaks, CA: Sage.

— (1998) 'Never too early, never too late: Risk factors and successful interventions for serious violent juvenile offenders', *Studies on Crime and Crime Prevention*, 7: 7–30.

Loeber, R., Farrington, D. P. and Petechuk, D. (2003, May) 'Child delinquency: Early intervention and prevention', *Child Delinquency Bulletin Series*, US Department of Justice.

Loeber, R., Slot, N. W., van der Laan, P. H. and Hoeve, M. (eds) (2008) *Tomorrow's Criminals: The development of child delinquency and effective interventions*, Farnham: Ashgate.

Loeber, R., Slot, N. W. and Stouthamer-Loeber, M. (2008) 'A cumulative developmental model of risk and promotive factors', in R. Loeber, N. W. Slot, P. H. Van der Laan and M. Hoeve (eds) *Tomorrow's Criminals: The development of child delinquency and effective interventions*, pp. 133–61, Farnham: Ashgate.

MacKenzie, D. L. (2006) *What Works in Corrections: Reducing the criminal activities of offenders and delinquents*, Cambridge: Cambridge University Press.

MacKenzie, D. L., Wilson, D. B., Armstrong, G. S. and Gover, A. R. (2001) 'The impact of boot camps and traditional institutions on juvenile residents: Perceptions, adjustment, and change', *Journal of Research in Crime and Delinquency*, 38: 279–313.

Martinson, R. (1974) 'What works? Questions and answers about prison reform', *Public Interest*, 10: 22–54.

McEachran, A. (2001) *The Predictive Validity of the PCL:YV and the SAVRY in a population of adolescent offenders*, Unpublished Master's thesis, Burnaby, British Columbia: Simon Fraser University. Available from: www.fmhi.usf.edu/mhlp/savry/SAVRY_Research.htm.

Moffitt, T. E. (1993) 'Adolescence-limited and life-course-persistent antisocial behavior: A developmental taxonomy', *Psychological Review*, 100: 674–701.

Moretti, M. M., Odgers, C. L. and Jackson, M. A. (eds) (2004) *Girls and aggression: Contributing factors and intervention principles, Perspectives in Law and Psychology Series, Volume 19*, New York: Kluwer Academic/Plenum.

Nicholls, T. L., Brink, J., Desmarais, S. L., Webster, C. D. and Martin, M. (2006) 'The short term assessment of risk and treatability (START): A prospective validation study in a forensic psychiatric sample', *Assessment*, 13: 313–27.

Offord, D. and Boyle, M. (1996) *Standard Client Information System*, Toronto: OACM.

Ogden, T. and Halliday-Boykins, C. A. (2004) 'Multisystemic treatment of antisocial adolescents in Norway: Replication of clinical outcomes outside of the US', *Journal of Child and Adolescent Mental Health,* 9: 77–83.

Ogden, T. and Hagen, K. A. (2006) 'Multisystemic therapy of serious behaviour problems in youth: Sustainability of therapy effectiveness two years after intake', *Journal of Child and Adolescent Mental Health*, 11: 142–49.

Olver, M. E., Stockdale, K. C. and Wormith, J. S. (2009) 'Risk assessment with young offenders: A meta-analysis of three assessment measures', *Criminal Justice and Behavior*, 36: 329–53.

Otto, R. K. and Douglas, K. S. (eds) (2010) *Handbook of Violence Risk Assessment*, New York: Taylor and Francis.

Pepler, D. J., Madsen, K. C., Webster, C. D. and Levene, K. S. (2005) *The Development and Treatment of Girlhood Aggression*, Hillsdale, NJ: Erlbaum.

Pepler, D. J., Walsh, M. M., and Levene, K. S. (2004) 'Interventions for aggressive girls: Tailoring and measuring the fit', in M. M. Moretti, C. L. Odgers and M. A. Jackson (eds) *Girls and Aggression: Contributing factors and intervention principles, Perspectives in Law and Psychology Series, Volume 19*, pp. 41–56, New York: Kluwer Academic/Plenum.

Pepler, D., Walsh, M., Yuile, A., Levene, K., Vaughan, A. and Webber, J. (2010) 'Bridging the gender gap: Interventions with aggressive girls and their parents' [Electronic version], *Prevention Science*, http://www.springerlink.com/content/.

Pollard, J. A., Hawkins, J. D. and Arthur, M. W. (1999) 'Risk and protection: Are both necessary to understand diverse behavioral outcomes in adolescence?', *Social Work Research*, 23: 145–59.

Rogers, R. (2000) 'The uncritical acceptance of risk assessment in forensic practice', *Law and Human Behavior*, 24: 595–605.

Romeo, R., Knapp, M. and Scott, S. (2006) 'Economic cost of severe antisocial behaviour in children', *British Journal of Psychiatry*, 188: 547–53.

Rutter, M. (2003) 'Crucial paths from risk indicator to causal mechanism', in B. B. Lahey, T. E. Moffitt and A. Caspi (eds) *Causes of Conduct Disorder and Juvenile Delinquency*, pp. 3–26, New York: Guilford.

Salekin, R. T. and Lynam, D. R. (2010) *Handbook of Child and Adolescent Psychopathy*, New York: Guilford.

Snyder, J. (2002) 'Reinforcement and coercion mechanisms in the development of antisocial behavior: Peer relationships', in J. B. Reid, G. R. Patterson and J. Snyder (eds) *Antisocial Behavior in Children and Adolescents: A developmental analysis and model for intervention*, pp. 101–22, Washington, DC: American Psychological Association.

Snyder, J. and Stoolmiller, M. (2002) 'Reinforcement and coercion mechanisms in the development of antisocial behavior: The family', in J. B. Reid, G. R. Patterson and J. Snyder (eds) *Antisocial Behavior in Children and Adolescents: A developmental analysis and model for intervention*, pp. 65–100, Washington, DC: American Psychological Association.

Stouthamer-Loeber, M., Wei, E., Loeber, R. and Masten, A. S. (2004) 'Desistance from persistent serious delinquency in the transition to adulthood', *Development and Psychopathology*, 16: 897–918.

Stouthamer-Loeber, M., Loeber, R., Wei, E. H., Farrington, D. P. and Wikström, P.-O. H. (2002) 'Risk and promotive effects in the explanation of persistent serious delinquency in boys', *Journal of Consulting and Clinical Psychology*, 70: 111–23.

Walsh, M., Yuile, A. and Jiang, D. (2004) *Early Assessment Risk List for Girls (EARL-21G): Predicting antisocial behaviors and clinical implications*, Presentation Child Development Institute. Toronto, Canada.

Walsh, M. M., Pepler, D. J. and Levene, K. S. (2002) 'A model intervention for girls with disruptive behaviour problems: The Earlscourt Girls Connection', *Canadian Journal of Counselling*, 36: 297–311.

White, S. F. and Frick, P. J. (2010) 'Callous-unemotional traits and their importance to causal models of severe antisocial behavior in youth', in R. T. Salekin and D. R. Lynam (eds) *Handbook of Child and Adolescent Psychopathy*, pp. 135–55, New York: Guilford Press.

10 Working with women

Towards a more gender-sensitive violence risk assessment

Vivienne de Vogel and Michiel de Vries Robbé

Compared to their male counterparts, women are less likely to perpetrate violent acts. Gender is one of the best predictors of violent and criminal behaviour (Monahan, et al., 2001). However, although women are only a minority in the penitentiary system and in forensic psychiatry, it seems that worldwide, in the past two decades, female violence is on the rise, especially among young girls (Heilbrun, et al., 2008; Odgers, et al., 2005). In addition, certain types of violence, such as intimate-partner violence and inpatient violence by psychiatric patients, are as common in women as in men (Magdol, et al., 1997; Nicholls, et al., 2009). Some scholars have stated that changes in policies, police efforts, or changes in societal toleration for the behaviour of girls and women may partially explain the increased female violence (Hawkins, et al., 2009). Nevertheless, criminal behavior, and more specifically violent behaviour towards others by women, is a significant problem that cannot be ignored. Consequently, there are growing concerns about whether the theoretical knowledge we have on violence in men and on violence risk assessment and management in men is sufficiently valid and useful for violent women.

In this chapter, the literature on violence by women and violence risk assessment and management with women is reviewed and it is concluded that more gender-sensitive guidelines for violence risk assessment are necessary. Subsequently, an initiative is presented towards more gender-sensitive violence risk assessment in women with a history of violence towards others with the aim of providing mental health professionals working with women with more practical guidelines for risk management. This *Female Additional Manual* (FAM; De Vogel, et al., 2011), an additional manual to the HCR-20 for adult women, was developed on the basis of a literature review, clinical expertise and the results of a pilot study. This development process will be described and a case study will be presented in order to illustrate the additional value of using the FAM.

Violence by women

Research has shown that in general, the nature, severity, frequency, and victims of violent offences committed by women are significantly different from those committed by men. Overall, female violence is more often reactive and relational and less often characterized as instrumental. Violence by women less often results in serious injuries and is less visible and subtler, for instance, in intimate-partner violence, child abuse, and violence against relatives (Monahan, et al., 2001; Nicholls, 2001; Odgers, et al., 2005). Intimate-partner violence is the most studied form of violence committed by women. Research has demonstrated that the prevalence rate of intimate-partner violence by women is comparable to or even higher than that by men (Adams, 2002; Magdol, et al., 1997). Some scholars state that violence by women in intimate relationships is less likely to lead to serious injury and that violence occurs mainly in reaction to male violence (Swan and Snow, 2006). Others, however, found few differences between men and women regarding prevalence and motives for intimate-partner violence (Carney, et al., 2007).

The literature on sexual violence by women is rather limited. Research has demonstrated that women form only a small proportion of the total sex-offender population (between 4–5 per cent; Cortoni, et al., 2010; Logan, 2008). Female sexual offenders compared to male sexual offenders are more likely to be in a caretaking position and less likely to abuse strangers (Rudin, et al., 1995). The majority of female sexual offenders commit sexual assaults against young people (Logan, 2008). Another gender difference regarding type of offences is that women compared to men are more likely to be charged with or convicted of arson and to have previous histories of firesetting behaviour (Coid, et al., 2000). With respect to inpatient violence, it has repeatedly been demonstrated that female psychiatric patients cause as many violent incidents as male psychiatric patients (Newhill, et al., 1995; Nicholls, et al., 2009; De Vogel and De Ruiter, 2005). However, it has also been found that violent incidents by female psychiatric patients are less likely to result in serious injury compared to violent incidents by male psychiatric patients (Krakowski and Czobor, 2004).

Violence risk assessment in women

Research has demonstrated that unstructured clinical judgement relating to violence risk is sensitive to sex-based biases; mental health professionals of both genders tend to underestimate the risk of violence in female psychiatric patients (Skeem, et al., 2005). Use of structured risk assessment instruments is recommended to avoid these types of biases; however, widely used structured risk assessment instruments such as the *Historical-Clinical-Risk Management-20* (HCR-20; Webster, et al., 1997) were developed based on violence risk research conducted primarily in male samples. Moreover, research into the psychometric properties of these instruments has been carried out almost exclusively on men. Some scholars have taken the position that there is no reason to assume that male-based instruments do not apply to women because most risk factors are considered valid for both sexes (Loucks and Zamble, 1999; Newhill, et al., 1995), also referred to as the 'gender-blind' perspective (Garcia-Mansilla, et al., 2009). However, recent research results and reviews on risk factors and risk assessment in female offenders suggest that – although many violence risk factors seem to be valid for both men and women – the assessment and formulation of violence risk differs at least to a certain degree between men and women, and consequently, that there is a need for more gender-sensitive risk assessment (Funk, 1999; Garcia-Mansilla, et al., 2009; Logan and Blackburn, 2009; McKeown, 2010; Odgers, et al., 2005; Van Voorhis, et al., 2010).

There are some risk factors that are specifically found valid for women, such as prostitution, self-harm and pregnancy at young age (Blanchette and Brown, 2006; Messer, et al., 2004; Morgan and Patton, 2002). Furthermore, several risk factors that have been proven valid for both sexes seem to have a stronger effect on women than on men; for example, childhood abuse, adult victimization, disruptions in relationships and families, and economic disadvantages (Benda, 2005; Bottos, 2007; Odgers, et al., 2005). Many mental health professionals who are working with women on a daily basis recognize these differences and have expressed the need for more gender-sensitive assessment of factors explaining and managing violence risk in female offenders (Adams, 2002; Odgers, et al., 2005). Better risk assessment and management in women is also important from a public mental health perspective because research has demonstrated an intergenerational transfer of risk of violence between mothers and children; mothers with a history of violent offences are more likely to raise disruptive, aggressive children (Serbin, et al., 1998).

Despite the many important advances in the field of violence risk assessment in the past thirty years and the fact that many risk assessment tools have become available for different ages and different types of violence, almost no specific tools have been developed for the assessment of risk of antisocial or violent behaviour in female offenders. One exception is the *Early Assessment Risk List for Girls* (EARL-21G; Levene, et al., 2001) for girls between 6 and 12 years old. Besides the risk factors valid for boys and girls, this instrument contains two items specific to girls: *Caregiver–daughter interaction* and *Sexual development*. However, there is no such instrument available for violence risk assessment in adolescent girls or adult women.

Violence risk assessment tools in women

Garcia-Mansilla and colleagues (2009) reviewed the literature on different methods of violence risk assessment in a range of female populations. They concluded that structured methods of risk assessment are more accurate than unstructured methods, but that overall, the research supporting applicability of violence risk assessment instruments in female populations remains equivocal.

Several studies have been conducted into the value of the widely used HCR-20, a violence risk tool exemplifying the structured professional judgement (SPJ) approach to clinical risk assessment and management, in female samples. Guy and Douglas (2006) examined a large set of HCR-20 data from aggregated samples with Item Response Theory and found no big differences between men and women in how the items are relevant to the construct. Strand and Belfrage (2001) compared the HCR-20 scores of female and male forensic patients and found no significant differences in mean subscale scores and total scores. Nicholls and colleagues

(2004) examined the HCR-20 in female and male civil psychiatric patients and found good predictive validity for inpatient violence for men and women. Regarding violence in the community, they found modest levels of predictive accuracy for the occurrence of 'any violence' for both sexes. Predictive accuracy for 'physical violence' in the community was significant for men, but not for women, except for the *Historical* subscale. De Vogel and De Ruiter (2005) examined the HCR-20 in a group of female forensic patients and a matched group of male patients. For men, the HCR-20 total score demonstrated good to excellent predictive validity for violent outcome. For women, only the HCR-20 final risk judgement, but not the HCR-20 total score, demonstrated significant predictive validity for violent outcome. Thus, while a simple addition of individual HCR-20 risk factors was not adequate in predicting violence risk in female patients, the SPJ method based on the HCR-20 seemed to perform well. Schaap and colleagues (2009) examined the predictive validity of the HCR-20 in female patients from two Dutch forensic hospitals[1] and found no significant predictive accuracy for HCR-20 scores for violent outcome. The same was found in a group of incarcerated women (Warren, et al., 2005) and in a group of female short-term psychiatric inpatients (Strub, 2010). McKeown (2010) did a literature review into violence risk assessment with the HCR-20 in women and concluded that for now, the research supports the use of the HCR-20 with female populations, but that more research is needed and that a particular focus on extra risk factors that may further inform violence risk assessment in women would be valuable. In conclusion, the results are equivocal and the predictive accuracy of the HCR-20 items in female samples has not convincingly been proven. It is worth noting here that good predictive validity of scores is not the only criterion for a valuable risk assessment tool (see Cooke and Michie, this volume); the usefulness/social validity and value in an individual case with respect to risk management and prevention of harm are at least as important (see also Hart and Logan, 2011).

Protective factors in women

Gender-responsive assessment should not only consider risk factors but also evaluate strengths and signs of resilience. It has been suggested that each sex may respond differently to protective factors (Rumgay, 2004). For example, Hawkins and colleagues (2009) found that family connectedness and religiosity provided significant protection for girls, but not for boys. Positive social relationships were found to have a stronger protective effect for adolescent girls compared to boys (Hart, et al., 2007). In a Dutch study into gender differences in risk assessment using the *Structured Assessment of Violence Risk in Youth* (SAVRY; Borum, et al., 2006) in adolescent girls and boys, it was found that scores on the protective factor *Positive attitude towards interventions and authority* were significantly higher for girls compared to boys (Lodewijks, et al., 2008). For adult women, it has been found that marriage of good quality, employment, and adequate social capital, reduce recidivism (Holtfreter and Cupp, 2007). A protective factor for adult women that is often mentioned in the literature is dedication to their children;[2] this factor could be an important incentive for treatment (Benda, 2005), although this can also be an extra risk factor (see FAM item R7 *Problematic child care responsibility*).

Recently, an SPJ instrument was developed for protective factors intended to be used in conjunction with SPJ risk assessment instruments such as the HCR-20: the *Structured Assessment of PROtective Factors* for violence risk (SAPROF; De Vogel, et al., 2009; also De Vries Robbé and De Vogel, this volume). Although the SAPROF was not specifically developed from a gender-sensitive point, it was found that the predictive validity of the SAPROF for not committing inpatient violence was good for both men and women. However, there were some differences in which factors were the most valuable. For men, the items *Self-control, Attitudes towards authority* and *Work* were the best predictors for not committing violent incidents during treatment. For women, the items *Coping, Intelligence* and *Financial management* were the strongest predicting factors (De Vries Robbé and De Vogel, 2011).

Gender-responsive treatment

During the past ten years, several authors have recognized a number of specific treatment needs of female offenders, often referred to as gender-responsive approaches (e.g. Bloom, et al., 2003; Bottos, 2007; Heilbrun, et al., 2008; Morgan and Patton, 2002). In general, these treatment models stress the importance of using gender-sensitive risk assessment and addressing issues such as trauma, (sexual) abuse, and the role of social relations and disruptions in these relations in treatment. A central concept in North American treatment programmes for women is empowerment; i.e., increasing women's self-esteem and internal locus of control (Salisbury, et al., 2009). It has been stated that the practice of violence risk management in women should respond to the observed high levels of psychiatric comorbidity, especially Axis I/II comorbidity (Logan and Blackburn, 2009). Lewis (2006) recommends a treatment model for incarcerated women that recognizes gender differences but also gender challenges, i.e., the acknowledgement that working with female offenders is in some respects harder than working with male offenders. Foley (2008) reviewed twelve gender-specific programmes for delinquent girls and concluded that most of these programmes did not yet sufficiently incorporate relevant theories and gender-specific risk and protective factors into their curriculum. Hubbard and Matthews (2008) studied the 'what works' literature and the literature on gender-responsive treatment and concluded that they are more complementary than competitive and that together they provide a blueprint for effective working with females.

Development of a more gender-sensitive risk assessment instrument

Considering the wish for more specific knowledge and research on violence risk assessment in women and the ambiguous results on the value of risk assessment tools for violence in women, we decided to formulate a more gender-sensitive risk assessment guideline and, subsequently, conduct studies into the psychometric properties and clinical value of this guideline. Because of the considerable level of similarity in risk factors for men and women (see also Guy and Douglas, 2006), we chose not to create a completely new risk assessment instrument for women but instead use the internationally most widely used risk assessment tool for violence, the HCR-20, as a basis.

In 2007, a draft version of the FAM was developed based on a literature review and clinical expertise (Van Kalmthout and Place, 2007). In a previous study, mental health professionals working in forensic psychiatry were specifically asked to consider case-specific risk factors that do not fit within the HCR-20 item descriptions (see De Vogel and De Ruiter, 2005). The three most frequently coded other considerations for women were 1) (pattern of) problematic partner choice; 2) problems with child-care responsibilities, especially the stress related to this; and 3) prostitution, particularly the often accompanying maladaptive lifestyle and vulnerability of the woman. Furthermore, interviews with mental health professionals were conducted which revealed additional risk factors specific for women: covert behaviour, like stirring things up and hiding or concealing the truth; manipulative way of dealing with sexuality, like exploiting her sexuality for personal gain; and low self-esteem. The FAM draft version was implemented at the end of 2007 for all female patients in the Van der Hoeven Kliniek, a Dutch forensic psychiatric hospital admitting both men and women (women make up about 20 per cent of the population). In 2010, we revised the tool and made improvements based on user feedback and experiences with coding procedures of other tools, specifically the SAPROF and the *Short-Term Assessment of Risk and Treatability* (START; Webster, et al., 2004). The revised tool was named the *Female Additional Manual: Research Version* (FAM:RV). In 2010, a prospective pilot study was carried out on the FAM:RV in the Van der Hoeven Kliniek. The results of this pilot study, as well as an updated literature review, were incorporated in the present FAM.

The FAM

The FAM consists of 14 items: additional guidelines for women for five HCR-20 items and nine new items with specific importance for women (see Table 10.1 and Table 10.2). Together with the other 15 HCR-20 items, the FAM makes up risk assessment guidelines specifically for women. Some of the additional guidelines to HCR-20 items are minor changes in the item description or notes aiming to pinpoint a different interpretation or implication of the item in women. The additional guidelines to the items *Early maladjustment* and *Personality disorder* aimed at better differentiation may also be valuable for men (see also the revision of the HCR-20 in preparation, the *Historical-Clinical-Risk Management-Version 3* – HCR:V3; Douglas, et al., in preparation).

Next to the additional guidelines for five HCR-20 items and the nine new items, we added three new coding aspects to the FAM based on clinical experiences with

Table 10.1 Additional guidelines in the FAM for HCR-20 items

HCR-20 items		Additional guidelines
H6	Major mental illness	Disorders that are specifically or predominantly prevalent in women are also included, such as postpartum depression, postpartum psychosis or Munchausen by Proxy Syndrome.
H7	Psychopathy	0 = Nonpsychopathic. Score of under 14 on the PCL-R, or under 11 on the Psychopathy Checklist-Revised: Screening Version (PCL:SV);
		1 = Possible/less serious psychopathy; score of 14–23 on the PCL-R, or 11–15 on the PCL:SV;
		2 = Definite/serious psychopathy; score of 24 or more on the PCL-R, or 16 or more on the PCL:SV.
H8	Early maladjustment	8a) Problematic circumstances during childhood (e.g., victim of abuse, witness of parental violence);
		8b) Problematic behaviour during childhood (e.g., antisocial behaviour, violence).
H9	Personality disorder	0 = No cluster B personality disorder or personality disorder with traits of suspiciousness;
		1 = Possible/less serious cluster B personality disorder(s) or personality disorder with traits of suspiciousness;
		2 = Definite/serious cluster B personality disorder(s) or personality disorder with traits of suspiciousness.
H10	Prior supervision failure	Supervision failure during voluntary stay in general psychiatric institutions is also included. A pattern must be observable.

Table 10.2 Specific risk factors for women in the FAM*

		Brief description	Literature
Historical items			
H11	Prostitution	Has worked as a prostitute for a substantial period of time. Often maladaptive living circumstances/lifestyle of a prostitute are seen as risk factor. Moreover, the vulnerability of a woman forced into prostitution makes her also vulnerable to be dragged into offences.	Morgan and Patton, 2002
H12	Parenting difficulties	Serious parenting difficulties, for instance, abuse or emotional neglect of children. Information is needed from official institutions like the Child Welfare Council.	Messer, et al. 2004; Van Voorhis, et al. 2010
H13	Pregnancy at young age	Serious impact of pregnancy at young age (before the age of 20). Abortions or miscarriages can also be included.	Messer, et al. 2004; Serbin, et al. 1998
H14	Suicidality/ self-harm	Serious and/or repeated suicide attempt(s) and/ or self-harm. As level of suicidality increases, so does the frequency of externalizing violence. Suicide is also seen as motive for some violent offences like filicide and arson.	Benda, 2005; Blanchette and Brown, 2006; Morgan and Patton, 2002

		Brief description	Literature

Historical items

| H15 | Victimization after childhood | Serious victimization after childhood (after the age of 17), such as sexual abuse and intimate-partner violence. Traumatization may also have an indirect effect: may lead to psychiatric disorders and substance abuse. | Benda, 2005 |

Clinical items

| C6 | Covert/ manipulative behaviour | Serious indications of covert or manipulative behaviour. Examples of covert behaviour are concealing or hiding the truth, stirring things up, gossiping, lying about relations, blackmailing others. Examples of manipulative behaviour are utilizing her sexuality in order to obtain power or other gains or utilizing somatic complaints in order to avoid treatment programme. | No empirical evidence |
| C7 | Low self-esteem | Negative beliefs and emotions about her own worth that may result in feelings of despair, hopelessness, having nothing to lose and consequently acting violently towards herself and/or others. | Van Voorhis, et al. 2010 |

Risk management items

| R6 | Problematic child-care responsibility | Serious problems because of the (desired) care for children. Raising children might be too stressful considering the woman's own problems/pathology. Also, grief over the loss of child(ren) through termination of parental rights, anger towards others for questioning her skills and/or taking away her parental rights. | Greene, et al. 2000; Van Voorhis, et al. 2010 |
| R7 | Problematic intimate relationship | Problematic (anticipated) intimate relationship, e.g., living with a criminal partner, intimate-partner violence. | Benda, 2005; Messer, et al. 2004; Van Voorhis, et al. 2010 |

*The FAM was designed as an additional manual to the HCR-20, but it can also be applied as an additional manual to the HCR: V3 when this tool is officially published. The additional guidelines in the FAM to the HCR-20 items H8, H9 and H10 are likely no longer necessary for combined use with the HCR: V3. With respect to the new FAM items, the item *Victimization after childhood* will likely be addressed in the HCR: V3 proposed item *Traumatic experiences*, although this item will likely not distinguish between childhood victimization and victimization during adulthood (see Douglas, et al., in preparation).

other tools. First, the assessor is invited to mark critical items, that is, risk factors that are considered essential for the present case. Static critical items are essential risk factors for the case at hand that should be kept in mind as long-term vulnerabilities for the risk of future violence. Dynamic critical items are items that the assessor believes risk management should focus on in order to lower the risk of future violence. The possibility of coding critical items is also applied in the START and SAPROF and is highly appreciated by mental health professionals because it structures their thinking and helps them to focus and prioritize treatment goals.[3] Second, the assessor is invited to not only make a final judgement on the risk of *violent behaviour towards others* (including influencing others to commit violence or being accessory to violence), but also to judge the risk of *self-destructive behaviour,*[4] the risk of *victimization* and the risk of *non-violent criminal behaviour*. Although there is presently no empirical evidence supporting the assumption that the risk factors in the FAM are indeed related to these specific risks, at least the distinction between the different types of risk may be useful for clinical practice. These three judgements should thus be seen as experimental and future research will have to demonstrate their value. Third, in the FAM, the final judgements should be coded on a five-point scale instead of a three-point scale. The reason to apply a five-point scale is because it is easier to pinpoint nuances; in a forensic population where treatment progress is usually slow, it can be useful and motivating to be able to show small changes. In addition, research in the Van der Hoeven Kliniek showed higher predictive validities for five-point scales than for three-point scales (De Vries Robbé and De Vogel, 2011).

Research results FAM

In 2011, a prospective study was started on the clinical value and psychometric properties of the FAM in the Van der Hoeven Kliniek. In this study, the FAM, HCR-20 and SAPROF are scored on standard risk assessment moments for all female patients admitted to the Van der Hoeven Kliniek. The FAM was coded pro-spectively for 42 female patients and a matched group of 42 male patients (matched on phase of treatment, pathology and type of offence). Two independent researchers coded the clinical records of twenty women in order to examine the interrater reli-ability. Good interrater reliability was found for all FAM items, the total score of the FAM and the final risk judgement of violence towards others.[5] Furthermore, we compared the ratings of the women to those of the men in order to assess the spe-cific applicability of the FAM items for women. Women obtained significantly higher scores on most of the new items.[6] From a preliminary analysis in a group of 46 women[7] it was found that, overall, the FAM had good predictive validity for incidents of violence to others during treatment, but even more so for incidents of self-destructive behaviour during treatment (De Vogel and De Vries Robbé, 2011). Further research into the predictive validity of the FAM for incidents during treat-ment and recidivism after discharge will take place within the next years.

Case study: Lisa

Lisa is a 30-year-old woman who was sentenced to two years imprisonment and the TBS-order (Dutch judicial measure imposing mandatory inpatient psychiatric treatment) because of being accessory to rape. She had previously been convicted of assault, property offences, fraud, drug dealing, and traffic offences. As a young girl, Lisa constantly broke the rules, lied, stole, and truanted from school. At the age of thirteen, Lisa started using drugs and committing crimes, mainly property offences and drug dealing. Although her parents tried very hard, they were not able to control or structure her behaviour. When Lisa was 16 years old, she left home and started to work as a prostitute. She was accused of stealing money from her clients. Lisa was constantly involved in unstable, often mutually violent relationships and had an abortion at the age of 17. At the time of her index offence, Lisa did not have stable housing, was addicted to cocaine, and was in a very unstable relationship. She claimed to be scared of her boyfriend because he had been physically abusive to her. One day, she caught her boyfriend in bed with another woman. Lisa got furious, grabbed a knife and threatened to kill the woman. She physically assaulted the woman and cut off her hair. Subsequently, she forced the brother of her boyfriend to rape the woman.

Lisa was admitted to the Van der Hoeven Kliniek in 2007. She was diagnosed with antisocial, narcissistic and borderline personality disorders and obtained a score on the *Psychopathy Checklist-Revised* (PCL-R; Hare 2003) of 25. When she was admitted to the hospital, she appeared motivated to engage in treatment and seemed to have some insight into her problems. The first year of treatment, she was very cooperative and followed her treatment programme properly, although treatment staff believed she behaved in a rather superficial and detached way. Many of her fellow male patients saw Lisa as a vulnerable girl who needed to be protected. Lisa had several short-term relationships with male patients. In 2008, Lisa requested to go on leave outside the hospital. During a multidisciplinary staff meeting, it was highlighted that there were many uncertainties and much turmoil surrounding Lisa. There had been several violent incidents between male patients in her living-group and Lisa had played a central role in most of these incidents. She had been stirring things up and had been suggesting to several men that she would have sex with them in return for favours. After this all became clear, Lisa was refused permission to go on unsupervised leave. She reacted very emotionally and became angry; she strongly denied her manipulative behaviour and she threatened to terminate treatment. After a couple of weeks, Lisa reconsidered her position and made a new start in treatment. The treatment became more focused on her manipulative behaviour and lack of insight into her pathology. However, in 2009 Lisa got into a relationship with a male patient, which was seen by treatment staff as very unstable and interfering with the treatment of both patients. It turned out that Lisa and her boyfriend were involved in dealing in medication, drugs and cell phones on a large scale in the hospital. Again, Lisa strongly denied her involvement, but after being confronted with the evidence, she admitted being involved in the dealing and also having used drugs herself. After this incident, Lisa was controlled more frequently and stringently. The relationship was closely monitored by treatment staff.

In 2010, a multidisciplinary risk assessment was conducted in the context of the inpatient setting with a view to Lisa having leave outside the hospital under the supervision of staff. The FAM was coded in addition to the HCR-20 and SAPROF.

The consensus codings of the FAM are shown in Table 10.3. As can be seen, Lisa obtained high scores on several of the FAM items: *Prostitution, Pregnancy at young age, Victimization after childhood, Covert/manipulative behaviour,* and *Problematic intimate relationship*. In addition, by lowering the PCL-R cutoff score for women, the HCR-20 item *Psychopathy* became more salient in Lisa's case. The new differentiation in the HCR-20 item *Early maladjustment* showed that Lisa did not really experience severe circumstances or victimization in childhood, but that she had demonstrated maladaptive behaviour from a young age. This distinction between problematic circumstances and problematic behaviour might have different implications for treatment. The items *Psychopathy* and *Problematic behaviour during childhood* were judged as the most essential static risk factors for Lisa and were coded as critical items. The items *Lack of insight, Covert/manipulative behaviour* and *Problematic intimate relationship* were seen as dynamic critical items, i.e. the most important factors to work on in treatment. The overall risk judgement was that within the present, controlled context, Lisa poses a moderate risk of violent behaviour towards others (especially the risk of influencing someone else like her boyfriend to commit violence). The risk of self-destructive behaviour was considered low and the risk of victimization low to moderate. The risk of non-violent criminal behaviour, more specifically fraud, illegal dealing, or property offences, was assessed as high. Risk management strategies based on these findings could be to exert more stringent control and supervision; for example, frequent drug testing and very strict conditions for the supervised leaves. Coaching on her intimate relationship and social contacts – especially on abstaining from antisocial contacts – is important. In terms of covert behaviour, treatment staff should be better trained in recognizing Lisa's manipulative skills. During the cognitive-behavioural psychotherapy, Lisa may work on gaining more insight into her behaviour. However, given the high level of psychopathy and lack of empathy, the therapy should focus mainly on insight into the disadvantages of her maladaptive behaviour for herself. Furthermore, treatment should aim at attaining life goals that are prosocial but also appealing to Lisa, considering her need for excitement in life. Regarding the intimate relationship, Lisa and her boyfriend could start attending therapy together with the goal of supporting each other in developing prosocial behaviour. Overall, some of the dynamic FAM items seem to offer additional opportunities for improved risk management strategies for Lisa.

Table 10.3 The HCR-20 and FAM for Lisa (context: inpatient setting with supervised leave)

Historical items		Score	Critical
HCR-20 items			
H1	Previous violence	2	
H2	Young age at first violent incident	2	
H3	Relationship instability	2	
H4	Employment problems	2	
H5	Substance use problems	2	

Historical items		Score	Critical
FAM items			
H6	Major mental illness: *additional guidelines to the HCR-20*	0	
H7	Psychopathy: *additional guidelines to the HCR-20*	2	√
H8	Early maladjustment: *additional guidelines to the HCR-20*		
	H8a Problematic circumstances during childhood	0	
	H8b Problematic behaviour during childhood	2	√
H9	Personality disorder: *additional guidelines to the HCR-20*	2	
H10	Prior supervision failure: *additional guidelines to the HCR-20*	2	
H11	Prostitution	2	
H12	Parenting difficulties	n.a.	
H13	Pregnancy at young age	1	
H14	Suicidality/self-harm	0	
H15	Victimization after childhood	2	

Clinical items			
HCR-20 items			
C1	Lack of insight	2	√
C2	Negative attitudes	1	
C3	Active symptoms of major mental illness	0	
C4	Impulsivity	1	
C5	Unresponsive to treatment	1	
FAM items			
C6	Covert/manipulative behaviour	2	√
C7	Low self-esteem	0	

Risk management items			
HCR-20 items			
R1	Plans lack feasibility	1	
R2	Exposure to destabilizers	2	
R3	Lack of personal support	1	
R4	Noncompliance with remediation attempts	1	
R5	Stress	1	
FAM items			
R6	Problematic child-care responsibility	0	
R7	Problematic intimate relationship	2	√

Final risk ratings	
Violence to others	moderate
Extra risk ratings (experimental)	
Self-destructive behaviour	low
Victimization	low-moderate
Non-violent criminal behaviour	high
Protective factors (optional)	
Final judgment SAPROF (optional)	moderate

Discussion

This chapter has reviewed the literature on violence risk assessment and management in women and has presented an initiative for more gender-sensitive violence risk assessment in adult women with a history of violence towards others. It is concluded that there is a growing need in forensic mental health for violence risk assessment instruments that are more tailored to women. Based on a literature review, clinical experiences and a pilot study, we have formulated additional guidelines for women for five historical HCR-20 items and provided nine gender-sensitive items for women. We believe the FAM presented here may be clinically valuable to mental health professionals who are working with women. There should be no doubt, however, that the FAM is work in progress and that empirical and clinical studies will have to demonstrate if the additional guidelines are valuable in daily clinical practice and if they have good predictive utility in general. Nevertheless, since this proposed method of risk assessment in women with the FAM still considers all HCR-20 items, it is not likely to ignore important risk factors less than the HCR-20 and thus can be used with the same caution that is valid for the use of the HCR-20 in women. Considering the low base rate of new violent convictions for women and the fact that inpatient violence is more easily observable than community violence, the FAM might have stronger predictive utility for inpatient violence compared to violent recidivism. Possibly, the FAM could also be useful in general mental health settings, especially to assess the risk of inpatient violence.

The present FAM was intended for adult women who have been violent towards others in general, for instance, towards their intimate partner or relatives, but also to strangers. It would be interesting to consider adapting or developing a gender-sensitive risk assessment instrument specifically for women who have been violent towards their intimate partner (see also Adams, 2002) or for adolescent girls who have been violent (see also Odgers, et al., 2005). Furthermore, it has been suggested that psychopathy – an important risk factor for violence – is displayed in a different way by women and girls compared to boys and men; for example, in a more subtle, histrionic and sexual way (Forouzan and Cooke, 2005). The findings on the widely used PCL-R in female samples thus far are not sufficiently convincing to conclude towards a similarity of the PCL-R structure across gender (Logan, 2009). A measure that is more tailored to the assessment of psychopathy in women/girls could be valuable for forensic practice.

We would like to provide some brief general practical recommendations for applying violence risk assessment in women. Mental health professionals who are working with violent women should be mindful of the often different nature of violence committed by women, be aware of the fact that most current risk assessment instruments are developed for men, and keep up with literature on female violence. We advise mental health professionals to use the SPJ approach to clinical risk assessment and management, because it seems to be most effective for both men and women (Garcia-Mansilla, et al., 2009), especially when the risk assessment is performed according to a multidisciplinary consensus model (see De Vogel and De Ruiter, 2006). Furthermore, we recommend mental health professionals to also consider potentially protective factors in women (see also Hawkins, et al., 2009), for example, with the SAPROF.

Finally, we want to make some recommendations with respect to future research into women who have been violent towards others. Studies into female populations will encounter several difficulties, most importantly small sample sizes (see also Burman, et al., 2001). Given the relatively small number of female forensic patients in the judicial system, collaboration between different settings is essential. More research is needed on (theoretical models of) violence by women and gender-specific risk and protective factors for women and girls. It would be interesting to examine if there are distinctive factors related to different types of violence in women or girls, such as intimate-partner violence and gang violence in girls. Furthermore, more research is needed into the psychometric properties and the clinical value of commonly used and new risk assessment instruments in women. Researchers could consider studying different outcome measures. In addition to official violent reconvictions, self-report data and observational data are possibly more suitable to study repeated violent behaviour for women, for instance, on more subtle forms of violence, like verbal aggression. Finally, research is needed into the effects of gender-responsive risk-treatment programmes and into the relationship between risk assessment and risk management. Increased knowledge of gender-specific risk and protective factors and adequate gender-sensitive risk assessment will hopefully lead to treatment programmes that are more responsive to the needs and issues of female offenders with the ultimate goal of preventing repeated violent behaviour in women.

Acknowledgements

We kindly thank Willemijn van Kalmthout and Caroline Place for their work on the development of the FAM. Also thanks to all mental health professionals of the Van der Hoeven Kliniek who contributed to the FAM, especially to Ellen van den Broek for her feedback on this chapter.

Notes

1 The codings of 15 women from the study of De Vogel and De Ruiter (2005) were included in this study.
2 Dedication to children can also be a protective factor for men, but the effect is expected to be stronger for women.
3 The coding of critical items is likely also useful for violence risk assessment in men.
4 The FAM should not be seen as an instrument to assess the risk of suicide. There are more risk factors for these types of behaviour that are not included in the FAM.
5 ICCs for FAM:RV items ranged from $.63 - 1, p < .05$; ICC for total score $= .94, p < .001$; ICC for Final risk judgment $= .95, p < .001$.
6 Women had significantly higher scores on: *Prostitution, Pregnancy at young age, Suicidality/self-harm, Victimization after childhood, Covert/manipulative behavior, Low self-esteem* and *Problematic intimate relationship.*
7 This sample consists of the 42 women of the comparative study plus 4 newly admitted women.

References

Adams, S. R. (2002) 'Women who are violent: Attitudes and beliefs of professionals working in the field of domestic violence', *Military Medicine*, 167: 445–50.

Benda, B. (2005) 'Gender differences in life-course theory of recidivism: A survival analysis', *International Journal of Offender Therapy and Comparative Criminology*, 49: 325–42.

Blanchette, K. and Brown, S. L. (2006) *The Assessment and Treatment of Women Offenders: An integrative perspective*, Chichester: John Wiley and Sons.

Bloom, B. E., Owen, B. and Convington, S. S. (2003) *Gender-responsive Strategies: Research, practice, and guiding principles for women offenders*, Washington DC: National Institute of Corrections.

Borum, R., Bartel, P. and Forth, A. (2006) *Manual for the Structured Assessment for Violence Risk in Youth (SAVRY)*, Odessa, FL: Psychological Assessment Resources.

Bottos, S. (2007) '*Women and Violence: Theory, risk and treatment implications, Research report No. R-198*', Ottawa, ON, Canada: Research Brand Correctional Service Canada.

Burman, M., Batchelor, S. and Brown, J. (2001) 'Researching girls and violence: Facing the dilemmas of fieldwork', *British Journal of Criminology*, 41: 443–59.

Carney, M., Buttell, F. and Dutton, D. (2007) 'Women who perpetrate intimate partner violence: A review of the literature with recommendations for treatment', *Aggression and Violent Behavior*, 12: 108–15.

Coid, J., Kahtan, N., Gault, S. and Jarman, B. (2000) 'Women admitted to secure forensic psychiatry services: I. Comparison of women and men', *Journal of Forensic Psychiatry*, 11: 275–95.

Cortoni, F., Hanson, R. K. and Coache, M. (2010) 'The recidivism rates of female sexual offenders are low: A meta-analysis', *Sexual Abuse: A Journal of Research and Treatment*, 22: 387–401.

Douglas, K. S., Hart, S. D., Webster, C. D., Belfrage, H. and Eaves, D. (in preparation) *HCR:V3 (Historical, Clinical, Risk Management (Version 3): Assessing risk for violence)*, Vancouver, BC, Canada: Mental Health, Law, and Policy Institute, Simon Fraser University.

Foley, A. (2008) 'The current state of gender-specific delinquency programming', *Journal of Criminal Justice*, 36: 262–69.

Forouzan, E. and Cooke, D.J. (2005) 'Figuring out *la femme fatale*: Conceptual and assessment issues concerning psychopathy in females', *Behavioral Sciences and the Law*, 23: 765–78.

Funk, S. J. (1999) 'Risk assessment for juveniles on probation: A focus on gender', *Criminal Justice and Behavior*, 26: 44–68.

Garcia-Mansilla, A., Rosenfeld, B. and Nicholls, T. L. (2009) 'Risk assessment: Are current methods applicable to women?', *International Journal of Forensic Mental Health*, 8: 50–61.

Greene, S., Haney, C. and Hurtado, A. (2000) 'Cycles of pain: Risk factors in the lives of incarcerated mothers and their children', *Prison Journal*, 80: 3–23.

Guy, L. S. and Douglas, K. S. (2006) 'HCR-20 violence risk assessment scheme: Evaluating item bias with item response theory', Paper presented at the 6th Annual Conference of the International Association of Forensic Mental Health, Amsterdam, June.

Hare, R. D. (2003) *Manual for the Hare Psychopathy Checklist-Revised*, Toronto, ON: Multi-Health Systems.

Hart, S. D. and Logan, C. (2011) 'Formulation of violence risk using evidence-based assessments: The Structured Professional Judgment approach', in P. Sturmey and M. McMurran (eds) *Forensic Case Formulation*, Chichester: Wiley-Blackwell.

Hart, J. L., O'Toole, S. L., Price-Sharps, J. L. and Shaffer, T. W. (2007) 'The risk and protective factors of violent juvenile offending: An examination of gender differences', *Youth Violence and Juvenile Justice*, 5: 367–84.

Hawkins, S. R., Graham, P. W., Williams, J. and Zahn, M. A. (2009) *Resilient girls: Factors that protect against delinquency*, available at www.ojp.usdoj.gov/ojjdp, (accessed 26 January 2010).

Heilbrun, K., DeMatteo, D., Fretz, R., Erickson, J., Yasuhara, K. and Anumba, N. (2008) 'How "specific" are gender-specific rehabilitation needs? An empirical analysis', *Criminal Justice and Behavior*, 35: 382–1397.

Holtfreter, K. and Cupp, R. (2007) 'Gender and risk assessment: The empirical status of the LSI-R for women', *Journal of Contemporary Criminal Justice*, 23: 363–82.

Hubbard, D. J. and Matthews, B. (2008) 'Reconciling the differences between the "gender-responsive" and the "what works" literatures to improve services for girls', *Crime and Delinquency*, 54: 225–58.

Kalmthout, W. van and Place, C. (2007) '*Risicotaxatie bij vrouwelijke TBS patiënten. Een aangepaste versie van de HCR-20. Is het mogelijk het onvoorspelbare te voorspellen?* [*Risk assessment in female TBS patients. An adapted version of the HCR-20 for women. Is it possible to predict the unpredictable?*]', Amsterdam, VU University Amsterdam.

Krakowski, M. and Czobor, P. (2004) 'Gender differences in violent behaviors: Relationship to clinical symptoms and psychosocial factors', *American Journal of Psychiatry*, 161: 459–65.

Levene, K. S., Augimeri, L. K., Pepler, D. J., Walsh, M. M., Webster, C. D. and Koegl, C. J. (2001) *Early Assessment Risk List for Girls: EARL-21G Version 1 – Consultation Version*, Toronto, ON: Earlscourt Child and Family Centre.

Lewis, C. (2006) 'Treating incarcerated women: Gender matters', *Psychiatric Clinics of North America*, 29: 773–89.

Lodewijks, H. P. B., Ruiter, C. de and Doreleijers, Th. A. H. (2008) 'Gender differences in violent outcome and risk assessment in adolescent offenders after residential treatment', *International Journal of Forensic Mental Health*, 7: 133–46.

Logan, C. (2008) 'Sexual deviance in females: Psychopathology and theory', in D. R. Laws and W. O'Donohue (eds) *Sexual Deviance: Theory, assessment and treatment*, 2nd Edition, New York: Guilford Press.

— (2009) 'Psychopathy in women: Conceptual issues, clinical presentation and management', *Neuropsychiatrie*, 23, S. 25–33.

Logan, C. and Blackburn, R. (2009) 'Mental disorder in violent women in secure settings: Potential relevance to risk for future violence', *International Journal of Law and Psychiatry*, 32: 31–38.

Loucks, A. D. and Zamble, E. (1999) 'Canada searches for predictors common to both men and women', *Corrections Today*, 61: 26–32.

Magdol, L., Moffitt, T. E., Caspi, A., Newman, D. L., Fagan, J. and Silva, P. A. (1997) 'Gender differences in partner violence in a birth cohort of 21 years olds: Bridging the gap between clinical and epidemiological approaches', *Journal of Consulting and Clinical Psychology*, 65: 68–78.

McKeown, A. (2010) 'Female offenders: Assessment of risk in forensic settings', *Aggression and Violent Behavior*, 15: 422–29.

Messer, J., Maughan, B., Quinton, D. and Taylor, A. (2004) 'Precursors and correlates of criminal behaviour in women', *Criminal Behaviour and Mental Health*, 14: 82–107.

Monahan, J., Steadman, H. J., Silver, E., Appelbaum, P. S., Robbins, P. C., Mulvey, E. P., Roth, L. H., Grisso, T. and Banks, S. (2001) *Rethinking risk assessment: The MacArthur study of mental disorder and violence*, Oxford: Oxford University Press.

Morgan, M. and Patton, P. (2002) 'Gender-responsive programming in the Justice System: Oregon's guidelines for effective programming for girls', *Federal Probation*, 66: 57–65.

Newhill, C. E., Mulvey, E. P. and Lidz, C. W. (1995) 'Characteristics of violence in the community by female patients seen in a psychiatric emergency service', *Psychiatric Services*, 46: 785–89.

Nicholls, T. L. (2001) *Violence risk assessment with female NCRMD acquittees: Validity of the HCR-20 and PCL:SV,* unpublished master's thesis, Simon Fraser University, Vancouver, British Columbia, Canada.

Nicholls, T. L., Ogloff, J. R. P. and Douglas, K. S. (2004) 'Assessing risk for violence among male and female civil psychiatric patients: The HCR-20, PCL: SV, and VSC', *Behavioral Sciences and the Law*, 22: 127–58.

Nicholls, T. L., Brink, J., Greaves, C., Lussier, P. and Verdun-Jones, S. (2009) 'Forensic psychiatric inpatients and aggression: An exploration of incidence, prevalence, severity, and interventions by gender', *International Journal of Law and Psychiatry*, 32: 23–30.

Odgers, C. L. and Moretti, M. M. (2002) 'Aggressive and antisocial girls: Research update and challenges', *International Journal of Forensic Mental Health*, 1: 103–19.

Odgers, C. L., Moretti, M. M. and Reppucci, N. D. (2005) 'Examining the science and practice of violence risk assessment with female adolescents', *Law and Human Behavior*, 29: 7–27.

Rudin, M. M., Zalewski, C. and Bodmer-Turner, J. (1995) 'Characteristics of child sexual abuse victims according to perpetrator gender', *Child Abuse and Neglect*, 19: 963–73.

Rumgay, J. (2004) 'Scripts for safer survival: Pathways out of female crime', *The Howard Journal*, 43: 405–19.

Salisbury, E. J., Van Voorhis, P., and Spiropoulos, G. V. (2009) 'The predictive validity of a gender-responsive needs assessment', *Crime and Delinquency*, 55: 550–85.

Schaap, G., Lammers, S. and Vogel, V. de (2009) 'Risk assessment in female forensic psychiatric patients: A quasi-prospective study into the validity of the HCR-20 and PCL-R', *Journal of Forensic Psychiatry and Psychology*, 20: 354–65.

Serbin, L. A., Cooperman, J. M., Peters, P. L., Lehoux, P. M., Stack, D. M. and Schwartzman, A. E. (1998) 'Intergenerational transfer of psychosocial risk in women with childhood histories of aggression, withdrawal, or aggression and withdrawal', *Developmental Psychology*, 34: 1246–62.

Skeem, J., Schubert, C., Stowman, S., Beeson, S., Mulvey, E., Gardner, W. and Lidz, C. (2005) 'Gender and risk assessment accuracy: Underestimating women's violence potential', *Law and Human Behavior*, 29: 173–86.

Stam, J. (2010) '*Risicotaxatie bij vrouwen: kan het beter? Een onderzoek naar de psychometrische kwaliteiten van de Female Additional Manual* [Risk assessment in women: Improvement possible? A study into the psychometric properties of the *Female Additional Manual*]', Amsterdam: Universiteit van Amsterdam.

Strand, S. and Belfrage, H. (2001) 'Comparison of HCR-20 scores in violent mentally disordered men and women: Gender differences and similarities', *Psychology, Crime, and Law*, 7: 71–79.

Strub, D. S. (2010) *Evaluation of the performance of the HCR-20 across genders in a civil psychiatric sample*, unpublished master's thesis, Simon Fraser University, Vancouver, British Columbia, Canada.

Swan, S. and Snow, D. L. (2006) 'The development of a theory of women's use of violence in intimate relationships', *Violence Against Women*, 12: 1026–45.

Vogel, V. de and Ruiter, C. de (2005) 'The HCR-20 in personality disordered female offenders: A comparison with a matched sample of males', *Clinical Psychology and Psychotherapy*, 12: 226–40.

— (2006) 'Structured professional judgment of violence risk in forensic clinical practice: A prospective study into the predictive validity of the Dutch HCR-20', *Psychology, Crime and Law*, 12: 321–36.

Vogel, V. de, Ruiter, C. de, Bouman, Y. and Vries Robbé, M. de (2009) *SAPROF: Guidelines for the assessment of protective factors for violence risk, English Version*, Utrecht, The Netherlands: Forum Educatief.

Vogel, V. de and Vries Robbé, M. de (2011) '*Risk assessment in female forensic psychiatric patients. First results with new gender-sensitive risk assessment guidelines*', paper presented at the 11th Conference of the International Association of Forensic Mental Health Services, Barcelona, Spain, June.

Vogel, V. de, Vries Robbé, M. de, Kalmthout, W. van and Place, C. (2011) *Female Additional Manual (FAM): Additional guidelines to the HCR-20 for assessing risk for violence in women*, Utrecht, The Netherlands: Van der Hoeven Stichting.

Voorhis, P. van, Wright, E. M., Salisbury, E., and Bauman, A. (2010) 'Women's risk factors and their contributions to existing risk/needs assessment: The current status of a gender-responsive supplement', *Criminal Justice and Behavior*, 37: 261–88.

Vries Robbé, M. de and Vogel, V. de (2011) '*Assessing protective factors: The SAPROF*', paper presented at the 11th Conference of the International Association of Forensic Mental Health Services, Barcelona, Spain, June.

Warren, J. I., South, S., Burnette, M. L., Rogers, A., Friend, R., Bale, R. and Van Patten, I. (2005) 'Understanding the risk factors for violence and criminality in women: The predictive validity of the PCL-R and HCR-20', *International Journal of Law and Psychiatry*, 28: 269–89.

Webster, C. D., Douglas, K. S., Eaves, D. and Hart, S. D. (1997) *HCR-20: Assessing the risk of violence, Version 2*, Burnaby, British Columbia, Canada: Simon Fraser University and Forensic Psychiatric Services Commission of British Columbia.

Webster, C. D., Martin, M., Brink, J., Nicholls, T. L. and Middleton, C. (2004) *Short-Term Assessment of Risk and Treatability (START): Clinical guide for evaluation risk and recovery*, Ontario, Canada: St. Joseph's Healthcare Hamilton.

11 Clinical risk assessment and management with military personnel and veterans

The tip of a camouflaged iceberg

John Marham

Mental health is arguably one of the more stigmatizing medical conditions that we come across in our day-to-day lives; this is possibly even more of an issue for armed forces personnel who are on active service. The provision of mental health services for the armed forces has been openly ridiculed since time immemorial. Shephard (2000) describes the arrival of a newly appointed neurologist in 1914 to the British army on the Western Front who was greeted with derision and incredulity. A senior officer could not understand this appointment and asked if he was here to look after his soldiers' nerves. When informed that he was, the senior officer announced it to his troops, who then ridiculed the appointment with jeers and laughter.

In 1982, Argentina invaded the Falkland Islands. This was a short but ferocious campaign. It was widely documented that despite the extensive training, many soldiers found it difficult to cope with the realities of battle. The British armed forces invited psychiatrists to come along. However, they too were held in poor regard as it was felt that they spent most of their time dealing with domestic problems, minor psychiatric issues, and alcoholism. Obviously, the psychiatrists knew of trauma-related mental health problems in the soldiers they saw, but felt that this only happened to conscripts, not to a professional volunteer army. Publically, the British Government acknowledged the emotional aftereffects of war – but also felt that it was bad for recruitment. Mental health problems in armed forces personnel were very much regarded as the soldier's own business; only if senior officers felt he or she was beyond recovery did these problems become a charity or a civilian doctor's problem.

Fortunately, times have changed and mental health is now taken more seriously than ever before within military circles. It is still hard to talk about mental health in the armed forces, but it is acknowledged that it is vitally important that serving and former military personnel have access to the right services and a place to deal with these issues (Fawcett 2009). In February 2009, the National Health Service (NHS) in the UK opened a network of services aimed directly at caring for military personnel; this was in line with a report written by the Department of Health (DH) for the use of NHS facilities by this population (DH, 2004). The DH issued guidance to cover the arrangements between the Ministry of Defence (MoD) and the NHS for the treatment of military personnel in NHS hospitals (DH, 2005). The underpinning principles of this guidance are as follows:

The treatment of armed services personnel should align with the treatment of civilians where possible;

The MoD is able to secure higher levels of access for operational purposes from any NHS Trust in the UK in return for enhanced payment, as negotiated by the MoD and NHS;

Armed services personnel will benefit from the provision of health care and improve operational effectiveness;

Defence Medical Services (DMS) personnel should be fully integrated into the NHS Trusts; and

Host NHS Trusts in the UK should not be financially disadvantaged when hosting DMS personnel or by the provision of treatments for armed forces personnel.

Mental health services for military personnel

There are currently 15 Departments of Community Mental Health (DCMH) for the use of military personnel, as well as several overseas departments (Palmer, 2009a). These military-run facilities are similar to NHS Community Mental Health Teams in the UK in that they offer specialist psychiatric services that include psychiatrists, clinical psychologists, community psychiatric nurses (CPNs), and mental health social workers. The NHS, in close liaison with their military counterparts, provides inpatient mental health care in the UK.

There are currently seven NHS Trusts in the UK that provide dedicated inpatient services for military personnel; that is, there is a contract between the MoD and the NHS to provide so-called tri-service cover or cover for the Army, the Royal Navy and the Royal Air Force. These units provide assessment and treatment for servicemen and women of the armed forces who are experiencing mental health difficulties requiring an inpatient admission (Abbott and Jones, 2009). These seven contracted NHS Trusts are within easy reach of the 15 military DCMH; they are self-contained, and they provide four dedicated beds operating on a 24-hour basis. It is vital that all NHS standards are maintained whilst implementing all the military frameworks and documentation. Collaboratively, common care pathways are agreed and maintained across the entire network. All these units were encouraged to share examples of best practice, learning and professional development (Palmer, 2009b).

These pathways are reviewed quarterly to ensure the care and treatment provided are appropriate for the patient's needs. The Nursing and Midwifery Council (2007) and the DH (2004) highlight the need for effective collaborative working because it helps achieve efficient patient-centred care. It is widely acknowledged that there are benefits to all disciplines working together efficiently to build understanding and achieve effective outcomes. Close links with military counterparts are essential; NHS staff establish close professional working relationships with all the Service Liaison Officers (SLO), who are pivotal members of the military multidisciplinary team (MDT). SLOs are experienced, senior practising mental health nurses (RMN or RN:MH) who work at the DCMH. They act as a conduit between the DCMH and the hospital inpatient unit, and they advocate for the soldier during their stay in hospital. Familiarization with the military language, paperwork, and procedures was the priority in order to communicate effectively with both the NHS and MoD MDTs.

The NHS review on military mental health (National Health Service, 2009) recognizes mental illness as a serious and disabling condition – but one that can be treated. It acknowledged that the main focus of treatment for those with mental health problems is recovery and rehabilitation. Jenkins (2005) details the background to how mental health care should be provided to armed forces personnel. He acknowledges mental health as a common phenomenon in the civilian population that is generally managed and cared for by a general practitioner. Care is more likely to be effective when specialist mental health services support the primary care team in order to provide integrated care. There are clearly parallels between civilian and military life.

However, what is required by civilian personnel with serious and enduring mental illness is fundamentally different from what is required by military personnel. Arguably, military personnel will have fewer serious and enduring mental health problems – they are unlikely to have been recruited if they did – but in terms of impact on safety, capability and effectiveness, mental health problems that develop following recruitment or as a consequence of the particular stressors of military life are just as disabling on a day-to-day basis as the range of mental health problems are for their civilian counterparts. Mental wellbeing is a dynamic state in which the individual works both productively and creatively with the aim of fulfilling their own potential (NHS, 2009). Work is very important in promoting mental wellbeing. However, it can also have a negative effect on the individual in the form of stress. Pressure may encourage better performance and even motivate the individual, but it becomes a negative force if it exceeds the ability of the individual to cope with it. It is widely felt that as forces personnel do their best to carry out their duty, it is vitally important that appropriate healthcare is provided. Whilst it is acknowledged that the overall number of those with mental health problems is low, it is important that both they and their families know that professional help is available because the consequences of limited or problematic access are likely to be significant, not just for the individual but for all involved with him or her (Greenberge, et al., 2009).

Greenberg, et al. (2009) states that within the UK armed forces, there are approximately 190,000 personnel: 100,000 in the Army, 50,000 in the Royal Air Force (RAF), and 40,000 between the Royal Navy and Royal Marine Commandos. These services all have their own medical facilities, which are run much like the NHS. The range of serious mental health problems is on first appearance much lower than that of the civilian population – because any armed service personnel with a severe illness would be unable to continue their service. It is generally accepted that military personnel are expected to be both physically and mentally robust and to have a high tolerance for adversity.

However, the British military has been operationally deployed more in the last twenty years than ever before, which is exposing our troops to the brutalities of combat (Alexander and Klein, 2007). When the NHS Network had been active for one year, January 2009 – January 2010, it published an Annual Performance and Activity Report (Palmer, 2010). Their military counterparts referred all the patients seen by NHS providers. The number of referrals received between January 2009 and January 2010 was 254: 151 from the Army, 49 from the Navy/Marines, 53 from the RAF, and one from the Territorial Army. This represents a rate of 16.1 per 1,000 with a mental disorder (UK Defence Statistics 2009).

Jones and Wessely (2001) researched psychiatric battle casualties from the nineteenth century through to the present day and concluded that psychiatric casualties are an inevitable feature of modern warfare. Mcallister and Hughes (2007) reported that 85 per cent of military personnel returning from active service with mental health problems had an adjustment disorder, which is described as a gradual and prolonged response to a stressful event. However, there is much debate as to the degree of the problem because of the military's reticence to report psychiatric casualties.

There has always been a resistance to mental health care by military personnel due to the 'stiff upper lip mentality' of the forces; it is very much seen as a sign of weakness to admit problems, despite high-profile health-promotion campaigns by military mental health services (Gould, et al., 2008). Azhar (2003) claims only a third of people with mental health problems come forward for treatment. During his research, Azhar (2003) discovered a widely accepted prejudice against the users of mental health services. He discovered that if someone has a broken leg, they are not told 'to get on with it'. However, if a patient has depression, they are told to 'go and exercise', to 'cheer up' or to 'get over it'. Obviously, this has some benefit, but we have all heard people express sentiments like this that simply exacerbate the stigma for the individual involved. A soldier who was admitted onto one of the network wards explained that as a soldier, if you have a sore leg or ankle, you 'just strap it up and push on, but when you are depressed there are no bandages for your head so what can you do?' He went on to state that if you tell someone you have mental health problems, you are generally regarded as a weak link. Author and former Special Air Service (SAS) soldier Andy McNab discusses the mental health problems suffered by several of his former colleagues and describes their feelings of guilt and unworthiness in relation to treatment (McNab, 2008). He explains that until recent times, receiving any kind of treatment was a sign of weakness and there was stigma attached to this. They would never admit to suffering because they didn't want their colleagues to think they were 'mad' or weak or not to be relied upon. There remains a stigma associated with going to see mental health services, both in the military and the civilian population. However, military personnel voice very particular fears about the possible negative impact on career development and actively hide their problems from colleagues, friends and family.

Mental health services for military veterans

Arguably, the most obvious risk to a soldier's mental health is combat itself, a violent and disturbing experience that may lead to future mental health problems. During research, it was discovered that 22 per cent of Falkland War veterans had symptoms of post-traumatic stress disorder (PTSD). This is much higher than is usually found in the general population. Similarly, troops deployed to the first Gulf War (1991) were suffering higher than normal levels of psychological distress many years after the conflict (Fox, 2009).

Around 18,000 armed service personnel return to civilian life each year. Once this happens, they lose access to the mental health services provided by the military. Only 50 per cent seek medical help from the NHS, and of those that do seek help, most will be prescribed antidepressants. Very few are advised to seek specialist help. Parish (2010) concurs with these claims and highlights the fact that younger veterans – that is, those under 24 years of age – are two to three times more likely to kill themselves than those in the civilian population and, consequently, need to be protected. Alcohol misuse, depression, and anxiety disorders are the most common difficulties suffered by military veterans; barriers to care and stigma prevent unwell veterans from coming forward to access civilian services. It is hoped that by making access to services easier, and with new initiatives, veterans will be encouraged to seek out the help they need (Murphy, et al., 2008).

Fox (2009) highlights the failure of care given to troops and describes it as a national scandal. It was claimed that, as a country, we focus on the things we can see (physical injury) and miss the things we cannot (psychiatric problems). More people who served in the Falklands War have committed suicide than were killed by the enemy: 255 were killed in action and an estimated 264 have committed suicide to date (Anon, 2009). The Centre for Suicide Prevention at the University of Manchester in England reviewed suicide rates in the military discharge data between 1996–2005 and discovered that of 233,803 respondents, 224 took their own lives. Kapur suggests that those joining the military at an early age were already vulnerable to suicide after it was identified that many who join the forces are already from high-risk categories (e.g., young, male, having low educational attainment, and coming from areas of social deprivation) (Kapur, While, Blatchley, Bray and Harrison, 2009; Needs, Hodgman and Pollard, 2011).

Beckford (2010) cites a study by the University of Manchester in which it is observed that the average age of those military personnel who took their lives was 22 years of age, and the author concurs with the shocking statistic that the risk of suicide of those under 24 years is up to three times higher than in the general population or among serving troops. Morris and Sengupta (2009) also highlight mental illness and suicide in younger veterans and describe it as a 'ticking time bomb' because of the suicide figures from past conflicts; unless you have served yourself, you cannot begin to imagine the stress involved in combat. Morris and Sengupta go on to cite David Hill, the Director of Operations for Combat Stress, who claims that it takes around 14 years for veterans to seek help for PTSD and they often harbour suicidal thoughts. Hill claims military training itself makes it less likely these people will ask for help because by definition they are trained to be resilient.

Many of the mental health issues and risks of these 'younger' veterans are increased after leaving the forces because younger service personnel who leave find it difficult to settle into civilian life. They can experience difficulty finding work or somewhere decent to live, making them vulnerable to homelessness. Leavers who have completed longer or full service cope more easily with life after the forces (BBC News, 2008). The MoD provides extensive help in the form of resettlement courses but admits that those who have served less than six years receive a much lower level of support and may 'slip through the net'. Those who have completed their career prepare for the transition into civilian life because they receive a pension and a lump sum of cash that cushions the impact of leaving, whereas those who leave early do not have this luxury (Ibid.).

Iverson, et al. (2005) contacted 496 veterans who were in touch with mental health services whilst they were still serving. Forty-four per cent of those who responded (64 per cent of all those contacted) had a formal psychiatric diagnosis. Iverson and colleagues reported two key findings. First, serving and ex-personnel are reluctant to seek help, and the military should continue to encourage a culture whereby anyone with mental health problems is accepted in order to garner change. Second, individuals who do seek help should be provided with high quality, effective treatments, delivered as quickly as possible.

Soldiers receive extensive training to try and help them deal with combat and the obvious potential mental health problems associated with it. However, despite this, many find it difficult to deal with the realities of battle and may be at a higher risk of developing mental health problems. Trauma Risk Management (or TRiM) is a new peer-led support system that is being used by the military to identify potential risk factors 'on the ground' in colleagues who may be starting to experience the effects of trauma; i.e., those who have been subjected to traumatic events and may be starting to suffer due to this (Dorney cited Greenberg, et al., 2009; Kings Centre for Military Health Research, 2010). Greenberg, et al. (2009) reviewed TRiM and found it to be an innovative peer-led assessment of stress management, which was acceptable to those being assessed and interestingly found 'it could do no harm'. If TRiM is to be effective, it is essential that it is used correctly and that the assessors are the right people on the ground, and that their skills are regularly updated. It is widely felt that if an assessment is carried out by a fellow soldier, there will be less stigma and the assessed person will be able to open up and express their true feelings after a traumatic event.

In recent years, there has been a groundswell of support for the military as the public have realized the pressures of being at war and, to a lesser extent, of returning from active service and adjusting back to the mundane day-to-day activities we all take for granted. The care of both serving soldiers and veterans will fall directly on the NHS, alongside charitable agencies like the Royal British Legion, the Soldiers Sailors and Airmen's Association (SSAFA), and Combat Stress, the ex-services mental welfare society. These organizations perform an invaluable service and are being accessed by veterans. But once again, stigma prevents many needy individuals from doing so – and they are grossly underfunded and need support. As identified, there are increasing numbers of specialist beds and treatment available to serving forces personnel. However, once someone has left the forces, they no longer have access to the new network and have to go through the usual assessment processes to gain the support and help they need. The ongoing war on terrorism is taking a dreadful toll on the military, with many young men and women being placed in terrible and dangerous situations, which may increase their potential for developing mental health problems. These soldiers are leaving the military earlier than they may have in more peaceful times and will require support to adjust to normality. Also, their families need support so they can help care for their loved ones, who may be suffering with trauma-related mental health issues.

Combat Stress is the leading charity in the UK that specializes in the care of veterans who have been traumatized as a result of their military service. At this time, they are receiving 1,000 plus new referrals each year on top of the 4,300 existing veterans they currently care for. January 2010 saw a new strategic partnership between the MoD, the NHS and Combat Stress, which will mean direct working relationships between all the parties. Chief Executive David Hill explains the need for this initiative and is pleased there is recognition of his staff throughout the country (Combat Stress News, 2010). Such a partnership will ensure collaborative working relationships and (hopefully) help to identify veterans with mental health problems.

The mental health problems of war veterans

Watson (2003, cited in Veterans World, 2006) discusses the strategy for assisting veterans and identifies several areas for improvement, including the following:

Recognition of the contribution made by the armed forces, both past and present;

The need to make ex-forces personnel aware of services available to them by statutory and charitable sectors; and

To ensure lessons learnt by veterans are fed back into the 'serving sector' as appropriate.

Watson describes a veteran as somebody who has served in the armed forces either as a regular or a reservist; this means the veteran's community is estimated to be over 10 million strong.

As alluded to earlier, one of the most obvious causes of potential mental health problems is service itself. Erlanger and Fothergill (2001) highlight the plight of veterans with PTSD and the changing of an individual's core beliefs through military training and service. Military training, from basic through to specialist training, de-civilizes the individual. It is designed to make the individual respond without question and to rely totally on their training so that they react instinctively and almost without thought. Whilst in training, new recruits are drilled by aggressive commands so that they act without question or thought. Eventually, everything becomes instinctive and automatic; it is felt the flow between fight and flight is numbed, leaving the individual at the extreme end (fight) at all times. They are constantly on standby and never truly turn off. Soldiers are taught to fight through an ambush and not to retreat. No one can predict an ambush, however. If you are caught in one, there is no time to discuss it and then react. They compare the civilian belief system as against the military beliefs, and the comparison is stark:

Civilian beliefs	Military beliefs
Flexible	Rigid
Forming	Fixed
Shades of grey	Black and white
Maybes	Yes or no

Therefore, if an individual's core beliefs are fundamentally changed, it is very difficult – arguably, impossible – to return to 'normal'. Erlanger and Fothergill (2001) ultimately conclude that by going through this training and surviving a trauma, the individual is almost set up to have PTSD.

The transition to civilian life is very difficult, even when a person is prepared to do so. Most will 'carry over' the military beliefs they had to live their lives by in order to succeed or even survive within the forces. These beliefs often lead to conflict with civilian society. Many veterans believe they have nothing in common with 'civvies' and, as such, hold onto their own – prejudiced – beliefs. It is felt veterans are likely to be well practised in avoidance, emotional numbing, and hypersensitivity as a result of surviving combat situations. These 'coping strategies' become an issue when taken into intimate or family situations (Scurfield, 2009, cited in Needs, et al., 2011). They are exacerbated by the excessive use or abuse of alcohol. Most veterans identify alcohol use as either a recreational activity or a way of coping with the stresses of military life (Frankland, 2009, cited in Fossey, 2010).

Alcohol has been a part of everyday life for a very long time; it is affordable, acceptable and almost encouraged as a way of being accepted by your peers. Many are the stories in the military of drinking until the early hours of the morning and then parading as 'normal' early the next day. A former patient at one of the NHS treatment centres explained 'they are then regarded as someone who can work hard and play hard without it affecting their work'. Fear, et al. (2010) discovered the armed forces consistently drank harmful amounts of alcohol. The authors observed that 36 per cent of 16–19 year olds and 32 per cent of 20–24 year olds drank dangerous amounts of alcohol, compared to 8 per cent and 14 per cent of civilians in the same age ranges. There are obvious risks involved as veterans are leaving the forces at much younger ages with an increased risk of mental health problems; it is felt that this risk is compounded alongside harmful levels of alcohol intake.

Palmer (2010) researched alcohol misuse in veterans and identified 30 per cent of those leaving the forces abusing alcohol at dangerous levels, resulting in 22.5 per cent of them coming into contact with the criminal justice system. Many of these veterans live with the consequences of this alcohol abuse, which increases the risk of domestic violence, homelessness, and suicide.

Military veterans and risk

Kent Police in the south east of England carried out a survey of military veterans who were arrested, and expressed surprise at the high frequencies observed. Before the study was carried out, it was thought that there could be around 30 veteran arrests per month. However, what they actually observed was an average of 232 veteran arrests over a two-month period, and of these, a third were involved in incidents of a violent nature. It was also suggested that this number may not be a true reflection of the actual scale of the problem after they identified a reticence to admit to being a veteran because they (the veterans) may lose their service pensions if convicted (Guardian, 2010). Back (cited in McVeigh, 2010), who pioneered the scheme for recording veteran arrests, stated that this growing trend is difficult to predict. However, if these figures are consistent across all police services in England and Wales, then this could mean as many as 60,000 veterans are being arrested annually.

Treadwell (2010) cites the MoD, who claim that there are approximately 2,500 veterans in prison, which is approximately 3.5 per cent of the prison population. However, the National Association of Probation Officers (NAPO, 2009) put this figure nearer 8,500, which is closer to 10 per cent of the prison population. Whichever of these figures is true, the numbers nonetheless mean veterans are the largest occupational group amongst offenders. NAPO claim veterans' offences are dominated by substance misuse and violence, especially domestic violence, and many appear to be suffering from mental health problems, including depression and PTSD. If you add to this number those on probation or parole, the total number of veterans involved within the criminal justice system is near 20,000. There is a huge variation in the figures offered but even if we consider the middle ground, the numbers are staggering. The Veterans In Prison Association (VIPA) is a charity that supports incarcerated veterans and they concur with these figures. VIPA Chief Executive David Wilson (VIPA, 2010), himself a former soldier and prison officer, suggests that VIPA is not about making excuses for offenders, but about rehabilitating them and helping to prevent reoffending.

Whether in the community, hospital or prison, assessing risk must be a priority for those involved with a veteran's care or treatment. Arguably, this represents more of a challenge than with civilians due to a natural resistance by veterans to share their experiences, either because of a perceived data-protection issue or simply because they will not talk with civilians because they lack understanding of what veterans have been through. Lester (2010) looked at the experiences of a soldier home on leave from active service in Afghanistan, and was surprised when a soldier explained how he 'has nothing in common with those about him in a crowded street and could not engage with them.' Lester discovered that once the euphoria of homecoming is over, many military personnel find life pointless and wish to return to combat because life seems flat.

Risk assessment, and ultimately risk management, is complex and is obviously affected by many factors, and the results of this process are guided by the assessor's own experiences and attitudes towards risk itself (DoH 2007). Bohr (cited Hart, et al., 2007) suggested prediction is very difficult, especially about future events; however, predicting if, when and how someone may become violent is one of the biggest clinical responsibilities we have. To do this informally or unaided can seriously limit the accuracy of the assessment and the resulting risk management plan. To help guide this process, there are many risk assessments in use (see earlier chapters in this volume). In addition, the Care Programme Approach (CPA) used across the UK has a generic risk assessment tool or screen, which enables the assessor to gain an overview of the risks posed by the service user in the key areas of risk of harm to self and others, as well as risk of self-neglect and vulnerability. The objective of this overview is to identify immediate risk issues in the context of a multidisciplinary setting, to detail the risks and the necessary risk management requirements to moderate risk or prevent harmful outcomes from occurring, to review the risk management plan and consider future measures, and to manage the ongoing issue of risk itself. The assessor attempts to ascertain if there are any current thoughts, plans or behaviours related to risk in these key areas and if there is a significant history of a risky behaviour. This broad assessment relies upon a good rapport between the assessor and service user, and it could be argued that such an assessment is rendered useless if this relationship fails. However, soldiers are fundamentally trained to do one thing – to respond, and in extreme circumstances, to kill if necessary. Soldiers are trained to be aggressive on command and, ultimately, to take life. Soldiers do not turn and run, they are taught to 'advance to contact', that is, to go forward and confront the enemy (Erlanger and Fothergill, 2001). Therefore, if the veteran discusses such a mentality during the assessment process – or past actions to this effect – alarm bells may well sound in the minds of the assessor and his or her colleagues. The resultant risk assessment may therefore not be a true reflection of the potential risks posed by the individual client. Clarke (2008) discusses the challenge of working with survivors of trauma and suggests there may be a potential for vicarious trauma to the staff or even retraumatizing the individual by reliving past incidents. She cites National Institute for Clinical Excellence (NICE) guidelines and highlights the need for experienced and appropriately trained and competent staff to work with individuals who may have trauma-related issues, including military veterans.

A more comprehensive guide for structuring the risk assessment process is the HCR-20 (Webster, et al., 1997; see also Douglas, et al., this volume). It is a sophisticated checklist of risk factors covering key historical, clinical and risk management areas relevant to risk of harm towards others. However, even this tool may have limitations if an individual's history is not known or they decide not to discuss the major issues or concerns in their lives, which may have preceded their current mental health problems. Many veterans will evidence risk factors for violence; for example, many may come from poor social and economical backgrounds in which abuse or neglect were common, many if not all have a history of violence, albeit their violence was a feature of their profession, many may have alcohol or substance-misuse problems that mask their presenting symptoms. Many veterans have little or no insight into their mental health problems, they are often ambivalent towards life and death, resulting in many impulsive and destructive acts of violence either towards themselves or towards others in response to a heightened – exaggerated – response to perceived threat. Many veterans socially withdraw and remove themselves from any potential support mechanism. Stress may be one of the biggest issues in a veteran's life, and an active part of their illness.

Whilst working in a secure psychiatric hospital, the author helped to nurse a veteran who did not believe he had a major mental illness; neither did he believe he had anything in common with his peers and, as such, he only related to members of staff, or socially isolated himself. When he became unwell, his risk of harm towards himself and others increased; he would begin punching walls whilst pacing up and down the ward, and attempts to engage him usually fell on deaf ears. Frequently, when a violence outburst was thought to be imminent, he was deemed suitable for medication without consent. On such occasions, a three-person team of nursing staff would 'form up' and attempt to de-escalate the situation, but the patient took any such approach, however considered and caring, as a direct threat and he would escalate, resulting in physical restraint being deemed necessary. However, due to his military training, he was able to escape from the approved holds and at times this resulted in members of staff being badly hurt. Even if the holds were main-tained, he would continue to 'fight' and almost took this as a challenge.

Upon reflection of this sad experience, it became obvious the patient was doing what he was trained to do – to fight and not to give in to what he perceived as an enemy. The act of restraint itself may trigger painful memories of past violent experiences and almost reinforce aggressive behaviour. Sturrock (2010) suggests more effective communication between staff and patients will help to improve the management of violence and aggression; we found that veterans responded well to a very structured approach, mapping out the week's activities in advance, so they knew where they should be and when.

Conclusions

Rogers (cited in Norman and Ryrie, 2004) promoted patient-centred treatments and claims they are fundamental in establishing and sustaining effective therapeutic relationships. The three main interventions are well known in our day-to-day work: empathy, genuineness and unconditional positive regard. I believe that, whilst looking after veterans, some recognition of the extraordinary things they have been involved in must be acknowledged – to do so would not be to the detriment of good practice. Arguably, one of the simplest low-visibility skills we can offer is time. This simple commodity is so valuable and, at times, so difficult to give. However, with veterans I find it a precious tool in my toolbox. If we can do something as simple as give time, promote self-worth, and listen to our patients, then it may help us discover the true person beneath the illness or the trauma (Kitwood and Bredin, 1994). The forthcoming military covenant requires us to recognize the sacrifices the armed forces have made and we have a duty to help them readjust to civilian life and to help them cope with the traumas relating to their time in the forces (VIPA, 2010).

Whilst researching this area of need, huge variations in the number of veterans involved have been highlighted. However, one thing is obvious, namely, veterans need to come forward in order to help agencies identify the complexity of their needs and respond accordingly. Whatever the scale of the problem and the related risk, it seems obvious we are seeing the tip of the – camouflaged – iceberg.

References

Abbott, D. and Jones, K. (2009) *Armed Forces: Mental health*, available at: http://www.theyworkforyou.com.

Alexander, D. and Klein, S. (2007) 'Combat-related disorders: A persistent chimera', *Journal of the Army Medical Corps*, 152: 96–101.

Allen, D. (2005) 'Simple steps to a quiet life', *Mental Health Practice*, 19: 3.

Anon (2009) *The Military and Mental Health*, available at: http://www.hamlet-trust.org.uk/articles/military-mental-health.html.

Azhar, M. (2003) 'Stigma in psychiatric patients: Current status', *Malaysian Journal of Psychiatry*, 11: 1–3.

BBC News (2009) 'Veterans at "higher suicide risk"', available at: http://news.bbc.uk/1/hi/7918654.stm.

— (2009) 'Ex-soldiers "struggle on leaving"', available at: http://newsvote.bbc.co.uk/mpapps/pagetools/print/news.bbc.co.uk/1/hi/uk/7511987.stm.

Beckford, M. (2010) 'Combat Stress appeal: Veterans found to be at risk of alcoholism and suicide', *The Telegraph*, available at: http://www.telegraph.co.uk/news/newstopics/onthefrontline/7428944/Combat-Stress-appeal-Veterans-found-to-be-at-risk-of-alcoholism-and-suicide.html

Clarke, V. (2008) 'Working with survivors of trauma', *Mental Health Practice*, 11: 14–17.

Combat Stress News (2010) *Newsletter of the Ex-Services Welfare Society*, available at: http://www.combatstress.co.uk.

Defence Analytical Services and Advice. 2009 edition of UK Defence Statistics. London: United Kingdom Defence Statistics.

Department of Health (2004) *The Ten Essential Shared Capabilities*, London: Department of Health.

— (2005) *Health Service Guidance Covering Arrangement Between the Ministry of Defence and the NHS*, London: Department of Health.

— (2007) *Best Practice in Managing Risk: Principles and Evidence for Best Practice in the Assessment and Management of Risk to Self and Others in Mental Health Services*, Department of Health, London. Accessed at webarchive.nationalarchives.gov.uk/+/www.dh.gov.uk/en/Publicationsandstatistics/Publications/PublicationsPolicyAndGuidance/DH_076511.

Erlanger, H. and Fothergill, N. (2001) *You're Not in the Forces Now*, Vietnam Veterans Counselling Service: Australian Government.

Fawcett, G. (2009) *Talking About Mental Health Problems*, available at: http://www.mod.uk/DefenceInternet/DefenceNews/PeopleInDefence/TalkingAboutmentalhealth.

Fear, N., Iverson, A., Meltzer, H., Workman, L., Hull, L., Greenburg, N., Barker, C., Browne, T., Earnshaw, M., Horn, O., Jones, M., Murphy, D., Rona, R. J., Hotopf, M. and Wessely, S. (2010) 'Patterns of drinking in the UK Armed Forces', *Society for the Study of Addiction*, 102: 1749–59.

Fossey, M. (2010) *Across the Wire: Veterans, mental health vulnerability*, London: Centre for Mental Health.

Fox, L. (2009) 'Troops mental care failings "national scandal"', Mental Health Foundation, accessed at: http://www.mentalhealth.org.uk/information/news/?EntryId17=73744.

Gould, M., Sharpley, J. and Greenberg, N. (2008) 'Patient characteristics and clinical activities at a British military department of community mental health', *Psychiatric Bulletin*, 32: 99–102.

Greenberg, N., Fear, F. and Jones, N. (2009) 'Medically unexplained symptoms in military personnel', *Psychiatry Journal*, 8: 170–73.

Guardian (2010) 'Forces consider Kent military veterans scheme', available at: http://www.guardian.co.uk/uk/2010.

Hart, S. D., Michie, C. and Cooke, D. J. (2007) 'Precision of actuarial risk assessment instruments: Evaluating the "margins of error" of group versus individual predictions of violence', *British Journal of Psychiatry,* Supplement, 49: 60–65.

Iversen, A., Dyson, C., Smith, N., Greenberg, N., Walwyn, R., Unwin, C., Hull, L., Hotopf, M., Dandeker, C., Ross, J. and Wessely, S. (2005) '"Goodbye and good luck": The mental health needs and treatment experiences of British ex-service personnel', *British Journal of Psychiatry*, 186: 480–86.

Jenkins, I. (2005) *Provision and Management of Defence Mental Health Services*, London: Defence Medical Services Department.

Jones, E. and Wessely, S. (2001) 'Psychiatric battle casualties: An intra- and inter-war comparison', *British Journal of Psychiatry*, 178: 242–47.

Kapur, N., While, D., Blatchley, N., Bray, I. and Harrison, K. (2009) 'Suicide after leaving the UK armed Forces – a cohort study', PLoS Med 6 (3): e1000026. doi: 10.1371/journal.pmed. 1000026.

Kings Centre for Military Health Research (2010) 'Health and well-being survey of UK armed forces personnel', *KCMHR Newsletter*.

Kitwood, T. and Bredin, K. (1994) 'Charting the course of quality care', *Journal of Dementia Care*, 2: 22–23.

Lester, N. (2010) 'The power of emotion', *Mental Health Practice*, 13: 7.

McAllister, P. and Hughes, J. (2007) 'The symptoms and recognition of post-traumatic stress reactions', *Journal of the Army Medical Corps*, 154: 107–9.

McNab, A. (2008) *Seven Troop*, London: Bantam Press.

McVeigh, K. (2010) 'New arrests data for veterans reveals "massive problems"', *The Guardian*, available at: http://www2.le.ac.uk/departments/criminology/research/current-projects/jt146soldiers.

Morris, N. and Sengupta, K. (2009) 'Shocking suicide toll on combat veterans', *The Independent*, available at: http://www.independent.co.uk/news/uk/home-news/shocking-suicide-toll-on-combat-veterans-1746475.html.

Murphy, D., Iversen, A. and Greenberg, N. (2008) 'The mental health of veterans', *Journal of the Army Medical Corps*, 154: 136–39.

National Association of Probation Officers (2009) *Armed Forces and the Criminal Justice System*, London: National Association of Probation Officers, available at: http://www.napo.org.uk/about/veteransincjs.cfm.

National Health Service (2009) *Promoting Mental Wellbeing Through Productive and Healthy Working Conditions: Guidance for employers*, London: National Institute for Health and Clinical Excellence, PH22:2009.

Needs, A., Hodgman, G. and Pollard, E. (2011) *UK Veterans in Prison: An exploration of current symptoms and contextual issues*, available at: http://www.veteransinprison.or.uk.

Norman, I. and Ryrie, I. (2004) *The Art and Science of Mental Health Nursing*, England: Open University Press.

Nursing and Midwifery Council (2007) *The Code*, London: NMC.

Palmer, C. (2009a) *MoD Patient Survey*, South Staffordshire and Shropshire NHS Foundation Trust: National Health Service.

— (2009b) *The Provision of Inpatient Services for Military Personnel*, Version 3, South Staffordshire and Shropshire NHS Foundation Trust: National Health Service.

— (2010) *MoD Inpatient Services Performance and Activity Report January 2009-January 2010*, South Staffordshire and Shropshire NHS Foundation Trust: National Health Service.

Parish, C. (2010) 'Call to improve care for ex-service personnel with mental illness', *Mental Health Practice*, 13: 1–36.

Shephard, B. (2000) *A War of Nerves*, London: Jonathan Cape.

Soldier, Magazine of the British Army (2009) *Contract Enhances Mental Care*, Aldershot: St. Ives Roche Limited.

Sturrock, A. (2010) Restraint in inpatient areas: The experience of service users, *Mental Health practice*, 14: 3.

Treadwell, T. (2010) *Ex-soldiers in Prison*, available at: www2.le.ac.uk/departments/criminology/research/current-projects/jt146soldiers.

Veterans In Prison Association (2010) Veterans In Prison Association, available at: www.veteransinprison.org.uk.

Veterans World (2006). Veterans Strategy Review Complete: MoD Issue 4. Pg 2. www.veteransagency.mod.uk/vetstrategy/vetstrategy.pdf. Accessed: Jan 2011.

Webster, C., Douglas, K., Eaves, D. and Hart, S. (1997) *HCR-20 Assessing Risk for Violence*, Version 2, British Columbia, Canada: British Columbia Forensic Psychiatric Services Commission.

Part IV

Key practice skills

12 Risk assessment

Specialist interviewing skills for forensic practitioners

Caroline Logan

Introduction

In mental health settings, clinical interviews are the principal point of contact between clients and the various practitioners involved in their care (Craig, 2005; MacKinnon, Michels and Buckley, 2009; Morrison, 2008; Shea, 1998). In the course of clinical interviews, the client's problematic personal characteristics and situational factors – such as their mental health needs, their relationships with others, their current circumstances and developmental influences – are discussed. The ultimate purpose of such an engagement and any subsequent similar meetings is to understand and then do something positive to address the needs identified. Therapeutic progress is encouraged through the practitioner's application of a sophisticated framework of information giving and enquiry, empathy and the nurturance of change, evaluation and reflection. The structure and component parts of this framework are – or should be – almost imperceptible to the client, and the client's participation in the encounter is largely being controlled by the practitioner in order to ensure that the time spent together is used in the most efficient way to promote the gradual relief of distress. Where clinical interviews fail to result in the hoped-for change, client ambivalence or lack of motivation may be to blame. However, a lack of skill on the part of the practitioner in the application of appropriate assessment and therapeutic techniques may also play a part, as could deficiencies in the conduct of the clinical interview itself. Practitioners, therefore, must attend not only to the motivation of their clients to engage and to their assessment and therapeutic skills, but also to those relating to the highly sophisticated task of clinical interviewing. Clinical interviewing skills are the focus of this chapter.

Clinical interviews in forensic settings present practitioners with challenges additional to those present in interviews conducted in more mainstream mental health services (Meloy, 2005). For example, forensic clinical practitioners must gather information relevant to the purpose of their assessment, but often relating to subjects that some clients may be reluctant to talk about in detail (e.g., offending behaviour). Therefore, practitioners have to address the resistance of their clients *at the same time as* acknowledging their individual choice as to whether to engage in the evaluation or not. Also, as the client is not the principal 'customer' in forensic clinical evaluations – the assessment and treatment of forensic clients is frequently at the request of courts, the parole board, or multi-agency public protection services, for example – confidentiality is limited or non-existent and the purpose of the encounter is to inform and assist others, as much as if not more so than the client. Therefore, motivating the client to take part in a forensic clinical interview, the long-term outcome of which may be more rather than less distress for the client, can be a substantial component of the time taken to undertake them as well as a challenge to the ethical values of the practitioner. Such tasks as these, in which multiple and often conflicting objectives are being juggled from the start, require the flexible application of a broad range of very specialized clinical skills. Yet, in spite of this, clinical interviewing skills are a modest component of most professional practitioner-training courses. Consequently, the specialist skills required by forensic practitioners are often only acquired through experience – trial and error – and on the availability of good-quality clinical supervision by a more experienced practitioner who knows the value of interview technique and prioritizes its development in junior colleagues. This is unfortunate and increases the risk that clinical interviews in forensic settings may not achieve the outcomes envisaged by practitioners, regardless of their skills in more general clinical interviewing techniques and in specific assessment and therapeutic processes.

Therefore, the specific focus of this chapter is the clinical interviewing skills required by practitioners working with clients in forensic services and dedicated to understanding and changing problematic patterns of behaviour through the medium of the clinical interview. The chapter will begin with a lengthy overview of core skills in forensic clinical interviewing. As the aim of this book is to aid in the development of practice specifically relating to risk assessment and management, the particular skills and techniques relevant to forensic clinical interviews addressing risk of harm to self and others will then be highlighted.

General practice in forensic clinical interviewing

What distinguishes forensic clinical interviewing from clinical interviewing more generally?

The basic principles of clinical interviewing emphasize the skills required to obtain a large volume of accurate information relevant to the purpose of the interview, in the course of establishing and maintaining a good working relationship with the client, and all in the shortest time possible (e.g., Morrison, 2008; Shea, 1998). Introductory texts in clinical interviewing emphasize a number of critical stages or components: (a) openings and introductions; (b) establishing the chief complaint; (c) developing, expressing and maintaining rapport with the client in the course of exploring the nature of their complaint and its origins; (d) using a variety of specialist techniques for encouraging the provision of details about the complaint, drawing on more specialized skills if ambivalence or resistance are encountered; (e) affirming the client's feelings and opinions or sensitively testing where necessary; and (f) closing individual interviews and preparing for subsequent meetings. Methods of sensitively and clearly communicating findings in letters and reports are generally – although not always – a consideration also.

Specialist techniques for encouraging a client to say more about their difficulties include the choice and range of questioning styles (e.g., use of open and closed questions, soundings), the application of listening skills (e.g., reflective listening, use of silence), and the use of various methods of overcoming resistance to engagement by identifying and challenging its causes (e.g., managing projection by the use of counter-projection) (Havens, 2007; Othmer, Othmer and Othmer, 2007; Shea, 2007b). Additional specialist techniques include making use of non-verbal communications (e.g., of interest and understanding), managing transference and counter-transference between client and interviewer, unobtrusive note-keeping and information recording during the interview, as well as the incorporation of more formal assessment techniques such as the *Mental Status Examination* or psychometric tests (e.g., Kosson, Gacono and Bedholdt, 2000; MacKinnon, Michels and Buckley, 2009; Morrison, 2008; Shea, 1998). Depending on the purpose of the encounter, interviews may emphasize different aspects of the problems discussed, such as exploring signs and symptoms in diagnostic interviewing (e.g., Bögels, 2000; Morrison, 2008), assessing and building motivation to change in ambivalent or resistant clients using motivational interviewing techniques in therapeutic interviews (e.g., Miller and Rollnick, 2002; Rosengren, 2009), and specialist skills for interviewing children, couples and families, or clients who are cognitively impaired (e.g., Milne, 2000; Sommers-Flanagan and Sommers-Flanagan, 2007).

Forensic clinical interviewing is the process of engaging with a client in the context of legal proceedings (e.g., in preparation for sentencing or a parole board hearing) in order to address a specific psycholegal question (e.g., what kind of risk does this person pose towards others, therefore how restrictive does his or her community supervision have to be?) (Meloy, 2005). The interview – the purposeful encounter of practitioner and forensic client – is also the forum in which therapies are delivered and their effects eventually evaluated. Forensic clinical interviewing may be distinguished from more routine or general clinical interviewing and from forensic or investigative interviewing. The latter has a fact-finding focus and is a style of interviewing often used by police officers and social workers (e.g., Ackley, Mack, Beyer, et al., 2011; Bull, Valentine and Williamson, 2009; Milne and Bull, 1999; Shepherd, 2007; Yeschke, 2002), while the former is more oriented towards the assessment of need and the delivery of therapy (e.g., Craig, 2005; Morrison, 2008; Shea, 1998, 2007a). While there are many aspects of routine clinical and investigative interviewing that are relevant to forensic clinical interviewing – and some of those features will be identified and discussed shortly – there are important ways in which forensic clinical interviews represent a particularly specialized undertaking. Meloy (2005) identified six distinguishing features of the forensic clinical interview.

First, forensic clinical interviews take place in the context of coercion – the client has little choice but to engage because of the fear of the negative consequences of not engaging. Meloy described the context of coercion as the 'ubiquitous core characteristic' of the forensic clinical interview (Meloy, 2005, p. 423), requiring practitioners to identify the factors perceived as most coercive in order to try to minimize the impact they may have on the validity and reliability of the information obtained, on the observations made, and on the quality of any interventions intended to be delivered.

Second, forensic clinical interviews are not confidential, which, like the coercive context, is a major departure from routine clinical interviews. Forensic practitioners must endeavour to engage often very complex, troubled and distrusting clients sensitively and empathically in the knowledge that the security of the confidential encounter does not exist for them. The consequences of this situation for the quality of the information gathered have to be negotiated with the client and factored into the practitioner's overall judgement about the value of the encounter in relation to its objectives.

Third, practitioners have a duty to the courts and to the client to produce an account of their work with the client that is understandable and meaningful for the purpose for which it was requested. That is, the output of forensic clinical interviews is a piece of admissible evidence that must be clearly communicated and free of the technical jargon that can obscure meaning. Further, it must be simply worded and structured such that it can be understood by at least averagely intelligent individuals, yet sufficiently detailed to address the psycholegal questions asked. The letters and reports describing forensic clinical interviews should go beyond their mere description to offer new knowledge or interpretations oriented towards supportive future actions with the client. The opinions expressed should reflect the (ideally considerable) expertise of the practitioner based on all evidence and not just the client's self-report, and all the information contained in communications about the client should be relevant to the psycholegal questions posed or matters addressed. Because such documents are evidence of effort to address important issues, they must be smartly presented and free from casual and unnecessary error.

Fourth, Meloy (2005) suggests that some form of distortion 'must be assumed to exist in all forensic interviews until it is disproven' (p. 428); the client in the forensic clinical interview may restrict or control the information they provide or manipulate the practitioner in order to gain some form of advantage, either in the long term (e.g., a more favourable judgement of future risk) or the short term (e.g., the pleasure of deceiving the interviewer). Thus, clients may distort information by exaggerating or inventing feelings or events in which they have played a role. Alternatively, they may minimize or deny symptoms or experiences, or change their meaning intentionally or unconsciously, in order to alter the way in which they are judged by others. As a consequence of the presence of some degree of distortion in forensic clinical interviews, evaluations must rely on collateral sources of information also. Planning and preparation are therefore essential to the forensic clinical interview in order to anticipate the distortions most likely to be observed and the reasons for their application in addition to the evidence likely to be required from elsewhere.

Fifth, at all stages, the practitioner must be ready for clients who will challenge him or her and who will watch the practitioner closely for evidence of how the interviews are progressing in relation to their hopes and expectations for the encounter. Disagreements and evidence that interviews are not going according to plan are likely to threaten the client, resulting in further and potentially more combative challenges. Practitioners have to be prepared to defend their approach and to protect themselves without jeopardizing the interviews as a whole. However, disagreement and scrutiny may also come from colleagues and from external services, including the courts and other criminal justice agencies, even years after original reports were submitted, requiring practitioners to be considerate at all times of their professional reputation and the quality of their work. Meloy cautions practitioners against being 'narcissistically insulted' when criticism is directed towards them and recommends instead a neutral, behaviourally scientific response to critical comment, regardless of the temptation to respond otherwise (Meloy, 2005, p. 434).

Finally, the forensic clinical interviewer has to maintain an impartial and objective stance throughout their work with clients, which requires clarity about their role and the avoidance of role conflicts (see also Hart, 2001). For example, practitioners should avoid providing assessments for the courts relating to clients to whom they have previously delivered therapy. Similarly, practitioners should avoid working as an expert for solicitors who are also family members, friends or acquaintances.

Therefore, forensic clinical interviewing has some very specific characteristics and demands that distinguish it from the form of clinical interviews conducted in other areas. What can we usefully learn from techniques developed in the forensic field more generally?

Models of interviewing relevant to forensic clinical practice

Forensic or investigative interviewing practice is used by police officers among others when working with witnesses and the suspects of criminal behaviour. Investigative interviewing practice has improved substantially since the development of the cognitive interview (Fisher and Geiselman, 1992). Specifically oriented to the collection of facts from witnesses who require assistance in retrieving important observations about events they have experienced or from suspects who are reluctant to recall information for fear of incriminating themselves, the cognitive interview has provided important structure and form to the interviews of investigators for almost two decades (Bull, et al., 2009). Cognitive interviewing focuses on interviewing structure and technique. Interviews are structured to start with an introduction, an invitation to freely recall the incident witnessed or experienced, followed by targeted recall (e.g., describing the incident starting from the end and working backwards), followed by interview closure. Interviewing techniques include the use of open rather than closed questions, the pursuit of detail, encouraging the client to take an active role in the interview (such as by avoiding any kind of interruption to the client's account), developing rapport and communicating empathy, active listening, and consideration in manner and tone of voice. Studies demonstrate the efficacy of cognitive interviewing techniques in police enquiries with witnesses and suspects (Fisher and Castano, 2008; Fisher and Perez, 2007), including those who are made vulnerable by youth or older age (Holliday, Brainerd, Reyna, et al., 2009). A more refined approach, developed specifically for the interviewing of suspects, is the conversational management approach developed by Eric Shepherd (Shepherd, 2007). In this approach, the interviewer is encouraged to be more controlling of the encounter than they may be with a witness, because of the particular challenges posed by a reluctant interviewee, which is what a suspect often is. Consequently, a number of resistance-reducing techniques have been delineated for use in investigative interviews, all based on the principles of *p*lanning and preparation, *e*ngagement and explanation, *a*ccount clarification and challenge, followed by *c*losure and *e*valuation (easily recalled using the mnemonic PEACE). Many of the conversation management techniques suggested by Shepherd, and the principles of cognitive interviewing suggested by Fisher and colleagues, have applications to interviews conducted by practitioners in forensic settings. In the following section, the most relevant aspects of investigative and clinical interviewing practice will be pooled and the key tasks in forensic clinical interviewing described.

Key tasks in forensic clinical interviewing

Preparations and objectives

All clinical interviews in forensic settings must be planned in advance (Ackley, et al., 2011; Kosson, et al., 2000; Shepherd, 2007). Prior to the very first interview with a client, and based on file information and guidance from collateral sources, consideration should be given to the following: (a) what to expect of the client, namely his or her personality and expectations of the interviews and, therefore, his or her likely response to the interview and interviewer; (b) the objectives of the interviews, which will relate to the requirements of the referrer, the legal context in which the objectives need to be addressed, and the professional and ethical rules governing the practitioner; (c) an initial view on the strategies that should be prepared to maximize the potential that the interview objectives will be met whilst maintaining some level of rapport with the client; (d) who should conduct the interview (including how many people should be present in the room, most likely related to the risks posed by the client towards the interviewer) and how observations should be recorded; (e) the arrangement of the interview room itself; (f) issues relating to consent and confidentiality, and how they will be introduced and recorded; and (g) how the objectives of the interviews will be arranged into a sequence of topics to be covered during the (ideally multiple) meetings to come. The assumption underlying this and all subsequent stages is that the client has the capacity to engage in the interview process, that is, he or she can make the decision to take part unimpeded by acute mental illness, severe cognitive impairment, or intoxication. Forensic clinical interviews should not proceed if the client lacks this capacity. Instead, they should be postponed until the person's capacity is restored or until appropriate supportive measures have been put in place.

Therefore, practitioners should commence interviews with clients having already examined their clinical records and formed a preliminary view of the issues in hand and how they will be addressed in the course of the following hours. At a minimum, the objectives of the encounter between practitioner and client should include (i) gathering information relevant to the reason for the interviews during the course of an open dialogue between practitioner and client in which the client's continued engagement is prioritized, (ii) detecting and monitoring patterns of defensive responding and self-preservation, (iii) managing resistance and minimizing its impact on information-gathering, (iv) addressing, including challenging, inconsistencies within and between interviews and between the client's self-report and the reports and observations of others, and (v) staying in control.

Multiple interviews should be planned for – they afford more opportunities to achieve objectives than single interviews. Topics covered should be arranged to ensure minimally contentious subjects are discussed at the beginning of the interviews, moving onto more contentious subjects, before the most demanding topics towards the end. An arrangement in this way will allow the practitioner the opportunity to observe the client in a comparatively more relaxed state before the more demanding questions begin.

Forensic clinical practitioners who fail to undertake such preparations or to formulate their objectives ahead of their first and each subsequent meeting with the client put at risk their control over the engagement. If the interviewer is not in control, the client is likely to dominate proceedings and the interviews fail to fulfil their purpose.

Who conducts the interview

A critical part of preparing for a forensic clinical interview is determining who is most suitable to conduct that interview (Ackley, et al., 2011). In many instances, there will be no choice of interviewer; the referral is sent to a particular psychologist or psychiatrist because of their expertise in the area and availability to do the assessment within the time frame required. However, there may on occasion be opportunities to select one interviewer from several available who may be optimally suited to the requirements of the clients. What does this mean? Through a careful review of materials on the client during the preparation phase, it may be possible to hypothesize about some of the key aspects of the client's personality (Ackley, et al., 2011). The choice of interviewer where several are available should be based on the matching of the client to the interviewer in terms of both personality and physical attributes (e.g. gender), where the objective would be to minimize opportunities to clash in a way that might damage the progress of the encounter. For example, a male client who is grandiose and hostile towards women may not respond to a female interviewer, even though her attempts to establish a rapport between them are extremely skilled. However, such a client may be more responsive to a male interviewer, and one that he thinks he might be able to dominate (e.g., one who is comparatively young and quietly spoken) more so than one by whom he could feel challenged and threatened (e.g., one who is physically bigger than the client and with evident self-confidence).

In the event that there is no discretion in the allocation of interviewer to client, it is the responsibility of interviewers to be aware of how their personal characteristics are likely to impact on the client (e.g., how they are perceived by others, what they wish to communicate about themselves to others through their choices in terms of conduct and appearance), given what they understand each client to be like. On the basis of that self-awareness, the interviewer should tailor their manner to their client's characteristics in order to discourage disengagement; forensic clinical interviewers should aspire to present themselves as an 'ambiguous stimulus' (Meloy, 2005, p. 431). For example, a socially avoidant client may be overwhelmed and inhibited by a self-confident and sharply dressed interviewer. In such a scenario, the interviewer could consider dressing casually for the encounter and ensuring tone of voice and manner are somewhat muted throughout. The client may not feel so overwhelmed and be more rather than less encouraged to engage. In the event that more than one interviewer is required, the same sensitivity should be exercised by all.

The interview setting

Minimum requirements of the settings in which forensic clinical interviews take place should be that they are as neutral as possible (i.e., they contain as little in the way of distracting information about the interviewer or the service as possible), warm, private (i.e., only those who must be present are present and within earshot), and quiet (i.e., away from telephones, bells, toilets, and banging doors) (Meloy, 2005). As a key objective is to ensure the interviewer maintains as much control as possible over proceedings, the interviewer should avoid doing anything that will antagonize the client towards him or her. Therefore, the interviewer should make an issue of catering for the client's physical comfort in order to show that it matters. Also, the setup of the interview space within such a private room should be influenced by the practitioner's understanding of the personality of the client to be interviewed (Ackley, et al., 2011). Consequently, a client who likes to feel in control of their environment or whose anxiety about the forthcoming interview would be made more manageable if they had a choice of where to sit, should be given just such a choice.

As much as possible and to the extent that it is safe to do so, the interviewer should avoid placing a significant physical barrier (e.g., a table) between themselves and the client, and instead opt for an arrangement whereby they sit opposite one another – between 90° and 180° apart – with sufficient legroom to avoid encroaching on the personal space of the other. Of course, forensic clinical interviews will be restricted if they have to be carried out in a public area (e.g., a seclusion room where multiple nursing staff or prison officers are present) or where a physical barrier is necessarily in place (e.g., a door, where the interview is conducted through the pill hatch or window). However, for safety reasons, there is sometimes no alternative but to conduct interviews in such conditions and they should be kept short but frequent in such circumstances until better conditions can be managed. Also for safety reasons, interviewers should place themselves between the door of the interview room and the client and ensure they are familiar with local practice for the rapid evacuation of the room in the event that risk of harm to the interviewer quickly escalates.

Introductions and orientation

At the commencement of the first interview with a client, practitioners should spend as much time as is required to explain who they are, why they are there, what the forthcoming interviews are for, who has asked them to conduct the interviews and why, the client's legal rights with respect to the forthcoming interviews, how the interviews will proceed and the nature of the procedures to be employed – setting goals collaboratively, if possible – the form of any report or other outcome, and who will see its contents (Lyon and Ogloff, 2000; McClanahan, 2000; Meloy, 2005; Shepherd, 2007). Interviewers need to impart a lot of information at this stage and they should be sure to do so in a way that does not overwhelm the client and gives them the opportunity to ask questions and discuss concerns. This stage should be considered an investment in the client's cooperation from this point on and should not be rushed. Clients who are particularly suspicious of others may need extra information or more opportunity to ask questions, and the time this requires should be factored into the interview plan. This introduction phase is also an opportunity to test hypotheses about the client's personality style and to identify ways in which the interview plan may have to be tailored to take this and the dynamic between the interviewer and the client into account.

At the conclusion of the information-giving section of the interview, the interviewer may wish to ask the client to describe their understanding of the structure and purpose of their forthcoming meetings (Meloy, 2005). This test of comprehension is one means by which the client's informed consent might be judged to be present and a consent form, which both parties would sign, may consolidate that understanding and approval to commence. Forensic clinical interviews should not proceed without the interviewer first obtaining the client's informed consent (Lyon and Ogloff, 2000). In the event of a dispute about the extent to which consent was informed prior to the commencement of an assessment or therapeutic engagement, the adequacy of the disclosure from both the practitioner and the client will be examined, in addition to the client's competence – and capacity – to give consent and the extent to which consent was voluntary as opposed to coerced. Practitioners should consider each of these factors and proceed only when each can reasonably be assumed to be present and evident to others as well as themselves (Lyon and Ogloff, 2000).

Aside from explaining its purpose and seeking informed consent, key tasks at the beginning of any engagement with a new client include controlling the client's anxiety, developing a rapport, establishing the centrality of the client's role in the interviews to come, maximizing their recall, and encouraging them to communicate accurately what they can remember and what they believe about themselves and others. Addressing such tasks as these will help to promote the appropriate psychological mood in the client and the most helpful social dynamics between the interviewer and the client (Fisher and Gieselman, 1992). Shepherd (2007) summarizes these key tasks in relationship-building as the promotion of *r*espect, *e*mpathy, *s*upportiveness, *p*ositiveness, *o*penness, *n*on-judgemental attitude, *s*traightforward talk, and *e*quals talking 'across' to each other (or RESPONSE).

Shepherd (2007) describes some conversation fostering behaviours whose use is critical from the start of any engagement with a client. These behaviours include the demonstration of signs of sincerity (e.g., smiling, appropriate facial expressions), the use of an open posture, a forward lean and touch (e.g., a handshake at the commencement and conclusion of individual interviews), eye contact where appropriate (i.e. not in a dominating way), and nods of the head and supportive sounds to indicate active and interested listening. McClanahan (2000) similarly advocates the display of a respectful attitude towards the client, such as by asking the client how he or she would like to be addressed or asking them to indicate when they need a break, to be demonstrated regardless of his or her attitude towards the practitioner.

Interview strategy

An interview strategy should be prepared following the first meeting with the client and should be the practitioner's plan for managing the interviews to come given the overall objectives of the encounter. The strategy should cover a number of points. It should begin with a statement of the practitioner's expectations of the client's approach to the interviews and to the practitioner (e.g., willing and cooperative, or suspicious and guarded), which may be influenced by the client's experience of forensic clinical interviews in the past and what he or she thinks they have to gain or lose by engaging now. The interview strategy should then detail what techniques the client may deploy to resist making progress (e.g., denial, minimization, obfuscation, talking too little or too much, anger), and a set of options for how the practitioner may cope with each technique in order to reduce their influence on the interview objectives. The interview strategy should then contain a list of topics to be covered – or tasks to be addressed – in the interviews to come, each with a set of introductory questions and follow-up probes. Topics and tasks should then be arranged in order of the extent to which they might be demanding of the client, that is, the least threatening topics (e.g., education or employment history) should be addressed first, working through to the most threatening topics (e.g., offending behaviour) towards the end, when challenges will also be undertaken as required.

Such a strategic approach to interviews – to the interviews as a whole as well as to each interview individually – has been described as a process of 'successive approximation' towards the objectives of the engagement (McGrath, 1990). A strategic approach, applied with discretion and flexibility, facilitates the practitioner's potential to detect opportunities taken by the client to challenge their control and to understand the purpose of them doing so in relation to the topics or tasks being considered at the time.

Rapport-building and empathy

In most texts on forensic and clinical interviewing, building a rapport with the client and demonstrating empathy are invariably prioritized as key activities likely to enhance cooperation and information-giving (e.g., Barone, Hutchings, Kimmel, et al., 2005; Morrison, 2008). Carl Rogers (1959) defined empathy as the ability 'to perceive the internal frame of reference of another with accuracy, and with the emotional components and meanings which pertain thereto' (p. 210). Empathy appears to involve both a cognitive process of emotion recognition and an emotional responsiveness that is commensurate with the emotions detected. The presence of empathy suggests a degree of felt emotion on the part of the empathic person for the person in distress. In a forensic clinical interview setting, where the client is likely to experience a degree of coercion in respect of his or her engagement with the process, demonstrations of regard for the situation faced by the client may make them feel more understood and less resistant to collaborating. Therefore, it is in the interests of the practitioner to demonstrate such regard and to make their demonstrations as realistic as possible, if not genuinely felt. Evidence of empathic feeling can help to maintain a positive impression of the practitioner in the mind of the client and make it easier for the client to provide more information in subsequent interviews, or to change an account on realizing that there are more, rather than fewer, advantages to being truthful. Further, a genuine feeling of empathy on the part of the practitioner increases the possibility that he or she will understand the reasons for resistance in the client and act promptly and sensitively to counter them and without the client losing face.

Questioning style

Shepherd (2007) describes poor interviewers as habitually demonstrating the following qualities: they talk too much, thus denying the client time to think and contribute; they don't pay sufficient attention to what the client says; they follow their own agenda rather than one agreed with the client; they limit the client's latitude to contribute freely to the discussion by dominating the conversation and interrupting the client; they make pre-emptive assertions, assuming and even telling the client they already know the answer; they ask constraining questions, and fill gaps in the conversation; and they change topics unpredictably and rush through questions, interrupting the client, both disrupting their concentration and allowing them not to have to recall important information. Such poor practice will elicit little useful or novel information from a client, and the interview will have been a waste of time. How could it be different?

Questioning style in interviews of any kind is critical to eliciting a steady flow of useful and relevant information (e.g., Fisher and Geiselman, 1992; Morrison, 2008; Shepherd, 2007). In respect of the forensic clinical interview, a number of techniques are recommended. First, use open rather than closed questions. That is, use questions such as 'What happened then?' that invite a lengthy response rather than questions such as 'Did you leave the house after you hit her?', which invites only a brief yes or no response. Second, avoid leading questions in which the practitioner's expectations of the client's answer – and what happened during key events – are revealed: 'She told you to get out, didn't she?' As much as possible, questions should be phrased in such a way that they reveal little of what the practitioner knows or assumes about the client; that is, the emphasis of questions should be neutral (Fisher and Geiselman, 1992). Third, avoid wording questions negatively – 'You didn't expect her to be there?' – because positively worded questions are easier to understand and therefore to answer: 'Did you expect her to be there when you arrived?' Fourth, avoid asking multiple questions because they suggest that the practitioner doesn't really know what they want to know. That is, instead of the first set of questions below, asked all at once, ask the second set of short, simple and phased questions.

Q: 'Why did you go to the house that day? What I mean is, did you expect trouble when you went there? Did you expect her to be there and for there to be a row, or did you think it was just going to be an ordinary visit with no surprises?'

and so on

Q: 'Why did you go to the house that day?'
     [Pause for answer]
Q: 'Who did you expect to be there when you arrived?'
     [Pause for answer]

and so on

Fifth, pace questions to allow for a pause between the client's completed response and the next question (Shepherd, 2007). Do not use such pauses just to write notes because broken eye contact relieves pressure on the client to provide more information. Instead, maintain eye contact during pauses and communicate non-verbally the expectation that more information is both welcome and expected. Consider pausing for between three to five seconds and anything up to 15 to 20 seconds between the client's response and the next question, where the duration of pauses will be dependent on the importance of the subject under discussion (e.g., a more important topic may warrant more extended pauses) and the client's response to those pauses (e.g., if they cause the client to become agitated or to feel oppressed and so threaten to make him or her disengage, pauses should be shorter rather than longer). The general guidance is to keep the interview as slow to moderately paced as it is safe to do so in order to create space for the provision of important details that both inform the practitioner and give him or her time to think and to stay in control.

Sixth, incorporate reviews into sessions to give the practitioner the opportunity to reflect on what has been covered – and what has not yet been covered or what has not been covered in sufficient detail as yet; 'Okay, so what we have just been talking about is . . . Is there anything important I forgot to ask about? I'd like to go on to talk about . . . Is that okay with you?' Some writers on the subject of investigative interviewing have advocated the use of a 'quick-fire' questioning style, which makes the client have to think on their feet and increases the chances of detecting inconsistencies and therefore attempts at deception (e.g., McGrath, 1990). In forensic clinical interviews, however, such a style is not recommended where interviews are intended to elicit a collaborative and detailed review of personal problems and lead to more long-term engagement with services.

Seventh, in order not to be personally confrontational or challenging, keep the tone of your voice soft and relatively quiet, regardless of the subject or of the tone of voice used by the client. Positive feedback – 'Thank you for helping me to understand things from your point of view. This is very helpful for me in our work together' – in a gentle tone of voice, even in response to aggression from the client, can further promote participation or, at the very least, it is unlikely to discourage it. A calm, gentle tone can also model for the client a helpful approach to the interview.

Eighth, the client may not understand the importance of the questions the practitioner asks and may not initially provide all the detail sought. Therefore, repeat questions either sequentially or at different points in the interview to ensure that all the detail required has been obtained. Repeating questions, perhaps rephrased ('I want to be sure I've got this right. What *exactly* happened when you got to the house?') or preceded by an apology or a reason for the repetition ('I'm very grateful to you for your patience in helping me to understand and I'm sorry if I'm taking a little while to do so, but this really is important. What *exactly* happened when you got to the house?'), will allow the client to understand the need for detail and the reason for the question being repeated.

Ninth, write only brief notes throughout the interview and always ensure there is time after the client has left and before the next client is due, or before the escort arrives to transport you off the unit, to write more detailed recollections of the interview and a summary of observations and impressions. During the interview, if the practitioner is anxious about missing important detail, a comment could be made about making a note of what is being said, so that the note-taking is explicit and doesn't inadvertently interrupt the flow: 'That's an extremely important point you have just made. I'll make a note of it right away because I don't want to forget it . . . What I've just written down is this . . . Have I got that right?'

Finally, when asking clients to recall events, such as when looking at offending behaviour for the purpose of a risk assessment, ask them to recall their experiences in a different order than from beginning to end (for example, backwards) or to recall what they felt emotionally or physically, or what they remember hearing, seeing or smelling. Requests for non-typical recollections can generate both more detail than has hitherto been provided and get away from recollections that sound like scripts, which can raise questions about how genuine the experienced emotions were and are. Such aided recall is core to the cognitive interview (Fisher and Geiselman, 1992) and of assistance in helping practitioners both gain detail and detect deception (e.g., Vrij, et al., 2011). The detailed information that will hopefully be elicited could be plotted on a diagram of the scene or a timeline to which both the practitioner and the client contribute in order to record what is being said and to spot missing information (Shepherd, 2007).

Listening

Listening well is an art form (Morrison, 2008; Shea, 1998; Yeschke, 1997). Good listening means setting up and maintaining interviews that encourage the client to say the kinds of things a forensic clinical practitioner is most interested in hearing about. Good listening also means attending to the client while he or she speaks, with good eye contact and body language that communicates interest and attention, an implicit encouragement to say more. Good listening is done quietly, and silence is golden in the effective forensic clinical practitioner. What does good listening look like?

When uncertain or nervous, or when trying to understand, it is easy to talk too much, as if feeling one's way through the information in order to gain confidence. However, talking too much – and therefore not listening – creates the risk that the client will feel excluded, or used solely to confirm what the practitioner has decided to believe, or relieved because they can see that the practitioner is unlikely to stop talking long enough to realize the questions the client might find difficult to answer. Further, the practitioner is explicitly controlling the encounter by talking too much when a more implicit form of control – such as by using expectant pauses between paced questions – could encourage a more collaborative encounter. Shepherd (2007), discussing the investigative interviews conducted by police officers with suspects, recommends that officers aim to talk no more than 20 per cent of the interview time. This may be difficult to achieve in forensic clinical interviews, with the many different types of agendas to be negotiated there. However, practitioners should be extremely conscious of the extent to which they are talking and ensure that over the course of interviews, it does not exceed 50 per cent; ideally, practitioners should talk for less than two thirds of the interview time. And when not talking, practitioners should ensure that the quality of their listening is good.

Non-verbal communication

A number of observations have been made already about the importance of non-verbal communications in forensic clinical interviews – in the form of signs of active listening, interest, and therefore rapport development and empathy promotion. Practitioners must be vigilant throughout interviews as to the more general messages they are communicating to their clients about their own attitudes, beliefs and expectations about the interview and about the client in order to ensure that those communications are within their control and that they promote the objectives of the interview rather than inadvertently thwart them (e.g., when a practitioner communicates verbally that she wants to know more whilst communicating disinterest or distaste in the arrangement of her face). Practitioners should also pay attention to their appearance. Individual differences are to be embraced, but practitioners should think about the potential for aspects of their appearance to interfere with the interview with a client. For example, a male practitioner who habitually wears a formal suit to work communicates to his colleagues and to the service as a whole that he is a professional person who wishes to be taken seriously. However, for some clients in some forensic services, a suit may communicate that the practitioner is wealthy and privileged with little in common with the client, making efforts to establish a rapport and build empathy a great deal harder. In their pre-interview research on clients, practitioners should determine whether there is evidence to suggest such sensitivity and they should pay attention to what they wear and to the message their choices may communicate. For the status-conscious client, a more informal mode of dress may be regarded as more neutral and may interfere less with what the practitioner hopes to achieve by the encounter.

In order that they become more self-conscious about such communications, and more informed about their individual interviewing style, it is recommended that practitioners seek opportunities to have interviews with clients videotaped in order that they can be reviewed and self-awareness improved. In the absence of video-recorded interviews, a second and trusted interviewer could be relied upon on occasion to provide impartial feedback on interview style. Morrison (2008) offers some excellent guidelines on judging the quality of clinical interviews.

Control

Control has been referred to throughout this chapter – practitioners should endeavour to be and to remain in control of their interviews with clients in forensic settings at all times, but their exercise of such control should be as imperceptible as possible. Paradoxically, being in control looks like encouraging the client to take control: 'What would you like me to call you?'; 'Just let me know when you need a break'; 'May I come to see you again in order that we can finish this assessment?' By giving the client control over small things, their efforts to take control over more substantial parts of the interview may be diminished.

A number of clients, however, may seek to take control from the practitioner – because they want to be heard or because they have a fundamental need to be in command or because they are afraid of what the outcome of the interviews might be and regard taking control as a way of guaranteeing a particular, more favourable, outcome. Pre-interview research should alert the practitioner to this possibility and the interview strategy should incorporate this expectation as well as an understanding of its purpose and a selection of techniques to ensure that its impact is minimized, both on the interview and on the practitioner.

Note-taking

Note-taking should not impede the interview. Note-taking requires the practitioner to break eye contact with the client usually just at a time – at the end of an answer to a question – when continued eye contact could be useful to encourage the production of further information. Broken eye contact is an opportunity lost to ensure the client knows that their information is of the utmost importance. Practitioners should acquire useful habits such as writing briefly in formal or informal shorthand and using breaks between interviews to compile more detailed notes covering the contents of the discussion and impressions of the client and the interview dynamics. As suggested above, drawing attention to note-taking as a way of ensuring a written record that is confirmed by the client is a further useful strategy.

Incorporating formal assessments

Some forensic clinical practitioners, such as psychologists, will require the client to complete a formal psychometric assessment (e.g., a self-report personality questionnaire, assessments of cognitive functioning) during the interview. Such assessments should be introduced at the beginning of the interviews and discussed again just prior to their administration. Avoid having the interview dominated by tests or interview schedules such that the practitioner dare not step away from their pre-prepared script. Practitioners should also avoid using assistants to administer these evaluations if at all possible. Introducing a second person to the client is potentially confusing and disruptive to the relationship being formed with the practitioner. In addition, using an assistant means an opportunity has been missed to gather additional information from the client regarding their attitudes towards testing, fear of failure or poor performance, their thoughts in relation to the specific questions asked, and so on. Where it is avoidable, findings should not be fed back to the client immediately but delayed until a following session in order to observe the client's longer-term response to testing and their views about their performance, all of which could be revealing about his or her personality in the event that this is important to the reason for the interviews.

Concluding the interview

Ideally, practitioners conclude interviews at a time and point agreed with the client. The final minutes of the interview are just as important as the first minutes because in that ending time, the session is winding down and the client should be more relaxed than at the start – perhaps the client is relieved because the encounter didn't go as badly as feared. This time is frequently when clients will raise an issue of significance, which they were anxious about raising earlier or have decided to raise now in order to prolong a session from which they are deriving some benefit. It is also a time when clients are so relaxed they may make unscripted or unprepared comments that can be informative and revealing. Either way, the practitioner is advised to leave sufficient time to manage whatever might arise in this segment of the interview.

In the event that the client leaves the room ahead of any preparation to conclude the interview, or alternatively, the client tries to delay the end of the session, practitioners should spend time with the client – or subsequently if they have already left the room – trying to establish the reason why concluding the interview by mutual agreement has been problematic. Either way, the practitioner has failed to maintain control over the interview and the interview objectives are at risk.

The practitioner needs to enquire why this happened in order to understand better what the client objected to in the interview, why the practitioner did not manage such objections before the client left, and whether the practitioner or the client was responsible for being unable to end the interview in a timely way.

Protecting yourself

Forensic clinical practitioners deal with distressing information on a regular basis and the negative impact upon them over time should not be underestimated (e.g., Willmot and Gordon, 2011). Practitioners must have access to good and regular clinical supervision in which opportunities are given to reflect upon interviews with clients and their ongoing engagements with them. Such a facility should also be offered to researchers whose needs in this respect may be overlooked because their involvement with the client is regarded as less intense or personally meaningful (e.g., Urquiza, Wyatt and Goodlin-Jones, 1997). Failure to address the potential for negative effects may impact upon the quality of the assessments being undertaken and the information gathered, the willingness of the client to cooperate with future assessments, as well as the mental health of the interviewer in the medium to long term.

Communicating your findings

The written communications of forensic clinical practitioners are probably the most important feature of their employment: 'In no other mental health speciality is one's "paper trail" more important to professional standing in the community', it is the 'legacy' of the forensic clinician (Meloy, 2005, p. 426). The findings of forensic clinical interviews, whether communicated in the form of clinical notes or reports for the use of the holding authority (e.g., forensic hospital, prison, probation services) or the courts, should share a small number of common features (e.g., Carlin, 2010; Meloy, 2005). Reports should ensure that the objectives of contact in general and individual interviews are clear (and repeated). Reports should be clearly written (i.e., with sparing use of jargon and all jargon used should be explained) and completely free of grammatical and typographic errors. Reports should be brief and to the point (to ensure that they are read), with extra information (e.g., psychometric test findings) placed in an appendix. Reports should be simply written (i.e., they should be comprehensible by someone of average intelligence), they should be thorough and detailed (every issue is explored if it is relevant to the forensic issue being addressed). Further, they should communicate new information about the client in the form of a formulation, and they should recommend action of some kind. Practitioners should take account of the client's self-perception but avoid relying exclusively on their self-report: 'Nothing discredits a forensic clinician more than mere regurgitation of the interviewee's perspective in the report or through testimony' (Meloy, 2005, p. 427). Always discuss any limitations relevant to the current or ongoing assessment and explain or hypothesize on the relevance of inconsistencies between the client's account of him or herself and the observations of others, presently and in the past. And always see written communications as opportunities to inform and educate colleagues as well as the client.

In respect of representing and defending findings in courts and tribunals, Lyon and Ogloff (2000) suggest that mental health professionals offering opinion evidence are of greatest service to the courts when their testimony is framed around the applicable legal standards. Therefore, professionals should be familiar with the relevant law and legal nomenclature – they need to become 'a comfortable guest, if not an insider, in the legal system' (Melton, 1987, p. 494).

Special considerations

Finally, practitioners will be required to take account of the age of the client, their gender, their ethnicity or cultural background, disability and first language, and their level of cognitive ability when preparing interview strategies. Such considerations will inform the practitioner's use of physical and eye contact, and also the choice of practitioner to conduct the interviews. Specialist guidance in forensic clinical interviewing for such situations is limited but is available in Aklin and Turner (2006), Holliday, et al. (2009), Lamb, Sternberg, Orbach, et al. (2000), Milne (2000), Milne and Bull (1999), Poole and Higgo (2006), and Suzuki and Ponterotto (2008).

Specialist techniques in risk assessment interviewing

Forensic clinical practitioners preparing to interview clients about future risk face a challenging prospect. A client may be wary or reluctant to engage because of probably quite realistic fears about what the findings of the assessment may lead to in terms of restrictions on their liberty. Clients who do not trust themselves to say the right thing or who fear what the practitioner knows or might find out from them during an incautious moment might reasonably conclude that to cooperate minimally or not to cooperate at all is the best strategy for self-defence. The following section will address some points additional to those discussed above, which may assist the forensic clinical interviewer in undertaking a risk assessment.

Anticipating the client and staying in control

As suggested above, practitioners should endeavour to gain some understanding of the client's basic characteristics prior to the first interview, as a form of preparation (e.g., Kosson, et al., 2000; Morrison, 2008). For more specialist interviews, such as interviews about risk or psychopathy assessments, practitioners should seek in advance information relating to the personalities of the clients they are about to interview (Ackley, et al., 2011). This is in order that practitioners can more accurately anticipate how the client is likely to present and how he or she is likely to respond to the probing enquiries to come, and to allow them to prepare their detailed interview strategies accordingly (Widiger and Frances, 1985). Therefore, in their pre-interview research, practitioners should attend to information that allows them to prepare for (a) the client's likely presentation on interview, their apparent self-concept and their interpersonal style, (b) their most likely methods of self-defence or self-preservation, and (c) the most likely methods they will use to conceal relevant information or dissimulate. Practitioners who fail to attempt such preparations are at risk of allowing their clients to dominate interviews for which *they* are sure to be better prepared.

The client's likely presentation and their apparent self-concept

Antisocial, histrionic, narcissistic, paranoid and borderline personality pathologies are those likely to be most relevant both in criminal justice and forensic mental health settings and to discussions about future risk of harm to others or to self (Logan, this volume; Logan and Johnstone, 2010; McMurran and Howard, 2009). There are many overlaps among these quite poorly defined conditions, and the proposed revisions to the *Diagnostic and Statistical Manual of Mental Disorders* (DSM-5, and to the European equivalent classification system, ICD-11) (American Psychiatric Association or APA, 2011) may address some of the problems of the current diagnostic systems, not least by dispensing with the histrionic and paranoid disorders as distinct pathologies.

Key to the presence of personality pathology as it will soon be redefined is the identification of deficits in self and interpersonal functioning, specifically, problems with self-identity and self-direction, and problems with empathy and intimacy in relation to others (APA, 2011). In respect of problems with self-identity, personality dysfunction will be suspected if the client describes or demonstrates signs of a poor or absent sense of self, poor boundary definition, fragile self-esteem, a weak or distorted self-image, and/or emotions that are rapidly changing and incongruent with context. In respect of self-direction, personality difficulties will be the suspected cause where there is evidence of difficulties with goal-setting and achievement, unclear or lacking internal standards, and limited or absent self-awareness. Interpersonally, problems with empathy will be reflected in difficulties in understanding the thoughts, feelings and behaviour of others, problems with accepting the views of others to the point of being threatened by alternative opinions, a tendency to focus on interactions with others in terms of personal need fulfilment and harm-avoidance, and bewilderment or outright ignorance about the impact of one's own actions on others. Finally, problems with intimacy will be reflected in a lack of interpersonal skills, unrealistic beliefs about relationships and the role of sexual intimacy, and extreme variations in feelings towards others who are valued more for their (temporary) ability to fulfil the client's needs at any one time than because of any sense of mutual association. Antisocial personality pathology may be more specifically characterized by difficulties in respect of antagonism (manipulation, deceit, callousness, hostility) and disinhibition (irresponsibility, impulsivity, risk-taking). Narcissistic personality pathology may be characterized by difficulties with antagonism (specifically grandiosity and attention-seeking). And borderline personality pathology may be more specifically characterized by difficulties in respect of negative affectivity (emotional lability, anxiety, separation insecurity, depressivity), disinhibition (impulsivity, risk-taking), and antagonism (hostility). Practitioners should anticipate the very specific ways that a client with whom they are about to meet may present in that and subsequent meetings if they have aspects of the above characteristics (e.g., by being hostile, impulsive, by having limited self-awareness), especially if *in extremis*. The more specific the characterization, the more specific the interview strategy will be and the more likely the practitioner will be to anticipate problems and maintain control of the encounter.

The client's methods of self-defence and self-preservation

There are a number of common methods of self-defence that may be anticipated in the risk assessment interview involving antisocial, narcissistic or borderline individuals (e.g., Kosson, et al., 2000). First, splitting may be observed, that is, the active maintenance of a separation of the individual from negative objects. Splitting stems from existential insecurity or the instability of one's self-concept, and it creates instability in relationships because another individual can be viewed as either personified virtue or personified vice at different times, depending on whether he or she gratifies the client's needs or frustrates them. Challenging questions in the course of a risk interview, especially if posed by an empathic practitioner viewed by the client as virtuous, may produce a rapid and dramatic change in temperature within the exchange, from which it may be difficult to recover rapport. Challenging questions should therefore be left until later in the interview process in order that the lasting damage caused by a negative reaction to them does not impact on the remainder of the interview too greatly. Attitudes towards others may be unstable, extreme and dependent on immediate mood and circumstance. Therefore, information provided by a client may be unreliable and will have to be checked for this reason alone.

Second, a client may protect him or herself from criticism or embarrassment in a risk interview through a process of projection. Projection means that the client locates his or her own unwanted feelings or attributes in another person, possibly even the practitioner, creating inaccurate descriptions and accounts that are a reflection of the inner world of the client. The projections of the antisocial/narcissistic client are most often disparaging and provocative – 'You can't trust him' – and the projections of the borderline client are most often fearful and help-seeking – 'Nobody cares about me', 'You are the only one who listens to me.' Such comments are revealing about the client's self-concept and fears about others: 'Rather than reflecting either unusual insight by the patient or a plausible but mistaken inference, these opinions usually provide more information about the underlying dynamics of the interviewee' (Kosson, et al., 2000, p. 206). Practitioners should be especially cautious of endorsing the projection of positive qualities onto others, including themselves, as this is often a precursor to devaluation. Checking information provided by the client will be essential, as above, but identifying and noting when and how projection occurs will be an informative interview tool. In terms of an effective response to projection where its subject is the practitioner, Havens (2007) discussed the technique of counter-projection whereby anger or suspicion is deflected by identifying a common 'out-there' figure that is to blame for everything:

Client: You are useless. I don't know why I bother speaking to you.
Practitioner: You feel no one is helping you.

Third, projective identification offers clients a higher level of predictability in interpersonal exchanges but at the cost of much diminished relatedness (Kosson, et al., 2000). Projective identification occurs when a client projects onto another person their fears or anger, then reacts to that person as if they were genuinely the source of fear- or anger-inducing acts. For example, the antisocial client projects hostility, envy, or aggression onto the practitioner; the client experiences an illusory sense of connection to the practitioner; the client then interprets his or her own behaviour and emotions as having been caused or brought on by the practitioner's negative behaviour. The subjective experience of projective identification involves both a continued although altered experience of the projected impulse – e.g. anger – and often a conscious fear of the recipient of the projection (e.g., the practitioner, as when the client is angry with the practitioner but acts as if the practitioner is angry with him or her), which is nevertheless more tolerable than the original hostile impulse. When involved in a projective identification cycle, the practitioner is likely to experience the presence of alien feelings or thoughts that actually originate in the client. If unrecognized for what they are, such responses can influence the practitioner's view of the client, creating a mistaken impression. Instead, practitioners should remain affectively neutral while confronting the projective process, whether critical or flattering, because if the practitioner responds to the affective pull of the interaction, he or she has accepted the client's unconscious invitation to act out the part given them. Self-awareness is the key here, especially of one's own 'narcissistic snares' (Maltsberger and Buie, 1974; Watts and Morgan, 1994), along with good clinical supervision (Daykin and Gordon, 2011).

Fourth, devaluation is a common defence technique in antisocial, borderline and especially narcissistic clients. Devaluation in the form of usually public criticism or disregard reduces any potential real or perceived threat (such as from the practitioner) while allowing the client some comfort within his or her own grandiosity: 'That practitioner is rubbish and now he knows it.' The importance of the other has to be degraded, usually by devaluing their most prized assets (e.g., calling an intelligent, careful and respectful practitioner stupid, negligent and racist/sexually inappropriate), in order for the disordered client to maintain the experience of him or herself as special, unique and entitled. Devaluation also serves to prevent the experience of envy or the conscious awareness of what he or she lacks. Envy and shame underpin the narcissist's frequent use of devaluation, moving from person to person alternately valuing and devaluing each.

Practitioners should scrutinize clinical records and question collateral sources of information for evidence of basic defences such as those described above and how they are likely to manifest themselves in the interviews to come. By being ready for them and by having some strategies in place with which to manage their impact on the interview, the practitioner's control is more likely to be maintained.

Dissimulation

Ekman (2001) defines lying as a deliberate attempt to mislead, without the prior notification of the target of the lie. Thus, a person who provides factually incorrect information is not necessarily lying unless that person knows it will mislead. Truthful narratives feature more (a) contextual embedding, (b) reproduction of conversation, (c) unexpected complications, and (d) attribution of another's mental state (Lee, Klaver and Hart, 2008). The detection of lying and concealment will be dependent on interviewers identifying what is missing from an account as well as what is incorrect in the information provided (Vrij, 2000). Practitioners cannot reliably detect lies and deception by observing behaviour and listening to speech (Vrij, et al., 2011). Instead, practitioners have to ask questions that actively elicit and amplify verbal and non-verbal cues to deceit, for example, by increasing the cognitive load on liars (the cognitive lie-detection perspective). This can be done by the effective application of strategic questioning – phased and planned questions, some repeated, organized into a structure, covering topics systematically and incrementally – in other words, an interview strategy as discussed above. In addition, by asking clients to give their account of their offence or key events relevant to a risk assessment in an unanticipated order (e.g., backwards) and by maintaining eye contact with the client (because eye contact is distracting and more cognitive effort is required to maintain it and not be distracted from the task of lying or concealment, if this is what the client is doing), deceit may be more readily exposed. A good interviewer will detect deception by revealing inconsistencies in the client's account. An early interview phase of low-threat questioning (e.g., about educational or work history) is therefore essential to create a baseline against which to detect change (e.g., in tone of voice, physical movement, eye contact, and so on) as a result of potentially deceptive responding – so called 'hotspots', which can be followed up at leisure (Frank, Yarborough and Ekman, 2006; Shepherd, 2007).

Staying in control of the encounter

Morrison (2008) offered the following advice about staying in control of clinical interviews, which are particularly relevant to risk interviews. First, when resistance is encountered, switch from facts to feelings – resistance usually has an emotional basis – and emphasize the normal, that resistance is understandable. Second, reject the behaviour not the person and continue to use a low warm tone of voice, making more pronounced one's efforts at active listening, and making evidence of rapport-building activity clear. Third, focus on the client's interests or strengths as this is safe territory compared to the subject that triggered the resistance and bring the client around to that subject again once the reason for resistance has become clear and strategies to counter it developed. Fourth, look for parallels that might be safer to discuss – what happened in the past rather than what's happening now – and try to draw those parallels out. And finally, avoid meeting hostility with efforts to provoke guilt ('I'm only trying to help you'), anxiety ('If you don't talk about it, you'll never get out'), or more hostility ('Don't shout at me!')

Shepherd (2007) summarized for forensic interviewers a variety of problems frequently encountered in demanding interviews (recalled using the mnemonic ASSESS): *a*ccount problems (missing detail, gaps, jumps, absence of reasonably expected detail, non-specific detail, sidesteps, inconsistency, contradictions, too rehearsed, narrative contrast), *s*ense problems, as in the account doesn't make sense because it is improbable, impossible, non-sensical, or counter to reasonable behaviour, *s*truggling to give detail (the client struggles to go beyond the original story, they repeat minimal non-specific detail, they admit their inability to give further detail), *e*vasion (the client tries to change the topic, answers the question with a question, gives measured or evasive responses, blanks an echo probe, sidesteps), *s*abotaging behaviour (argues, becomes angry, becomes abusive, threatens, refuses to be helped, refuses to cooperate), and *s*ignificant expressive behaviour (speech has marked dysfluencies that didn't occur before, marked pauses before or when answering important questions, voice changes pitch, change from self-control to gabbling).

Some top tips for staying in control of the forensic clinical interview and the client, based loosely on the PEACE model (Milne and Bull, 1999; Williamson, 2006) of investigative interviewing, are listed in Table 12.1.

Anticipating yourself and staying in control

Working with clients motivated to present themselves favourably and as less of a risk of future harm than they might in fact be is cognitively and emotionally challenging for practitioners (Gacono, Nieberding, Owen, Rubel and Bodholdt, 2001). The amount of effort the interviewer will have to expend to detect and challenge inconsistencies and dissimulation will be correlated directly with the determination of the client to defend his or her position. In order to keep the demands on them to a minimum, practitioners should consider how their interpersonal style might interfere with the interview process and seek to control that negative influence. Therefore, practitioners should prepare for interviews by anticipating in themselves the following: (a) their own presentation and self-concept, and the interpersonal dynamic, (b) their own most likely methods of defence or self-preservation, and (c) the very personal challenge of confrontation.

The interviewer's presentation and self-concept

The presentation and self-concept of the interviewer is as relevant to proceedings as those of the client because the exchange between them is a dynamic of two

Table 12.1 Recommendations for forensic clinical interviews

Preparation	•	Anticipate the client – including personality and personality disorder, their likely defensive strategies
	•	Anticipate yourself – your personality, your defensive strategies, your least favourite forensic clinical interview scenarios, your strengths and weaknesses in interviews
	•	Prepare an interview strategy for the specific interviews to come
Engage and explain	•	Set the scene; limits on confidentiality; informed consent
Account	•	Baseline phase – neutral questioning
	•	Active account phase – information gathering about relevant topics; commit the client to an account of relevant events; use open questions; do not reveal own views or expectations; observe non-verbal communication; minimize the intrusiveness of note-taking; maintain eye contact; look for what's not present in account and demeanour as well as for what is present; repeated questioning in order to elicit detail on subjects whose understanding or recall is obscure; endeavour to talk less than 50 per cent of the time
	•	Challenge phase – address inconsistencies and contradictions within the client's account – 'hotspots'; robust questioning about the veracity of the client's account of his or her past harmful conduct and future potential; endeavour to talk less than 20 per cent of the time; detect changes in manner and demeanour from the baseline phase
Closure	•	Return to more neutral questioning – about future prospects
	•	Recap
Evaluate	•	Review findings against interview objectives
	•	Assess requirement for further interviews
	•	Determine quality of interview – strengths and weaknesses – and identify what can be learned from this particular interview encounter

(possibly more) people, each contributing equally. Practitioners should assess their own personalities – if necessary, they should undertake a formal assessment of personality using structured instruments like the *Neuroticism-Extroversion-Openness Personality Inventory-Revised* (NEO-PI-R, Costa and McCrae, 2008) or the *Minnesota Multiphasic Personality Inventory-2nd Edition* (Ben-Porath and Tellegen, 2008) or the *Young Schema Questionnaire* (Young, 1994). As suggested above, practitioners should also examine what others see of them – their clothes, their style, their jewellery, their cars or motorbikes, their homes – and ask themselves 'What do I reveal about myself in the possessions I wear and surround myself with?' On the basis of what they understand about themselves, practitioners should identify the key ways in which they influence the people around them, at home and at work – do you make others relaxed or wary, cooperative or competitive, loving or jealous, and what sorts of people habitually demonstrate what sorts of responses? By identifying commonly occurring responses, the practitioner is in a better position to speculate on some of the ways in which individual clients may react to their presence. Identifying possible reactions in advance means the more sensitive and accurate preparation of strategies to manage anything that might interfere with the smooth and managed order of the interview. As mentioned already, practitioners should endeavour to present themselves as 'ambiguous stimuli' in the forensic clinical interview (Meloy, 2005, p. 431).

The interviewer's methods of self-defence and self-preservation

Clients will understandably try to defend themselves in order to try to create in the practitioner's mind the impression of low risk and safety in conditions of lower security, if not the community. It is the duty of practitioners to challenge the impressions clients would have them believe, and in doing so, the client may react defiantly – with anger, silence, accusations, devaluation, by leaving the room, and so on. Practitioners are then put in the position of managing those reactions whilst not losing control of the interview. They should consider doing so by utilizing a combination of the following techniques.

First, practitioners should anticipate the interpersonal situations they generally find uncomfortable in their personal lives (e.g., another person crying because of something you have said or done, another person being verbally aggressive or confronting you with things you did wrongly or badly or not at all, another person being uninterested in you or made bored by you). They should then plan a variety of strategies for responding to the most challenging situations identified, in the event that they arise in forensic clinical interviews, as well as give consideration to how those strategies may be responded to by the client, all so that the practitioner is prepared and flexible in his or her responses. Similarly, practitioners should consider the kinds of offenders that they least like to interview (e.g., child sexual offenders) because of the intrusion of personal feelings of distaste that can be difficult to control during unguarded moments and which may be easily detected by the client.

Second, practitioners should attend to transference and especially counter-transference processes in their interview encounters. Countertransference refers to the direct and indirect responses that the practitioner has to the client. Indirect countertransference occurs when the practitioner unconsciously associates the characteristics of the client with central characters in his or her own life and, as a consequence, experiences emotions that do not originate in their relationship with the client. Direct countertransference occurs when a practitioner's own emotional reaction to the client influences their judgement of the client's characteristics. Common countertransference reactions relevant to risk interviews include denial and self-deception responses to clients (i.e., blindness to their harm potential, which can occur when the practitioner fears the client's rage and avoids setting limits for appropriate confrontation, Meloy, 1995), illusory therapeutic alliance (i.e., where the practitioner thinks their working relationship with the client is healthy and progressive when it is not, leading to the practitioner becoming vulnerable to exploitation, self-devaluation, and burnout), misattribution of psychological health (i.e., where the practitioner declares a dramatic improve-ment because of their input, which may not be obvious to others), and especially negative reactions to the client (such as helplessness or guilt, which may stimulate unconscious rage against the client, expressed passively through therapist withdrawal or actively through intensified efforts to treat; Strasburger, 1986). Self-reflection and quality clinical supervision should be used to identify the presence and meaning of such processes, and to use them to the benefit of the interview. Kosson, et al. (2000) described direct countertransference reactions, where recognized, as the 'silver of the photographic plate' (p. 214), highlighting the client's inner dynamics and an opportunity not to be missed.

Finally, practitioners should consider the forensic clinical interviews they have carried out across their careers and try to identify one or more that they are especially proud of and one or more of which they are embarrassed or ashamed. They should then try to identify what it was about the good interviews that made them good and what it was about the bad ones that made them bad. Practitioners are advised to get into the habit of judging the quality of their interviews and identifying in supervision their strengths and weaknesses in relation to this particular mode of client engagement. And within interviews and in their immediate aftermath, the following questions may help in determining the range and depth of countertransference (Morrison, 2008): What am I feeling now?; What do I feel about this client and why?; and Who does this client remind me of?

The challenge of confrontation

Unlike other sorts of forensic clinical interviews, the risk interview is likely to require the practitioner to challenge the client – about the accuracy of his or her recall of significant events, about his or her perceptions of their own risk of future harm, and about his or her engagement in the risk management process. It is not always necessary – some clients are very forthcoming and insightful about their risks. However, many clients are not, because they lack self-awareness or because they are motivated to conceal, or both. Therefore, forensic clinical practitioners are required to prepare for the challenge of confronting the client with the inaccuracies, distortions and misperceptions observed during the course of their meetings. Challenging the client may be prepared for using the following guidelines.

First, as already suggested, start the engagement with a client by asking about non-contentious subjects in order to obtain a baseline sample of interview performance. This opportunity will make it more possible for practitioners to detect any deviation from the baseline in response to more demanding questions. Therefore, delay challenges until the latter part of the interview or interviews with the client – ideally, until about two thirds of the way through the anticipated length of the engagement with the client.

Second, challenges may be ranked into at least three levels of explicitness. The practitioner can challenge the client's version of events by asking a question such as 'I'm sorry but I don't understand your account of what happened. Can you go through your account again for me?' This response requires the client to repeat their account and gives the practitioner licence to ask more probing questions than previously while assuming full responsibility for putting the client to the trouble of doing so. This is a relatively non-threatening level of challenge. The next level of challenge is more confrontational and shifts the responsibility for not being clear from the practitioner to the client. Here, the practitioner informs the client that he or she is not providing a logical explanation and requests their more detailed account: 'I'm sorry but your account doesn't make sense. Can you go through your account again?' This intermediate level of challenge is more likely to provoke a negative reaction in the client – anger, disengagement, and distress – when it is realized that the practitioner has not in fact been persuaded by the client's efforts to be believed. This level of challenge should be used with care and a negative response prepared for. The final level of challenge is to directly confront the client with evidence of their efforts to deceive: 'Your account of what happened is not the same as the account given by others. Why do you think that is?' or 'I think you have been lying to me.' A negative response should be anticipated and prepared for because this level of challenge directly communicates the practitioner's disbelief of the client's story. Practitioners should decide from the start of interviews which level of challenge is likely to be the safest to use with each client, and to prepare themselves to manage with care and consideration the consequences of their use.

The risk interview

The risk interview itself should encapsulate all of the guidance given in this chapter so far, from evidence of preparation and planning through to the topics to be covered, the manner in which the accounts of relevant events are obtained, challenges, concluding the interview, and reviewing its contents and checking them against collateral sources. Multiple interviews about risk are recommended in order to maximize opportunities to detect relevant information (Meloy, 2005). How should the interview be organized to ensure this quality of expertise?

Bögels (2000) distinguishes between skills focusing on the relational and communication aspects of the diagnostic interview (process skills) with skills focusing on information gathering (content skills). Process skills reflect the ability of the practitioner to show interest in the problems of the client, to elicit information in an open and natural way, to communicate their understanding of the problem to the client, and to provide the client with as much information as possible about the purpose of the interview; process skills aim to establish a working relationship with the client and much of this chapter has focused on just this range of skills. Content skills reflect the way interviewers handle their agenda, that is, the topics to cover during the interview, dictated by the interview objectives.

Practitioners should prepare for the content of interviews before they commence. Specifically, they should define an interview topic plan, and anticipate how and when the client might try to avoid any or all of the individual topics and how such avoidance might be managed (Ede and Shepherd, 1998). The interview topic plan provides the framework for the engagement, allowing the practitioner to see when and possibly why the client tries to avoid talking about particular subjects or demonstrates distress in the course of discussions. An interview topic plan also illustrates to anyone who scrutinizes the practitioner's work that they have a 'standard of care' and are interested in their own clinical reliability (Meloy, 2005, p. 435).

Each topic should be accompanied by a list of areas to be covered within that subject, and starter questions and follow-up probes prepared. Questions should be ethical, truthful, purposeful, truly enquiring, relevant, empathic, comprehensible and brief, and finish each topic and interview with a summary and a request for questions or queries from the client (Ede and Shepherd, 1998). Table 12.2 summarizes a possible risk interview topic plan, summarizing after Bögels (2000) the process and content skills required of the forensic clinical practitioner engaged in such an encounter.

Table 12.2 Recommendations for risk interviews conducted by forensic clinical practitioners

Content	Process	Cognitive task
Introduction • What this assessment is for • Who commissioned it • What will happen to the findings of the assessment • Plan for the assessment • Aims of the assessment • Limits on confidentiality • Consent	• Task-oriented: (a) information-giving; (b) explaining; (c) clarifying • Attending, listening • Respectful • Observing • Being vigilant for common ground • Rapport-building	• Detecting and recording patterns of verbal and non-verbal behaviour as a basis for identifying changes later in the interview • Forming preliminary views on personality style • Estimating challenges to assessor control of the interview
Problem clarification • Risk of what? • What is the client's view? • What does the client understand about the concerns of others?	• Enquiring • Attending, listening • Observing • Rapport-building • Respectful	• Detecting and recording patterns of verbal and non-verbal behaviour as a basis for identifying changes later in the interview • Forming preliminary views on self-awareness/insight as well as personality style • Forming preliminary views on attitudes towards risk management
Baseline evaluation • Work history • Plans and goals for the future	• Open questions • Enquiring • Attending, listening • Observing • Rapport-building • Respectful • Paraphrasing • Summarizing	• Detecting and recording patterns of verbal and non-verbal behaviour as a basis for identifying changes later in the interview • Forming preliminary views on self-awareness/insight as well as personality style

Content	Process	Cognitive task
History		
• Family history, your parents • School and education • Your life as a child and young person • Relationships with parents • Friends and social networks • Intimate relationships • Stress and coping • Mental health • Physical health • Substance use • Personality	• Open questions • Enquiring, looking for detail • Attending, listening • Rapport-maintaining • Psychological testing • Observing • Respectful • Paraphrasing • Summarizing	• Detecting and recording patterns of verbal and non-verbal behaviour and any changes from baseline as sensitive issues are discussed • Therefore, identifying sensitive issues (possible hotspots) • Forming preliminary views about patterns of self-defence • Forming more substantial views about personality, insight, attitudes as well as cognitive and interpersonal style and stress vulnerability • Forming views about possible diagnoses • Staying in control of the interview
Harmful behaviour		
• Explore index offence/most recent serious incident • Explore past similar incidents • Establish patterns across past and recent harmful incidents (functional analysis)	• Open questions • Enquiring, looking for detail • Exploratory • Attending, listening • Rapport-maintaining • Observing • Respectful • Paraphrasing • Summarizing • Challenging inconsistencies and patterns of self-defence in a manner tailored to suit the personality style of the interviewee • Managing resistance to collaboration in order to keep the interviewee engaged • Collaborative	• Monitoring changes in verbal and non-verbal behaviour • Identifying hotspots • Identifying predisposing factors • Identifying precipitating factors • Identifying protective factors • Identifying perpetuating factors • Forming more substantial views about personality, insight, interpersonal and cognitive style • Forming more substantial views about patterns of self-defence • Staying in control of the interview

(continued)

Table 12.2 (continued)

Content	Process	Cognitive task
Future risk • Under what circumstances might harmful behaviour recur and why?	• Open questions • Enquiring, looking for detail • Exploratory • Attending, listening • Rapport-maintaining • Observing • Respectful • Paraphrasing • Summarizing • Challenging more robustly inconsistencies and patterns of self-defence in a manner tailored to suit the personality style of the interviewee • Managing resistance to collaboration in order to keep the interviewee engaged • Collaborative	• Staying in control of the interview • Confirming predisposing factors • Confirming precipitating factors • Confirming protective factors • Confirming perpetuating factors
Formulation	• Collating, summarizing • Explaining • Respectful • Rapport-maintaining • Collaborative	• Formulating an explanation for future risk of harmful behaviour that is understandable to the interviewee and identifying shared understandings and areas of disagreement
Risk management • Treatment requirements • Supervision requirements • Monitoring requirements • Problems foreseen and why • Work required • Compliance	• Open questions • Enquiring, looking for detail • Exploratory • Attending, listening • Rapport-maintaining • Observing • Respectful • Paraphrasing • Summarizing • Challenging inconsistencies • Managing resistance • Collaborative	• Staying in control • Confirming formulation • Forming views about treatment and supervision compliance • Forming views about treatment, supervision and monitoring requirements
Recall and conclude • Recap on aims • Recap on what will happen to the findings of the assessment • Anything left unsaid or not discussed?	• Rapport-maintaining • Respectful • Summarizing • Observing	• Relinquish control (safely)

Concluding comments

In this chapter, the essential skills required in forensic clinical practitioners conducting risk interviews with clients in the criminal justice and forensic mental health systems have been outlined. Planning and preparation have been noted as essential foundations for the interviews to follow, and knowledge of the client and self-knowledge on the part of the practitioner have been identified as critical elements in the practitioner's quest to remain in control of the encounter, and therefore in control of the achievement of the interview aims and objectives. However, this element of control will sit uneasily in the repertoire of many practitioners. Just how ethical is it to exert so much control, to seek to stay in control of such exchanges with vulnerable clients subject to legal proceedings of one kind or another, to effectively manipulate the client in order to maximize the flow of relevant and useful information pertaining to future risk? This question should be answered by recalling the reason why the risk assessment was requested in the first place; its justification is both to promote the safety of others and to protect the client by limiting any potential to be harmful again (Logan, 2003). Further, a collaborative interview is more likely to ensure that the client's views and aspirations are represented than is one conducted without their fully informed consent and in an atmosphere of suspicion and fear (Logan, 2003). Nonetheless, the skills described here, to encourage clients to say things that they might not otherwise have said in the context of an encounter that might lead to recommendations relating to their liberty, are a most powerful set of skills indeed, and they are not to be used lightly – or abused.

Note

I would like to thank Professor David Cooke of Glasgow Caledonian University, and Dr Jayne Taylor and Dr Amy McKee of Greater Manchester West Mental Health NHS Foundation Trust for their comments on an early draft of this chapter.

References

Ackley, C. N., Mack, S. M., Beyer, K. and Erdberg, P. (2011) *Investigative and Forensic Interviewing: A personality-focused approach*, Boca Raton, FL: CRC Press.

Aklin, W. M. and Turner, S. M. (2006) 'Towards understanding ethnic and cultural factors in the interviewing process', *Psychotherapy: Theory, Research, Practice, Training*, 43: 50–64.

Barone, D. F., Hutchings, P. S., Kimmel, H. J., Traub, H. L., Cooper, J. T. and Marshall, C. M. (2005) 'Increasing empathic accuracy through practice and feedback in a clinical interviewing course', *Journal of Social and Clinical Psychology*, 24: 156–71.

Ben-Porath, Y. and Tellegen, A. (2008) '*The MMPI-2-RF: Manual for administration, scoring and interpretation*', San Antonio, TX: Pearson Assessments.

Bögels, S. M. (2000) 'Diagnostic interviewing in mental health care: Methods, training and assessment', in A. Memon and R. Bull (eds) *Handbook of the Psychology of Interviewing*, pp. 3–20, Chichester: Wiley.

Bull, R., Valentine, T. and Williamson, T. (eds) (2009) *Handbook of Psychology of Investigative Interviewing: Current developments and future directions*, Chichester: Wiley-Blackwell.

Carlin, M. (2010) 'The psychologist as expert witness in criminal cases', in J. M. Brown and E. A. Campbell (eds) *The Cambridge Handbook of Forensic Psychology*, pp. 773–82, Cambridge: Cambridge University Press.

Costa, P. T. and McCrae, R. R. (2008) 'The revised NEO Personality Inventory (NEO-PI-R)', in G. J. Boyle, G. Matthews and D. H. Saklofske (eds) *The Sage Handbook of Personality Theory and Assessment: Personality measurement and testing, volume 2*, pp. 179–99, London: Sage.

Craig, R.J. (ed.) (2005) *Clinical and Diagnostic Interviewing*, Lanham, ML: Jason Aronson Inc.

Daykin, A. and Gordon, N. (2011) 'Establishing a supervision culture for clinicians working with personality disordered offenders in a high secure hospital', in P. Willmot and N. Gordon (eds) *Working Positively with Personality Disorder in Secure Settings: A practitioner's perspective*, pp.200–209, Chichester: Wiley-Blackwell.

Ede, R. and Shepherd, E. (1998) *Active Defence: A lawyer's guide to police and defence investigation and prosecution and defence disclosure in criminal cases, revised first edition*, London: The Law Society.

Ekman, P. (2001) *Telling Lies: Clues to deceit in the marketplace, politics, and marriage*, New York: W. W. Norton and Company.

Fisher, R. P. and Castano, N. (2008) 'Cognitive interview', in B. Cutler (ed.) *Encyclopaedia of Psychology and Law*, Thousand Oaks, CA: Sage.

Fisher, R. P. and Geiselman, R. E. (1992) *Memory-enhancing Techniques for Investigative Interviewing: The cognitive interview*, Springfield, IL: Charles C. Thomas Publisher.

Fisher, R. P. and Perez, V. (2007) 'Memory-enhancing techniques for interviewing crime suspects', in S. Christianson (ed.) *Offender's Memories of Violent Crimes*, pp. 329–54, Chichester: Wiley.

Frank, M. G., Yarbrough, J. D. and Ekman, P. (2006) 'Investigative interviewing and the detection of deception', in T. Williamson (ed.) *Investigative Interviewing: Rights, research, regulation*, pp. 229–56, Cullompton: Willan Publishing.

Gacono, C., Nieberding, R., Owen, A., Rubel, J. and Bodholdt, R. (2001) 'Treating juvenile and adult offenders with conduct disorder, antisocial and psychopathic personalities', in J. B. Ashford, B. D. Sales and W. Reid (eds) *Treating Adult and Juvenile Offenders with Special Needs*, pp. 99–129, Washington DC: American Psychological Association.

Hart, S. D. (2001) 'Forensic issues', in W. J. Livesley (ed.) *Handbook of Personality Disorders: Theory, research, and treatment*, pp. 555–69, New York: Guilford Press.

Havens, L. (2007) 'Approaching the mind in clinical interviewing: The technique of soundings and counter-projection', in S.C. Shea (ed.) Clinical Interviewing: Practical tips from master clinicians, Special issue of *Psychiatric Clinics of North America*, 30: 145–56.

Holliday, R. E., Brainerd, C. J., Reyna, V. F. and Humphries, J. E. (2009) 'The cognitive interview: Research and practice across the lifespan', in R. Bull, T. Valentine and T. Williamson (eds) *Handbook of Psychology of Investigative Interviewing: Current developments and future directions*, pp. 137–60, Chichester: Wiley-Blackwell.

Kosson, D. S., Gacono, C. B. and Bodholdt, R. H. (2000) 'Assessing psychopathy: Interpersonal aspects and clinical interviewing', in C. B. Gacono (ed.) *The Clinical and Forensic Assessment of Psychopathy: A practitioner's guide*, pp. 203–30, Mahwah, NJ: Lawrence Earlbaum Associates, Publishers.

Lamb, M. E., Sternberg, K. J., Orbach, Y., Hershkowitz, I. and Esplin, P. W. (2000) 'Forensic interviews of children', in A. Memon and R. Bull (eds) *Handbook of the Psychology of Interviewing*, pp. 253–78, Chichester: Wiley.

Lee, Z., Klaver, J. R. and Hart, S. D. (2008) 'Psychopathy and verbal indicators of deception in offenders', *Psychology, Crime and Law*, 14: 73–84.

Logan, C. (2003) 'Ethical issues in risk assessment practice and research', in G. Adshead and C. Brown (eds) *Ethical Issues in Forensic Mental Health Research*, pp. 71–85, London: Jessica Kingsley Books.

— (this volume) 'Suicide and self-harm: Clinical risk assessment and management using a structured professional judgement approach', in C. Logan and L. Johnstone (eds) *Managing Clinical Risk: A guide to effective practice*, Oxford: Routledge.

Logan, C. and Johnstone, L. (2010) 'Personality disorder and violence: Making the link through risk formulation', *Journal of Personality Disorders*, 24: 610–33.

Lyon, D. R. and Ogloff, R. P. (2000) 'Legal and ethical issues in psychopathy assessment', in C. B. Gacono (ed.) *The Clinical and Forensic Assessment of Psychopathy: A practitioner's guide*, pp. 139–74, Mahwah, NJ: Lawrence Earlbaum Associates, Publishers.

MacKinnon, R. A., Michels, R. and Buckley, P. J. (2009) *The Psychiatric Interview in Clinical Practice*, Arlington, VA: American Psychiatric Press Inc.

Maltsberger, J. T. and Buie, D. H. (1974) 'Countertransference hate in the treatment of suicidal patients', *Archives of General Psychiatry*, 30: 625–33.

McClanahan, R. D. (2000) *The Impact of Therapist Values in the Culturally Diverse Clinical Interviewing Process: A Delphi study*, unpublished dissertation. Tennessee State University, USA.

McGrath, R. J. (1990) 'Assessment of sexual aggressors: Practical clinical interviewing strategies', *Journal of Interpersonal Violence*, 5: 507–19.

McMurran, M. and Howard, R. (eds) (2009) *Personality, Personality Disorder, and Violence: An evidence-based approach*, Chichester: John Wiley and Sons.

Meloy, J. R. (2005) 'The forensic interview', in R. J. Craig (ed.) *Clinical and Diagnostic Interviewing*, pp. 422–43, Lanham, ML: Jason Aronson Inc.

Melton, G. B. (1987) 'Bringing psychology into the legal system: Opportunities, obstacles, and efficacy', *American Psychologist*, 42: 488–95.

Miller, W. R. and Rollnick, S. (eds) (2002) *Motivational Interviewing: Preparing people for change*, 2nd edition, New York: Guilford.

Milne, R. (2000) 'Interviewing children with learning disabilities', in A. Memon and R. Bull (eds) *Handbook of the Psychology of Interviewing*, pp. 165–80, Chichester: Wiley.

Milne, R. and Bull, R. (1999) *Investigative Interviewing: Psychology and practice*, Chichester: John Wiley and Sons.

Morrison, J. (2008) *The First Interview*, 3rd Edition, New York: Guilford Press.

Othmer, E., Othmer, J. P. and Othmer, S. C. (2007) 'Our favourite tips for "getting in" with difficult patients', in S. C. Shea (ed.) Clinical interviewing: Practical tips from master clinicians, Special issue of *Psychiatric Clinics of North America*, 30: 261–68.

Poole, R. and Higgo, R. (2006) *Psychiatric Interviewing and Assessment*, Cambridge: Cambridge University Press.

Rogers, C. R. (1959) 'A theory of therapy, personality, and interpersonal relationships as developed in the client-centred framework', in S. Koch (ed.) *Psychology: The study of a science, Volume 3, Formulations of the person and the social context*, pp. 184–256, New York: McGraw-Hill.

Rosengren, D. B. (2009) *Building Motivational Interviewing Skills: A practitioner workbook*, New York: Guilford Press.

Shea, S. C. (1998) *Psychiatric Interviewing: The art of understanding*, 2nd Edition, Philadelphia, PA: Saunders.

— (ed.) (2007a) 'Clinical interviewing: Practical tips from master clinicians', Special issue of *Psychiatric Clinics of North America*, 30: 145–315.

— (2007b) 'My favorite tips for uncovering sensitive and taboo information from antisocial behavior to suicidal ideation', in S. C. Shea (ed.) Clinical interviewing: Practical tips from master clinicians, Special issue of *Psychiatric Clinics of North America*, 30: 253–60.

Shepherd, S. (2007) *Investigative Interviewing: The conversational management approach*, Oxford: Oxford University Press.

Sommers-Flanagan, J. and Sommers-Flanagan, R. (2007) 'Our favourite tips for interviewing couples and families', in S. C. Shea (ed.) Clinical interviewing: Practical tips from master clinicians, Special issue of *Psychiatric Clinics of North America*, 30: 275–82.

Strasburger, L. (1986) 'Treatment of antisocial syndromes: The therapist's feelings', in W. Reid, D. Dorr, J. Walker and J. Bonner (eds) *Unmasking the Psychopath*, pp. 191–207, New York: Norton.

Suzuki, L. A. and Ponterotto, J. G. (eds) (2008) *Handbook of Multicultural Assessment: Clinical, psychological, and educational applications, 3rd edition*, Edison, NJ: Wiley/Jossey-Bass.

Urquiza, A. J., Wyatt, G. E. and Goodlin-Jones, B. L. (1997) 'Clinical interviewing with trauma victims: Managing interviewer risk', *Journal of Interpersonal Violence*, 12: 759–72.

Vrij, A. (2000) *Detecting Lies and Deceit: The psychology of lying and the implications for professional practice*, Chichester: John Wiley and Sons.

Vrij, A., Granhag, P. A., Mann, S. and Leal, S. (2011) 'Outsmarting the liars: Toward a cognitive lie detection approach', *Current Directions in Psychological Science*, 20: 28–32.

Watts, D. and Morgan, G. (1994) 'Malignant alienation: Dangers for patients who are hard to like', *British Journal of Psychiatry*, 164: 11–15.

Widiger, T. A. and Frances, A. (1985) 'The DSM-III personality disorders', *Archives of General Psychiatry*, 42: 615–23.

Williamson, T. (ed.) (2006) *Investigative Interviewing: Rights, research, regulation*, Cullompton: Willan Publishing.

Willmot, P. and Gordon, N. (2011) *Working Positively with Personality Disorder in Secure Settings: A practitioner's perspective*, Chichester: Wiley-Blackwell.

Yeschke, C. L. (1997) *The Art of Investigative Interviewing: A human approach to testimonial evidence*, Boston: Butterworth-Heinemann.

— (2002) *The Art of Investigative Interviewing: A human approach to testimonial evidence*, 2nd Edition, Boston: Butterworth-Heinemann.

Young, J. E. (1994) *Cognitive Therapy for Personality Disorders: A schema-focused approach*, Sarasota, FL: Professional Resource Press/Professional Resource Exchange.

13 Protective factors for violence risk

Bringing balance to risk assessment and management

Michiel de Vries Robbé and Vivienne de Vogel

In the past two decades, knowledge about risk factors for future violence has increased exponentially. Many instruments have been developed aiming to assess the risk of future violent behaviour and several are currently in widespread use (i.e., HCR-20, Webster, et al., 1997; LSI-R, Andrews and Bonta, 1995; Static-99, Hanson and Thornton, 1999). The evolution of structured risk assessment instruments over the past few decades has provided us with increasingly helpful tools, to not only assist the prediction of future violent behaviour but to also guide clinical intervention and decision-making (Douglas and Skeem, 2005; Webster, et al., 2002). Researchers and clinicians have gradually embraced these risk assessment tools and have come to appreciate their usefulness for clinical practice and violence prevention. More specifically, those factors in structured risk assessment instruments that are changeable or dynamic in nature serve as valuable targets for treatment goals, risk management strategies, and treatment evaluation (Douglas and Skeem, 2005), and their potential value for clinical practice has become more and more acknowledged in forensic mental health.

Despite major advances in everyday risk assessment procedures, there still appears to be a significant aspect of risk assessment that is generally overlooked: protective factors. Protective factors are those factors that can compensate for a person's risk factors and thus play an important part in the overall risk judgement. In his critique of risk assessment in forensic practice, Rogers (2000) stated that most adult-based studies are one-sided in their enumeration of risk factors, to the partial or total exclusion of protective factors. He argued that risk-only evaluations are inherently inaccurate and implicitly biased, often resulting in negative consequences to forensic populations. According to Miller (2006), the focus on risk factors in most risk assessment instruments is likely to result in the over-prediction of recidivism, which is costly both for the offender in terms of loss of personal liberties, and for society in terms of financial burden. Many researchers now agree that by focusing solely on risk factors, important information concerning the other side of the violence risk equation, the possible risk-reducing effect of protective factors, is wrongfully ignored and that including protective factors in risk assessment is vital for an accurate appraisal of the risk of relapse into violence (e.g., DeMatteo, et al., 2005; Gagliardi, et al., 2004; Haggård-Grann, 2005; Salekin and Lochman, 2008). However, as of yet, the specific assessment of protective factors remains understudied and the concept of protective factors is still ambiguous (Braithwaite, et al., 2010; De Vogel, et al., 2011).

In this chapter, the potential added value that protective factors have for the assessment of violence risk and for the treatment of violent offenders is discussed. The literature on protective factors is reviewed and the available assessment tools are described, focusing especially on a newly developed structured professional guideline for the specific assessment of protective factors: the *Structured Assessment of PROtective Factors* for violence risk (SAPROF, De Vogel, et al., 2007, English Version 2009). Recent research results and a case study on the SAPROF are presented in order to illustrate the strengths-based approach and its contribution to risk assessment, treatment planning, and risk management.

The concept of protective factors

Some authors interpret protective factors exclusively as the absence of risk factors (Costa, et al., 1999) or as the opposite of risk factors (Hawkins, et al., 1992; Webster, et al., 2004), suggesting that any risk factor can also be a protective factor and the other way around. Others propose that a protective factor may exist without a corresponding risk factor (Farrington and Loeber, 2000). For example, research has demonstrated that religiosity has a negative relationship to delinquency and conduct problems (Pearce, et al., 2003), however, the *absence* of religion does not constitute a risk factor. The positive effect of protective factors weighs against the negative effect of risk factors. Unfortunately, the exact mechanism of the interaction between risk and protective factors remains unclear.

Researchers have proposed several theoretical models about the direct and indirect effects of protective factors on favourable and unfavourable outcomes (Fitzpatrick, 1997; Jessor, et al., 2003; Turbin, et al., 2006). Three models have been outlined: (1) a *mediation* model, which implies the effect of protective factors directly on risk factors (and the other way around); (2) a *moderator* or buffer model, which suggests the interaction effect of protective factors on the relationship between risk factors and negative behaviour; and (3) a *main effect* model, in which protective factors impact directly on negative behaviour. The present authors believe that for the negative outcome of violent behaviour, it is likely to be the first two of these mechanisms that are primarily in effect: protective factors have a negative influence on risk factors directly (resulting in reduced or weakened risk factors), but they also have an influence on the association between risk factors and violent behaviour (resulting in a compensating effect on the risk factor–violence relationship). An example of a positive mediation effect is the favourable influence of the protective factor 'medication' on the risk factor 'active symptoms of major mental illness'. An example of a positive moderator or buffer effect is the impact on violent outcome of risk factors like 'substance abuse problems' or 'impulsivity' being diminished by the measured imposition of the protective factor 'external control'. Future studies that include the structured assessment of both risk and protective factors will have to provide more insight into the exact mechanisms of their interaction.

An exploration of protective factors

In recent years, researchers and clinicians in forensic mental health practice have started to acknowledge the presumed value of protective factors for more accurate risk assessment and more effective violence prevention in clinical practice (Douglas, et al., 2005; Farrington and Loeber, 2000; Heilbrun, 2003; Jones and Brown, 2008; Webster, et al., 2004). Protective factors for violence risk are defined as characteristics of an offender, or alternatively, his or her environment or situation, that reduce the risk of future violent behaviour (De Vogel, et al., 2009); protective factors therefore range across personal and situational variables. Research on protective factors has identified static and dynamic factors that can help offenders refrain from violent behaviour. Static protective factors include personal historical variables such as 'intelligence' (e.g., Kandel, et al., 1988) and 'secure childhood attachment' (e.g., Fonagy, et al., 1997). Dynamic or changeable protective factors are internal personal characteristics such as 'coping' (e.g., Vance, et al., 2002) and 'self-control' (e.g., Tangney, et al., 2004), motivational personal attributes such as 'work and leisure activities' (e.g., Gendreau, et al., 2000) and 'motivation for treatment' (e.g., Howells, et al., 2005), and external environmental factors such as 'social network' (e.g., Turbin, et al., 2006) and 'professional care' (e.g., Cooper, et al., 2006). Additionally, research on *desistance*, the refraining from criminal behaviour (Ezell and Cohen, 2005; Maruna, 2001; Vaughan, 2007), and *knifing-off*, which is the discontinuation of criminal opportunities (Maruna and Roy, 2006), has shown that reductions in violence risk over time can be the result of situational changes or due to the processes of aging and maturation.

It has been argued that treatment aimed at reducing violent recidivism should not only be focused on diminishing risk factors but also on reinforcing protective factors (Blum and Ireland, 2004; Resnick, et al., 2004). Encouragement of the healthy aspects of mentally disordered patients and their environment can provide a valuable contribution to their treatment and resocialization process. This concept of including positive factors in treatment is by no means new to forensic psychiatry (see for instance the good lives model of Ward and Brown [2004] and the positive psychology approach of Seligman [2002]) and many protective factors are often addressed during clinical intervention. However, linking this positive preventive approach to a specific structured evaluation of personal and situational strengths in risk assessment is a relatively new and potentially very promising development.

Tools assessing protective factors

To our knowledge, there are only a few risk assessment instruments that explicitly take protective factors into account (De Vogel, et al., 2011). The *Structured Assessment of Violence Risk in Youth* (SAVRY, Borum, et al., 2006), a structured professional judgement (SPJ) checklist for violence risk assessment in youth, contains six protective factors (e.g., 'prosocial involvement', 'resilient personality traits') in addition to 24 risk factors. Recent studies on the significance of the protective factors in the SAVRY in various samples of adolescents showed good predictive validity for refraining from violent reoffending for the summed ratings on the six protective factors (Lodewijks, et al., 2010; Rennie and Dolan, 2010). The *Inventory of Offender Risk, Needs and Strengths* (IORNS, Miller, 2006) also includes protective factors. The IORNS is a self-report risk assessment measure, which was developed to determine risks, needs and protective factors for all types of adult offenders. In a sample of American pre-release prisoners, several of the IORNS subscales, including the 'Protective Strength Index' and the 'Personal Resources Scale', were able to differentiate between offenders who were sent back to prison for half way house rule violations and offenders who did not violate any rules (Miller, 2006). Another increasingly widely used instrument containing protective factors is the *Short-Term Assessment of Risk and Treatability* (START, Webster, et al., 2004), a clinical guide for the dynamic assessment specifically of short-term risks. The 20 dynamic items are simultaneously coded on two three-point scales – first as a source of protection (Strength) and then for their operation as risk factors (Vulnerability) – because the instrument assumes all 20 characteristics can simultaneously influence vulnerability as well as strength. In recent studies, the START Strength scale (i.e., the sum of all strength ratings) has been shown to be significantly predictive of short-term inpatient violent behaviour (Braithwaite, et al., 2010; Nonstad, et al., 2010; Wilson, et al., 2010).

The need for a new instrument

We have just described instruments that seem promising for use with specific groups of patients. The SAVRY was developed specifically for the assessment of risk in juvenile offenders. The IORNS is a self-report assessment tool. However, given the risk of socially desirable responding in the users of forensic psychiatric services, a self-report measure on its own does not seem sufficient for the structured assessment of protective factors. The START is designed specifically for the short-term (1 to 8 weeks) assessment of imminent risk in (forensic) psychiatric patients (see Webster, et al., 2004, p. 30). As such, it is less suitable for the medium-term assessment (months to years) of more persistent risk and protective factors. As the pathology of long-term forensic psychiatric patients is generally persistent, the risk assessment time frame in forensic psychiatry is often longer.

The most widely used instrument for the assessment of violence risk in forensic psychiatric patients, the HCR-20 (Webster, et al., 1997), has a medium-term focus (six months to a year). As the HCR-20 includes solely risk factors, the addition of protective factors for this same time frame seems a valuable and positive counterpart to all risk assessments with the HCR-20 or other risk tools with this time frame. Complementing the risk assessment procedure with a structured assessment of factors that may compensate the risk level would provide a more balanced overall assessment. However, an instrument with a specific focus on protective factors for the medium-term prediction and prevention of violence risk has not yet been developed. Considering this, and at the same time noticing the mental health professionals' need for guidelines in this area, a structured guideline was developed to assess protective factors for medium-term violence risk in adult (forensic) psychiatric patients: the SAPROF.

Development of the SAPROF

The SAPROF is designed according to the structured professional judgement (SPJ) approach (see Douglas, et al., this volume, for an overview) and intended as a positive, dynamic addition to structured risk assessment tools, such as the HCR-20 and related SPJ instruments. The aim of the instrument is to identify protective factors that can compensate for risk factors in order to create a more balanced assessment of future violent behaviour. Moreover, insight into the presence or absence of protective factors may give a more complete view of the individual in his or her context and may offer additional guidelines for treatment and risk management. The positive approach of the assessment of protective factors may also inspire positive risk communication and have a motivating effect on patients and treatment staff. Therefore, the idea behind developing the SAPROF was to create an instrument that was both empirically founded and clinically useful.

The construction of the SAPROF started with extensive literature reviews on protective and contextual factors for violent behaviour. Subsequently, to acquire additional indications for factors that might protect against relapse into violent behaviour, the clinical expertise of mental health professionals at the Van der Hoeven Kliniek, a Dutch forensic psychiatric hospital, was tapped by asking clinicians to specifically consider protective factors during case conference risk assessment meetings (see De Vogel, et al., 2009). Based on both the literature review and this clinical expertise, a pilot version of the SAPROF was constructed. Subsequently, a study was conducted with the pilot version in two Dutch forensic psychiatric hospitals and one forensic outpatient setting, in which mental health professionals and researchers rated the SAPROF and were asked to comment on the item descriptions and the instrument in general. The inclusion of clinical feedback at different stages in the development process made the instrument more practically applicable. Together with an updated review of the literature, the feedback on the pilot version was incorporated into the present version of the SAPROF, which first came out in Dutch in 2007. Based on additional user feedback, the Dutch version was slightly revised and the English version was published in 2009. Subsequently, the English version was translated into several different languages over the past years.

The SAPROF

The SAPROF is a checklist that includes 17 protective factors (see Table 13.1). Factors are scored on a three-point rating scale, in order to be easily compatible with three-point rating risk tools (e.g. the HCR-20), and are organized into three scales based on the face-value origin of their protection: *Internal factors*, *Motivational factors* and *External factors*. Two items are historical and were included based on empirical evidence of their protective significance ('intelligence'

Table 13.1 The SAPROF checklist and expected changes during treatment

	Possible key factor	*Possible goal factor*	*Expected change during treatment*
Internal factors			
1. Intelligence	Yes	No	Static
2. Secure attachment in childhood	Yes	No	Static
3. Empathy	Yes	Yes	Improving
4. Coping	Yes	Yes	Improving
5. Self-control	Yes	Yes	Improving
Motivational factors			
6. Work	Yes	Yes	Improving
7. Leisure activities	Yes	Yes	Improving
8. Financial management	Yes	Yes	Improving
9. Motivation for treatment	Yes	Yes	Improving
10. Attitudes towards authority	Yes	Yes	Improving
11. Life goals	Yes	Yes	Improving
12. Medication	Yes	Yes	Improving
External factors			
13. Social network	Yes	Yes	Improving
14. Intimate relationship	Yes	Yes	Improving
15. Professional care	Yes	Yes	Decreasing
16. Living circumstances	Yes	Yes	Decreasing
17. External control	Yes	Yes	Decreasing

and 'secure attachment in childhood'). The other 15 factors are dynamic, which means they could serve as targets in risk management and treatment interventions and could be valuable for treatment evaluation. Additionally, the SAPROF offers the opportunity to mark factors as particularly important for a specific individual, either in terms of present protection (*key* factors) or in terms of treatment goals (*goal* factors). The instrument concludes with a final judgement. Since the SAPROF has a focus on protection rather than on risk, the final judgement concerns the level of protection available to the individual for the specific assessment situation: the *Final Protection Judgement*. The findings from the SAPROF are then combined with the results from an SPJ risk measure, such as the HCR-20, to arrive at an overall *Integrated Final Risk Judgement*.

Since most of the research that underlies the SAPROF was based mainly on populations of male violent offenders, the SAPROF was initially developed to assess protective factors for adult males with a history of violence who suffer from a mental or personality disorder. The SAPROF can also be used with women; however, the assessor should be careful when drawing conclusions based on the SAPROF for women, as little research has been conducted on protective factors for females. In general, limited support is available regarding the applicability of commonly used risk assessment instruments for women (see also De Vogel and De

Vries Robbé, this volume). The few studies that have included protective factors for adult women suggest it is especially the interpersonal relationship factors which may be potentially valuable protective factors for women (Benda, 2005; Holtfreter and Cupp, 2007). A preliminary clinical study on the predictive validity of the SAPROF for not committing inpatient violence showed equally good results for men and women. Best predictors for women were the factors 'financial management', 'intelligence', and 'attitudes towards authority' (De Vries Robbé and De Vogel, 2010). Furthermore, very little research has been conducted into protective factors specifically for sexually violent behaviour. Almost no specific factors for sexual offenders were found from the literature reviews on protective factors or from the feedback collected from mental health professionals in the SAPROF development process. However, the SAPROF factors are regarded as appropriate for use with both violent and sexual offenders. Empirical research will have to determine precisely if this assumption is just and whether we may need to amend the instrument for use with sexual offenders (see also the research section of this chapter).

A case example: Jacob

Jacob is a 35-year-old man, who was sentenced to three years' imprisonment and the TBS-order (Dutch judicial measure implying mandatory inpatient psychiatric treatment) following his conviction for attempted murder. Jacob grew up as the oldest of two boys in a family that highly valued soccer competences. His parents had high expectations for him and, while Jacob's father was strict and rigid, his mother was gentle and spoiling. At a very young age, Jacob joined the youth team of a prestigious soccer club. After finishing high school and military service, he started playing high-level soccer for a living. At the age of 20 he got involved in a turbulent relationship with a 16-year-old girl and quickly moved in with her. After being unfaithful with a teammate's girlfriend, the relationship ended and his soccer team turned against him. Eventually Jacob stopped playing soccer altogether and his life went downhill from there. He started abusing alcohol and hard drugs, spent his money on flamboyant partying and got into financial trouble. He had many short-term relationships, sometimes several at the same time, and physically abused one of his girlfriends when she tried to leave him. One night, Jacob knocked at the door of a woman who lived in his building. He attempted to make sexual advances towards her, but when the woman asked him to leave, he suddenly stabbed her multiple times with a knife. After taking some money, he left the woman for dead. Despite her injuries, the victim survived the attack. Jacob was arrested soon after in a confused state.

After his prison sentence, Jacob was admitted to the forensic psychiatric hospital. His main problem areas were considered to be: low tolerance for frustration; lack of perseverance; problems with addiction; and inability to cope with emotions, criticism and authority. Although Jacob was impatient and his ability to change his behaviour was constantly overrated, both by himself and by others, he participated well in the hospital. He passed all random drug tests and there were no incidents of physical violence. After a year, Jacob was allowed outside the hospital on supervised leave, during which he always behaved appropriately. Two years after the start of his treatment, Jacob started his resocialization phase, which meant he lived and worked outside of the hospital but was still supervised closely by his inpatient treatment team. His increased freedom did not go without setbacks. Several (non-physical) conflicts and drug-related incidents showed his continuing vulnerability to addiction and his difficulty seeking help from others. Following alleged cocaine use, Jacob was readmitted to inpatient treatment in the hospital.

After this relapse, he seemed to become more aware of the seriousness of his problems. The central theme for him and his treatment team became his relapse-prevention plan, focusing especially on his impulsivity, his tendency to avoid difficult matters, and the lack of communication with his support system. After several months he was allowed to return to his own apartment outside the hospital. In the following year, Jacob managed to keep up his good intentions. He remained in close contact with his treatment team, was open about the difficulties he encountered in daily life and asked for help when needed. He finished his psychotherapy in the hospital and found a new therapist at an affiliated outpatient treatment setting. He emphasized his wish to continue this therapy on a voluntary basis in the future. Although Jacob still did not have many close friends, his relationship with his family improved and his parents became more involved in his treatment. Soon after his return to the resocialization phase he started going out with a girl, which turned into a serious relationship. With the work skills he learned at the hospital, he managed to find a stable job at a small company in a nearby town. As both Jacob and his employer were content with his work, he was offered a year contract. He succeeded in paying off the last part of his debts from the past and continued to manage his finances properly. In his spare time, Jacob joined an indoor recreational soccer team and started salsa dancing classes. His girlfriend proved to be supportive and understanding of the importance for him of complying with the agreements made with his treatment team. As their relationship continued to stand firm, they started making plans to move in together. Twelve months after his return to the resocialization phase, the treatment team feels Jacob might be ready to finish his mandatory treatment. Routinely, a careful multidisciplinary assessment of risk and protective factors is carried out, before officially proposing the termination of his mandatory treatment to the court.

Analysis of Jacob's protective factors

Jacob's risk assessment consists of independent codings on the SAPROF and the HCR-20 by three different raters and a final consensus rating, which is agreed upon during a case-conference meeting. Table 13.2 shows the consensus scores for the SAPROF. The first two items are static and thus not applicable as treatment targets. As Jacob has an IQ score of 90 on the *Wechsler Adult Intelligence Scales 3rd Edition* (WAIS-III), which according to this intelligence test is at the low end of the average range, the first static item 'intelligence' is scored 1. However, it is an important observation that Jacob's capabilities are easily overestimated. The second

Table 13.2 Case study: SAPROF scores and final judgements

Name: **Jacob**			
Assessment: **Unconditional discharge**	*Score*	*Key*	*Goal*
1. Intelligence	1	☐	
2. Secure attachment in childhood	1	☐	
3. Empathy	1	☐	☐
4. Coping	1	☐	☑
5. Self-control	1	☐	☐
6. Work	2	☑	☐
7. Leisure activities	2	☐	☐
8. Financial management	2	☐	☐
9. Motivation for treatment	1	☑	☐
10. Attitudes towards authority	2	☐	☐
11. Life goals	0	☐	☐
12. Medication	N/A	☐	☐
13. Social network	1	☐	☑
14. Intimate relationship	2	☑	☐
15. Professional care	1	☐	☐
16. Living circumstances	1	☐	☐
17. External control	0	☐	☑
Final Protection Judgment			moderate
Integrated Final Risk Judgment			moderate

Note: HCR-20 scores are not shown but are included in the Integrated Final Risk Judgment.

static item, 'secure attachment in childhood', is scored 1 since his parents were there for him when he was growing up, but were also rigid and spoiling. The other items of the SAPROF are all dynamic and therefore qualify as possible goals for further treatment intervention. They are rated based on information from the past six months to a year, but with the current situation in mind, which in Jacob's case is his unconditional discharge from mandatory treatment. The internal dynamic items 'empathy', 'coping' and 'self-control' are all scored as 1. 'Coping' and 'self-control' are especially important items for Jacob as, in the past, these were his weaknesses and caused his life to go downhill. Since his best coping mechanism during treatment has been seeking help from his treatment team, developing new coping skills is seen as an important target for future treatment.

Next, the motivational items are coded. Overall, they show a positive picture. Jacob's stable job brings him a good score on the item 'work'. The daily structure and life fulfilment that his job gives him make employment a key factor in keeping Jacob on the right track. His participation in a soccer team, together with his salsa dancing, gives him a score of 2 on 'leisure activities'. Since the soccer league he currently plays in is purely recreational, it is not seen as a potential stress factor like soccer has been for Jacob in the past. He also scores well on the item 'financial management' as he manages his finances well and has paid off all his debts. His 'motivation for treatment' is a difficult item to rate for treatment staff. They believe in his good intentions to seek voluntary treatment after his mandatory treatment has ended. However, not all members of the treatment team are convinced Jacob will be motivated to keep coming on a voluntary basis when problems arise in the long run. He therefore gets a score of 1, but as his voluntary treatment is seen as a very important protective factor for the near future, it is still marked as a key factor. The item 'attitudes towards authority' concerns whether or not Jacob will be able to keep to the rules and agreements. Since he has not had any problems with this in the past year, he gets a score of 2. Although Jacob is generally motivated not to fall back into his old behaviour, there is nothing out of the ordinary that gives him extra motivation in terms of 'life goals'. The development of personal ambitions or responsibilities that bring extra life fulfilment would be an additional incentive for him to stay on the right track. Since 'medication' was not considered necessary, this item is not applicable for Jacob.

Finally, the external items show a mixed picture. Jacob's relationship with his close family has been restored to some extent and they are willing to support him. However, he still has a hard time making new friends and does not have a wide supportive network. He therefore gets a score of 1 and extending his 'social network' is seen as a goal-item. Although he has not been with his girlfriend for that long, the 'intimate relationship' is an important factor for Jacob. His girlfriend is supportive and provides him with company and meaning in life. Maintaining this stable relationship is seen as a valuable protector for Jacob and thus 'intimate relationship' is marked as a key item. Since living together with a partner or family member is seen as a form of social control, Jacob also receives a score of 1 on 'living situation'. After mandatory treatment ends, Jacob will keep seeing his outpatient therapist voluntarily. The bi-weekly sessions with his therapist give him a score of 1 on 'professional care'. Lastly, the item 'external control' gets a rating of 0, as all mandatory supervision will be dropped when treatment is ended, and no further court conditions are being imposed on Jacob.

After analyzing the ratings on the SAPROF and weighing and integrating them for Jacob's specific situation, the conclusion on the *Final Protection Judgement* for the context of unconditional discharge is 'moderate' level of protection for future violent behaviour. Combining this with Jacob's risk ratings on the HCR-20 makes it possible to formulate an overall *Integrated Final Risk Judgement*. The overall judgment is rated as 'moderate' risk for relapse into violent behaviour if mandatory treatment is dropped altogether. Although Jacob has quite a few protective factors supporting him, it is especially the presence of several key protective factors that give him the protection he needs: his suitable job, his stable intimate relationship, and the continued voluntary outpatient treatment. It also becomes clear, however, that these key factors make Jacob's situation quite vulnerable: if his relationship was to break off, if he was to be fired from his job, or if his outpatient treatment was to end for some reason, an important part of Jacob's protection would be lost. Jacob's most likely path to violence seems to be through the loss of important protective factors, resulting in alcohol and drug abuse, financial problems, and a decrease in coping skills and self-control, which could eventually lead to possible violence, most likely towards women. Given the importance of his key protective factors, the treatment team feels the need for a closer monitoring of Jacob's situation after treatment ends and the factor 'external control' is marked as a goal item.

Following the outcome of the assessment, instead of proposing unconditional discharge, the treatment team decide to propose conditional discharge with outpatient treatment as a mandatory condition and supervision by the probation service, who will be able to intervene if Jacob's situation should start to deteriorate. The results of the assessment are discussed with Jacob and his outpatient therapist and suggestions are made for the further development of Jacob's goals within the continuing outpatient therapy: improving his coping skills and developing a more widespread supportive social network. With the outpatient therapist and probation service securely in place, the treatment staff feel confident that Jacob will be able to deal adequately with his risks and not fall back into his old behavioural patterns. As Jacob agrees with this plan and his motivation to work on a positive future without violence seems sincere, treatment staff are confident that Jacob will be able to safely return to society, albeit under court conditions.

Research with the SAPROF

The SAPROF was initially validated in two samples: violent offenders (De Vries Robbé, et al., 2011) and sexually violent offenders (De Vries Robbé, et al., in preparation). Both studies showed good results in terms of interrater reliability and of predictive validity for not committing new violent offences after treatment. As the positive effect of protective factors is expected to diminish, the negative effect of risk factors on violence risk, the total score of all present risk factors minus all available protective factors, is seen as the most accurate violence risk estimate for research. For both the violent-offender sample and the sexual-offender sample, this combined total score of HCR-20 scores minus SAPROF scores showed a significantly better predictive validity than the HCR-20 total score alone (see De Vries Robbé, et al., 2011). Both patient samples were combined to further establish the predictive validity of the SAPROF for the total group (de Vries Robbé, et al., in preparation). The sample consists of 188 discharged mentally disordered offenders who were followed up for at least three years after treatment (11 years average, ranging from 3 to 24 years). Table 13.3 shows the predictive validity for ratings on the SAPROF, the HCR-20 and the combined HCR-SAPROF measure for the total sample at different follow-up times. The SAPROF showed good predictive validity for all (1–11 year) follow-up periods. The combined HCR-SAPROF measure was the best predictor for the 1–3 year follow-up periods; for the long term the SAPROF alone was the best predictor. Moreover, for this follow-up both the SAPROF total score and the combined HCR-SAPROF measure were significantly better predictors than the HCR-20 total score alone. We believe on a group level this demonstrates the additional value of using the SAPROF in addition to the HCR-20. On the individual level the clinical value of the SAPROF factors is expected to be even greater as most SAPROF factors are dynamic and the indication of key and goal factors brings forth new connections to risk management. As for the final judgements, the *Final Protection Judgement* and the *Integrated Final Risk Judgement* had slightly lower predictive validity for violent recidivism than the total scores on both instruments for all follow-up times. An explanation for the absence of the additional value of both final judgements could be that this study was retrospective and thus final judgements were hard to make. Eleven out of the seventeen SAPROF factors had significant individual predictive power for violent recidivism. The best predicting factors were 'self-control', 'work' and 'attitudes towards authority'.

For 108 patients, assessment ratings were conducted at two different times: pre-treatment and post-treatment. The average treatment length was 5.6 years (range 1–15). Analyses on the complete sample of patients with multiple SAPROF ratings showed that overall post-treatment total scores were significantly higher than pre-treatment total scores. As shown in Table 13.1, for research purposes, the SAPROF can be divided into three categories depending on the expected direction of change in scores during treatment: 'static' (factors 1–2), 'dynamic improving' (factors 3–14) and 'dynamic decreasing' (factors 15–17). Figure 13.1 shows the differences between the pre- and post-treatment ratings for the three categories within the SAPROF. As expected, ratings for the 'dynamic improving' factors had increased significantly during treatment and ratings for the 'dynamic decreasing' factors were significantly reduced for the whole sample.

Subsequently, the sample was divided into two groups: those patients who had recidivated at any time after treatment with a violent offence (N = 33) and those patients who had not (N = 75). Comparisons between the two groups were carried out for the separate categories within the SAPROF on two different outcomes: (1) pre-treatment total scores, and (2) post-treatment total scores. Analysis of the pre-treatment scores only revealed significantly higher scores for non-recidivist on the 'static' factors category, yet for the start of treatment ratings no differences were found between recidivists and non-recidivists on the dynamic categories

Table 13.3 Area under curve (AUC) values for SAPROF and HCR-20 ratings upon discharge (N = 188)

Follow-up period	1 year	2 year	3 year	Long-term M = 11 year
SAPROF total score	.85**	.78**	.75**	.73**
HCR-20 total score	.84**	.77**	.73**	.64*
HCR total score – SAPROF total score	.87**	.80**	.76**	.70**
Final Protection Judgment	.83**	.75**	.71**	.67**
Integrated Final Risk Judgment	.84**	.77**	.72*	.68**

$** = p < .001, * = p < .01$

Note: The values for the HCR-20 total score, the HCR total score - SAPROF total score and the Integrated Final Risk Judgment concern violent recidivism, the values for the SAPROF total score and the Final Protection Judgment concern non-recidivism of violence.

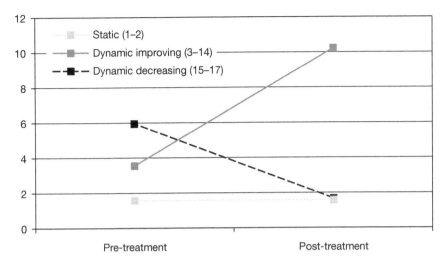

Figure 13.1 SAPROF mean pre- and post-treatment total scores by category: *Static* factors, *Dynamic improving* factors and *Dynamic decreasing* factors (N = 108)

within the SAPROF. The analysis of the post-treatment ratings, however, revealed significantly higher 'dynamic improving' scores as well as higher 'dynamic decreasing' scores for those patients who had not committed any new violent offences after treatment. Thus, patients who had not recidivated after treatment generally were equipped with more protective factors on all three SAPROF categories at the time of discharge, than those who did end up recidivating in violence. Moreover, as non-recidivists improved significantly more during treatment on their 'dynamic improving' protective factors than recidivists (see also De Vries Robbé and De Vogel, 2010), treatment progress as measured by the SAPROF was indeed predictive of violent recidivism after treatment. This demonstrates the usefulness of the SAPROF not only as a positive dynamic assessment tool but also as a treatment-evaluation instrument.

Discussion

With this chapter, the authors hope to increase awareness of the potential value of protective factors for risk assessment and their usefulness for treatment planning and risk management in forensic mental health services. The inclusion of protective factors will provide mental health professionals with a more balanced violence risk assessment and additional guidelines for strengths-based clinical interventions. This chapter provided information about the psychometric properties of the SAPROF, an instrument specifically designed for the assessment of protective factors.

First results with the SAPROF have shown that the instrument can be coded reliably and that protective factors can be as predictive for not recidivating in future violence as risk factors are predictive for violent recidivism. Complementing risk assessment with protective factors demonstrated an increase in the predictive accuracy of risk assessment. Moreover, it was shown that dynamic protective factors are able to measure change during treatment, which in turn proved predictive of future violence. Although these results support the value of including structured assessment of protective factors in risk assessment and clinical practice, more research is needed to further consolidate these findings. Prospective, international multi-centre studies with large samples of (forensic) psychiatric patients and offenders are necessary, as well as studies with specific groups of patients, such as female offenders and possibly juvenile offenders. Research on the SAPROF thus far has primarily been carried out at the Van der Hoeven Kliniek. Consequently, the sample that has been studied consisted of a relatively homogeneous group of male forensic psychiatric patients. Although the patient sample that was used for the construction of the SAPROF was different from the research sample, both samples originated from the same population of forensic psychiatric patients. Currently, several studies on the SAPROF are being carried out in Canada, Germany, Italy, the Netherlands and the United Kingdom, which all focus on different types of offenders.

In the Van der Hoeven Kliniek in the Netherlands, the SAPROF was implemented in clinical practice in 2007, in order to complement and balance risk assessment. The regular use of protective factors in forensic clinical treatment has since shown valuable potential. Frequent users of the SAPROF have stated that the instrument can be helpful in formulating treatment goals, phasing treatment and facilitating risk communication (Van den Broek and De Vries Robbé, 2008). Prospective studies into the qualitative value of complementing forensic treatment with the protective factors approach are currently ongoing. As many of the protective factors are dynamic in nature, repeated assessments of these factors are highly recommended. Especially when changes occur in a patient's situation or liberties, alterations on the dynamic protective factors should be assessed carefully as different factors can be of particular importance for different situations. At the start of clinical intervention, the external mandatory protection usually provides almost all of the available protection. During treatment the aim is to increase the 'dynamic improving' factors to such a level that eventually the protection from mandatory intervention is no longer necessary and the patient can be discharged. Accordingly, a *Final Protection Judgement* for a given situation is not based on adding up the scores on all protective factors, but consists of a personal protection profile that is subject to change as treatment progresses. At any moment, it is the combination of the present risk factors and the available protection that determines one's resistance against relapse into violence. The relevance of specific protective factors can vary greatly between patients. While one patient may benefit most from medication and the availability of mental health professionals, another may benefit more from structured daily activities and a supportive social network.

In terms of the implementation and application of protective factors in clinical practice, it may be valuable to attempt to link the results from protective factors assessments with strengths-focused treatment interventions, such as the good lives model approach (Ward and Brown, 2004). The inclusion of positive, strength-focused factors in treatment may lead to more elaborate and patient-adjusted risk management strategies and improved risk communication, which is motivating for both staff and patients. In conclusion, protective factors bring a valuable balance to risk assessment and provide new guidance in narrowing the gap between risk assessment and violence prevention. The additional use of protective factors offers a well-rounded approach to risk management and treatment interventions in forensic clinical practice.

Acknowledgements

We kindly thank Corine de Ruiter and Yvonne Bouman for their co-authorship in developing the SAPROF. Also thanks to all mental health professionals of the Van der Hoeven Kliniek who contributed to the development of and research on the SAPROF.

References

Andrews, D. A. and Bonta, J. (1995) *The Level of Service Inventory-Revised*, Toronto: Multi-Health Systems, Inc.

Benda, B. (2005) 'Gender differences in life-course theory of recidivism: A survival analysis', *International Journal of Offender Therapy and Comparative Criminology*, 49: 325–42.

Blum, R. W. and Ireland, M. (2004) 'Reducing risk, increasing protective factors: Findings from the Caribbean Youth Health Survey', *Journal of Adolescent Health*, 35: 493–500.

Borum, R., Bartel, P. and Forth, A. (2006) *Manual for the Structured Assessment for Violence Risk in Youth (SAVRY)*, Odessa, FL: Psychological Assessment Resources.

Braithwaite, E., Charette, Y., Crocker, A. G. and Reyes, A. (2010) 'The predictive validity of clinical ratings of the Short-Term Assessment of Risk and Treatability (START)', *International Journal of Forensic Mental Health*, 9: 271–81.

Broek, E. van den and Vries Robbé, M. de 'The supplemental value of the SAPROF from a treatment perspective: A counterbalance to risk?', paper presented at the eighth Conference of the International Association of Forensic Mental Health Services, Vienna, Austria, July 2008.

Cooper, C., Eslinger, D. M. and Stolley, P. D. (2006) 'Hospital-based violence intervention programs work', *Journal of Trauma-Injury Infection and Critical Care*, 61: 534–40.

Costa, F. M., Jessor, R. and Turbin, M. S. (1999) 'Transition into adolescent problem drinking: The role of psychosocial risk and protective factors', *Journal of Studies on Alcohol*, 60: 480–90.

DeMatteo, D., Heilbrun, K. and Marczyk, G. (2005) 'Psychopathy, risk of violence, and protective factors in a noninstitutionalized and noncriminal sample', *International Journal of Forensic Mental Health*, 4: 147–57.

Douglas, K. S. and Skeem, J. L. (2005) 'Violence risk assessment: Getting specific about being dynamic', *Psychology, Public Policy, and Law*, 11: 347–83.

Douglas, K. S., Yeomans, M. and Boer, D. P. (2005) 'Comparative validity analysis of multiple measures of violence risk in a sample of criminal offenders', *Criminal Justice and Behavior*, 32: 479–510.

Ezell, M. E. and Cohen, L. E. (2005) *Desisting from crime: Continuity and change in long-term crime patterns of serious chronic offenders*, New York: Oxford University Press.

Farrington, D. P. and Loeber, R. (2000) 'Epidemiology of juvenile violence', *Child and Adolescent Psychiatric Clinics of North America*, 9: 733–48.

Fitzpatrick, K. M. (1997) 'Fighting among America's youth: A risk and protective factors approach', *Journal of Health and Social Behavior*, 38: 131–48.

Fonagy, P., Target, M. and Steele, H. (1997) 'The development of violence and crime as it relates to security of attachment', in J. Osofsky (ed.) *Children in a violent society* (pp. 150–177), New York: Guilford Press.

Gagliardi, G. J., Lovell, D., Peterson, P. D. and Jemelka, R. (2004) 'Forecasting recidivism in mentally ill offenders released from prison', *Law and Human Behavior*, 28: 133–55.

Gendreau, P., Goggin, C. and Gray, G. (2000) *Case needs review: Employment domain*, Saint John, NB: Centre for Criminal Justice Studies, University of New Brunswick.

Haggård-Grann, U. (2005) *Violence among mentally disordered offenders: Risk and protective factors*, Stockholm, Sweden: Edita Norstedts Tryckeri.

Hanson, R. K. and Thornton, D. (1999) *Static-99: Improving actuarial risk assessments for sex offenders*, Ottawa, Ontario: Department of the Solicitor General.

Hawkins, J. D., Catalano, R. F. and Miller, J. Y. (1992) 'Risk and protective factors for alcohol and other drug problems in adolescence and early adulthood: Implications for substance abuse prevention', *Psychological Bulletin*, 112: 64–105.

Heilbrun, K. (2003) 'Violence risk: From prediction to management', in D. Carson and R. Bull (eds) *Handbook of psychology in legal contexts* (pp. 127–42), New York: Wiley.

Holtfreter, K. and Cupp, R. (2007) 'Gender and risk assessment. The empirical status of the LSI-R for women', *Journal of Contemporary Criminal Justice*, 23: 363–82.

Howells, K., Day, A., Williamson, P., Bubner, S., Jauncey, S., Parker, A. and Heseltine, K. (2005) 'Brief anger management programs with offenders: Outcomes and predictors of change', *Journal of Forensic Psychiatry and Psychology*, 16: 296–311.

Jessor, R., Turbin, M. S., Costa, F. M., Dong, Q., Zhang, H. and Wang, C. (2003) 'Adolescent problem behavior in China and the United States: A cross-national study of psychosocial protective factors', *Journal of Research on Adolescence*, 13: 329–60.

Jones, N. J. and Brown, S. L. (2008) 'Positive reframing: The benefits of incorporating protective factors into risk assessment protocols', *Crime Scène*, 15: 22–24.

Kandel, E., Mednick, S. A., Kirkegaard-Sorensen, L., Hutchings, B., Knop, J., Rosenberg, R. and Schulsinger, F. (1988) 'IQ as a protective factor for subjects at high risk for antisocial behavior', *Journal of Consulting and Clinical Psychology*, 56: 224–26.

Lodewijks, H. P. B., Ruiter, C. de and Doreleijers, Th. A. H. (2010) 'The impact of protective factors in desistance from violent reoffending. A study in three samples of adolescent offenders', *Journal of Interpersonal Violence*, 25: 568–87.

Maruna, S. (2001) *Making Good: How ex-convicts reform and rebuild their lives*, Washington, DC: American Psychological Association.

Maruna, S. and Roy, K. (2006) 'Amputation or reconstruction? Notes on the concept of "knifing off" and desistance from crime', *Journal of Contemporary Criminal Justice*, 22: 1–21.

Miller, H. A. (2006) 'A dynamic assessment of offender risk, needs, and strengths in a sample of general offenders', *Behavioral Sciences and the Law*, 24: 767–82.

Nonstad, K., Nesset, M. B., Kroppan, E., Pedersen, T. W., Nøttestad, J. A., Almvik, R. and Palmstierna, T. (2010) 'Predictive validity and other psychometric properties of the

Short-Term Assessment of Risk and Treatability (START) in a Norwegian high secure hospital', *International Journal of Forensic Mental Health*, 9: 294–99.

Pearce, M. J., Jones, S. M., Schwab-Stone, M. E. and Ruchkin, V. (2003) 'The protective effects of religiousness and parent involvement on the development of conduct problems among youth exposed to violence', *Child Development*, 74: 1682–1696.

Rennie, C. E. and Dolan, M.C. (2010) 'The significance of protective factors in the assessment of risk', *Criminal Behaviour and Mental Health*, 20: 8–22.

Resnick, M. D., Ireland, M. and Borowsky, I. (2004) 'Youth violence perpetration: What protects? What predicts? Findings from the National Longitudinal Study of Adolescent Health', *Journal of Adolescent Health*, 35: 424.el–424.e10.

Rogers, R. (2000) 'The uncritical acceptance of risk assessment in forensic practice', *Law and Human Behavior*, 24: 595–605.

Salekin, R. T. and Lochman, J. E. (2008) 'Child and adolescent psychopathy. The search for protective factors', *Criminal Justice and Behavior*, 35: 159–72.

Seligman, M. E. P. (2002) 'Positive psychology, positive prevention, and positive therapy', in C. R. Snyder and S. J. Lopez (eds) *Handbook of positive psychology* (pp. 3–9), New York: Oxford University Press.

Tangney, J. P., Baumeister, R. F. and Boone, A. L. (2004) 'High self-control predicts good adjustment, less pathology, better grades, and interpersonal success', *Journal of Personality*, 72: 271–324.

Turbin, M. S., Jessor, R., Costa, F. M., Dong, Q., Zhang, H. and Wang, C. (2006) 'Protective and risk factors in health-enhancing behavior among adolescents in China and the United States: Does social context matter?', *Health Psychology*, 25: 445–54.

Vance, J. E., Bowen, N. K., Fernandez, G. and Thompson, S. (2002) 'Risk and protective factors as predictors of outcome in adolescents with psychiatric disorder and aggression', *Journal of the American Academy of Child and Adolescent Psychiatry*, 41: 36–43.

Vaughan, B. (2007) 'The internal narrative of desistance', *British Journal of Criminology*, 47: 390–404.

Vogel, V. de, Ruiter, C. de, Bouman, Y. and Vries Robbé, M. de (2007) *Handleiding bij de SAPROF. Structured Assessment of Protective Factors for Violence Risk* [SAPROF Manual. Structured Assessment of Protective Factors for Violence Risk], Utrecht, The Netherlands: Forum Educatief.

— (2009) *SAPROF. Guidelines for the assessment of protective factors for violence risk. English version*, Utrecht, The Netherlands: Forum Educatief.

Vogel, V. de, Vries Robbé, M. de, Ruiter, C. de and Bouman, Y. H. A. (2011) 'Assessing protective factors in forensic psychiatric practice. Introducing the SAPROF', *International Journal of Forensic Mental Health*, 10:171–77.

Vries Robbé, M. de and Vogel, V. de (2010) *Addendum to the SAPROF Manual. Updated research chapter*, Utrecht, The Netherlands: Van der Hoeven Stichting.

Vries Robbé, M. de, Vogel, V. de and Spa, E. de (2011) 'Protective factors for violence risk in forensic psychiatric patients. A retrospective validation study of the SAPROF', *International Journal of Forensic Mental Health*, 10: 178–86.

Vries Robbé, M. de, Vogel, V. de and Douglas, K. S. (in preparation) 'The additional value protective factors: Violence risk assessment with the SAPROF and the HCR-20'.

Vries Robbé, M. de, Vogel, V. de, Koster, K. and Bogaerts, S. (in preparation) 'Protective factors for sexually violent offenders'.

Ward, T. and Brown, M. (2004) 'The Good Lives Model and conceptual issues in offender rehabilitation', *Psychology, Crime and Law*, 10: 243–57.

Webster, C. D., Douglas, K. S., Eaves, D. and Hart, S. D. (1997) *HCR-20. Assessing the risk of violence. Version 2*, Burnaby, British Columbia: Simon Fraser University and Forensic Psychiatric Services Commission of British Columbia.

Webster, C. D., Martin, M., Brink, J., Nicholls, T.L. and Middleton, C. (2004) *Short-Term Assessment of Risk and Treatability (START): An evaluation and planning guide*, Hamilton, Ontario: St. Joseph's Healthcare Hamilton.

Webster, C. D., Müller-Isberner, R. and Fransson, G. (2002) 'Violence risk assessment: Using structured clinical guides professionally', *International Journal of Forensic Mental Health*, 1: 43–51.

Wilson, C. M., Desmarais, S. L., Nicholls, T. L. and Brink, J. (2010) 'The role of client strengths in assessments of violence risk using the Short-Term Assessment of Risk and Treatability (START)', *International Journal of Forensic Mental Health*, 9: 282–93.

Postscript

14 Future directions in clinical risk assessment and management

Caroline Logan and Lorraine Johnstone

A great deal has been written about clinical risk assessment in correctional, forensic psychiatric, and community settings with individuals who harm others as well as themselves. Indeed, this book is founded on a considerable amount of that research and guidance. Practitioners now have the means to identify reliably a range of factors known to correlate directly – and indirectly – with adverse outcomes, such as violence or suicide (see Otto and Douglas, 2010). In addition to specific risk assessment protocols such as the HCR-20 (Webster, Douglas, Eaves, and Hart, 1997), forensic practitioners, by virtue of their core training, are able to access a range of meaningful heuristics in order to guide their daily pursuit of harm prevention or minimization. However, the process of converting the findings of a risk assessment into effectively and demonstrably managed clinical risk for individual clients is not straightforward. Spelling out that process has been a key objective of this book. We have endeavoured to do this by addressing two important issues in the context of discussing adverse outcomes – or risks – of different kinds (e.g., violence, sexual violence) in different populations (e.g., women, young people): the *structured professional judgement* (SPJ) approach to clinical risk assessment and management, which emphasizes *risk formulation* as the essential bridge between the risk assessment and risk management tasks. If nothing else, readers should take from this book the importance, or at least the relevance, of these tasks in their work with harmful clients. In this chapter, we summarize the main points made by each of the contributors to the book as they relate to these key processes and offer suggestions for future directions in both clinical practice and research.

Structured professional judgement

SPJ is an approach to clinical risk assessment and management that requires a practitioner to use their discretion – their professional judgement – in the process of making decisions about the risks posed by their clients (Hart and Logan, 2011); using this approach, practitioners identify which information to gather, how to weight it, and how to combine it. In this book, David Cooke and Christine Michie have reviewed the SPJ approach (Chapter 1) and demonstrated, we think compellingly, its advantages over commonly used non-discretionary approaches emphasizing risk prediction (for example, the *Risk Matrix 2000*, Thornton, 2003). Structure is added to professional judgement in the form of explicit guidelines that direct practitioners to the kinds of information relevant to specific decisions about, for example, violence risk (see Douglas, Blanchard, and Hendry, Chapter 2, this volume) as opposed to sexual violence risk (see Russell and Darjee, Chapter 4, this volume). The HCR-20 (Webster, et al., 1997) and the *Risk for Sexual Violence Protocol* (RSVP, Hart, Kropp, Laws, et al., 2003) are two examples of structured professional guidelines for the assessment of violence and sexual-violence risk respectively. Logan (Chapter 5, this volume) and Taylor and Thorne (Chapter 6, this volume) introduced sets of guidelines relevant to the assessment and management of suicidal behaviour and pathological firesetting in adults respectively.

The SPJ approach requires practitioners, once all the most relevant information about risk factors is before them, to attend to the *purpose* of harmful behaviour to the individual. Determined through the process of formulation, such an undertaking promises to discover the answer to the question 'Why?' in respect of a client's decision to be harmful (see Cooke and Michie, Chapter 1, this volume). Once it is clear what the client has gained or sought to gain from being harmful in the past and how the most relevant risk factors combined to make harmful behaviour a desirable objective then, it is possible to look to the future to determine the circumstances – or scenarios – in which the client might decide to be harmful again in pursuit of the same or a similar goal. Such an understanding, which goes well beyond simply listing risk factors that are present, then becomes the platform for risk management. Combining interventions relating to treatment, supervision, monitoring and, where relevant, victim safety planning, risk management is designed to weaken risk factors, strengthen protective factors, and overall influence negatively the decision-making sequences from which harm is a potential outcome.

The product of the assessment, therefore, is an improved understanding about the harm potential of the client and a set of strategies for intervention and monitoring based directly on this understanding. This is SPJ, and the revised worksheet for the HCR-20 (and the worksheet for the new version 3 of the HCR-20), and the worksheets for the RSVP and the *Suicidal Behaviours Risk Evaluation* (SBRE, Logan, chapter 5) set out each of the stages from beginning to end to ensure that none are missed and the outcome is a structured and informed professional judgement about risk. John Taylor and Ian Thorne (chapter 6, this volume) describe the application of such a process to pathological fire-setting in adults and David Cooke and Lorraine Johnstone apply it to situational and organizational factors that are a contribution to the violence of individuals (chapter 7, this volume), and in each of the chapters on key client groups – chapters 8 through to 11 – SPJ underpins the specialist assessment and intervention techniques described. Also, in a powerful tribute to the capacity of practitioners and clinical teams working together within and across services, Lorraine Johnstone demonstrates the application of SPJ guidelines and practice to work with clients presenting with complex comorbid disorders and social problems.

With others such as Douglas and colleagues (chapter 2), we contend, that the SPJ approach – and only the SPJ approach – assists the development of risk management plans based on an understanding of the causes of past harmful behaviour (see also Hart and Logan, 2011). Risk assessment in the absence of such an understanding has the potential to generate meaningless risk management plans because they may be based on variables that have little direct relevance to the risks posed by the individual. Therefore, risk management could be disproportionate – either too restrictive or not restrictive enough – and to us, this is unacceptable and unethical.

Risk formulation

In Chapter 1, David Cooke and Christine Michie suggested that the emphasis on risk formulation represented a 'fourth era' (p. 3) of risk assessment practice, and signalled how the field is developing and must develop further. The relevance of formulation to every chapter in this book is testament to this observation and aspiration. But what do we mean exactly by formulation within the SPJ approach to clinical risk assessment and management? First, the task of formulation is, on the basis of the information gathered about the risk and protective factors most relevant to the client, to determine those most influential in the client's decision to be harmful in the past. That is, a decision-theory framework is applied to relevant information about the client's past harmful conduct (Hart and Logan, 2011). Second, based on this analysis, future harmful behaviour is speculated through a process of scenario planning, that is, through the preparation of a story about the harm the client might do to him or herself or to others (Hart and Logan, 2011). Only by analysing the relevance and the connections and the meaning of harmful behaviour for the client will it be possible to anticipate how and why he or she might decide to be harmful again. This analytical process is formulation, in two stages, and the most rational and essential bridge between the relatively straightforward risk assessment stage and the purpose of the whole undertaking, namely risk management.

Formulation has a number of objectives (Hart and Logan, 2011; Hart, Sturmey, Logan, and McMurran, 2011). First, formulations must *organize* information about a person and his or her problems. This involves an appraisal of not only risk factors but also protective factors; a client's risk of harm will be related to the interplay of relevant risk factors (e.g., major mental illness, alcohol dependence, cognitive impairment), but also to changes in the functioning of protective factors (e.g., attitudes towards treatment, relationship with a care provider), with the assumption being that risk of harm will become an issue in an individual client when specific risk factors are very active or acute *and* when protective factors cease to work effectively. In this volume, in the section on key practice skills, Michiel de Vries Robbé and Vivienne de Vogel (Chapter 13) describe their work on the importance of protective factors and on the necessity of including their consideration in any judgement about future risk of harm. The work they describe is at a relatively early stage, but its focus on what usually works to keep clients safe is a critical consideration in any judgement about their risk of harm.

Second, formulations must create or generate a *mutual understanding* of problems and symptoms, that is, an understanding that is shared even to some extent between the practitioner and the client. Joint working like this is especially emphasized – and encouraged – in the work presented by de Vries Robbé and de Vogel in Chapter 13. However, collaborative working towards a shared understanding of risk is a feature of all chapters in this book, including the interview guidance offered in Chapter 12. Third, formulations should hypothesize *connections* between antecedents, the problems under study, and the consequences that maintain the problem over sometimes very long periods of time. This emphasis on connections that maintain risk over time is a particular feature of Lorraine Johnstone's chapter on mental disorder and violence (Chapter 3), where the complex interplay between personal and social problems is explored in detail.

Fourth, the purpose of formulations is also to assist with developing an *intervention plan* that will lead to the desired outcome. This is critical: formulation is an account of the underlying mechanism of risk and hypotheses about action to generate change (Logan, Nathan and Brown, 2011). This link between formulation and action is a marked feature of the chapters on key client groups – clients with cognitive impairment (by Suzanne O'Rourke, Chapter 8), young people (by Corine de Ruiter and Leena Augimeri, Chapter 9), women (Vivienne de Vogel and Michiel de Vries Robbé, Chapter 10), and serving and veteran military personnel (John Marham, Chapter 11). Finally, the purpose of formulation is to provide the basis and the language with which to *communicate* with other professionals, to make links across services to ensure continuity of care. In no other chapters is this made clearer than those by Katharine Russell and Rajan Darjee (on sexual offenders, Chapter 4) and Lorraine Johnstone (on complex cases, Chapter 3).

We assert that risk assessment without formulation is no risk assessment at all. Instead, a risk assessment that is simply a list of (present) risk factors, with no justification of their relevance to the individual or account of their interaction, is just that, a list of descriptive features of the client that offers no new knowledge and no call to action, and brings into question the professionalism of the practitioner as well as the ethics of his or her practice.

Future directions in practice

In the five or ten years to come, it is our shared hope that forensic practitioners will undertake risk formulations as a matter of routine. Further, it is our hope that the evidence base for the reliable and valid application of formulation skills (see Hart, et al., 2011) will be substantial such that when the term 'formulation' is used in clinical settings, there is at last consensus on what that means and what a good quality formulation looks like. It is also our hope, for all the reasons set down in Cooke and Michie's opening chapter, that risk prediction – the prediction of risk in the individual – will be generally seen as the futile exercise that we believe it to be and that practitioners will no longer base judgements about their clients on this misleading exercise. In addition, we propose to do what we can to ensure that the application of the SPJ approach in the areas of pathological fire setting and suicide and self-harm is consolidated because these are critical areas of forensic practice in which such an approach is valuable.

Further attention must be paid to one additional area of practice. In researching for the preparation of Chapter 12, Caroline Logan was surprised to find that there was comparatively – very – little already published in the area of forensic clinical interviewing. The literatures on clinical interviewing and forensic or investigative interviewing are considerable. But that for forensic practitioners – psychologists, psychiatrists, nurses, social workers, and occupational therapists – on interviewing skills for use when trying to engage with clients who are reluctant to commit to a working or even therapeutic relationship or whose engagement is intermittent or conditional on the practitioner's demonstration of a favourable opinion is only small. More publications on the topic of forensic clinical interviewing, more research on interviewing techniques, and more practice-developing courses on this particular skill are urgently required.

Future directions in research

It almost goes without saying that the principal areas in which we think further research is required are into the SPJ approach and risk formulation. Research into the SPJ approach will require attention to the measurement of prevented harm – whether the process of risk assessment itself leads to a reduction in the level of expected harm (Douglas and Kropp, 2002). Research on formulation will require more specific attention to be paid to the reliability and validity of the narratives made by practitioners working with the same cases. Hart and colleagues have set down a template for the evaluation of risk formulations, which researchers should consider closely if they are to contribute to this important area of development (Hart, et al., 2011). Otherwise, it is our observation that more empirical research is required in the areas of pathological fire setting risk to supplement and develop the important work presented by Taylor and Thorne (Chapter 6) and risk assessment and management with clients with cognitive impairment (O'Rourke, Chapter 8), especially if such impairment is comorbid with other mental health and social problems (see Johnstone, Chapter 3).

Finally, and on the basis of John Marham's passionate overview of armed forces personnel and the risks they pose to themselves and to others (Chapter 11), especially if they are veterans of active service, we regard it as a matter of priority that further research be carried out into the growing population of correctional and forensic mental health clients who have military and conflict experience. Correctional and forensic mental health services will be far better prepared to cope, in terms of the awareness and specific training of staff, if such a development is anticipated and understood.

Concluding comments

It has been a real pleasure to prepare and to contribute to this book. What we realized in the course of doing so, in our repeated requests to contributors to try to stay close to the word limit given for individual chapters, was that each surely had within them a whole and enthusiastic book on their subject alone. The SPJ approach is a remarkable model for the generation and organization of rational and practical ideas about clinical risk assessment and management, too long under the shadow of seemingly more scientific and objective risk prediction approaches. We think this imaginative and inspiring book represents a real break from the actuarial tradition, showing off the SPJ approach in its own right as a practical approach for practitioners in real-world clinical situations in which decisions about risk management – often relating to the curtailment of liberty – have to be justified to tribunals and the Courts, and to clients and their carers alike. We are proud of this work, and we hope that you will benefit from the knowledge contained within as much as we have benefited from being associated with it as its editors.

References

Douglas, K. S. and Kropp, P. R. (2002) 'A prevention-based paradigm for violence risk assessment: Clinical and research applications', *Criminal Justice and Behavior*, 29: 617–58.

Hart, S. D. and Logan, C. (2011) 'Formulation of violence risk using evidence-based assessments: The structured professional judgment approach', in P. Sturmey and M. McMurran (eds) *Forensic Case Formulation*, Chichester: Wiley-Blackwell.

Hart, S. D., Kropp, P. R., Laws, D. R., Klaver, J., Logan, C. and Watt, K. A. (2003) *The Risk for Sexual Violence Protocol (RSVP): Structured professional guidelines for assessing risk of sexual violence*, Burnaby, British Columbia: Mental Health, Law, and Policy Institute, Simon Fraser University.

Hart, S. D., Sturmey, P., Logan, C. and McMurran, M. M. (2011) 'Forensic case formulation', *International Journal of Forensic Mental Health*, 10: 118–26.

Logan, C., Nathan, R. and Brown, A. (2011) 'Formulation in clinical risk assessment and management', in R. W. Whittington and C. Logan (eds) *Self-harm and Violence: Towards best practice in managing risk*, Chichester, UK: Wiley-Blackwell.

Otto, R. K. and Douglas, K. S. (eds) (2010) *Handbook of Violence Risk Assessment Tools*, Abingdon, UK: Routledge.

Thornton, D. M. (2003) *Scoring Guide for the Risk Matrix 2000.4*. Unpublished work.

Webster, C. D., Douglas, K., Eaves, D. and Hart, S. D. (1997) *HCR-20 Assessing Risk for Violence* (2nd ed.), Vancouver: Simon Fraser University.

Afterword

Perhaps more than any other country in the world, the United Kingdom has embraced advances in violence risk assessment over the past two decades and incorporated them into daily practice in civil mental health, forensic mental health, and correctional settings. A number of researchers and research groups have made important contributions to the knowledge base. Moreover, agencies such as the National Health Service, the National Offender Management Service and Her Majesty's Prison Service in England and Wales, and the Scottish Prison Service and the Risk Management Authority in Scotland – to name but a few – have made major contributions to the dissemination of knowledge and enhancement of practitioners' skills with respect to violence risk assessment and management. It comes as no surprise, then, to see a book of this sort emerge from the UK.

It also comes as no surprise to see a book of such high quality result from the efforts of Drs Logan and Johnstone. In addition to being knowledgeable about the topic, they have tremendous practical experience. And they had enough good judgement to assemble a team of contributors that could write authoritatively about a range of topics relevant to clinical practice. Speaking professionally, I thank Caroline and Lorraine for their great contribution to the field; speaking personally, I congratulate my friends on a job well done.

What is surprising to me is that this book succeeds despite – or, perhaps, because of – its narrow focus on a single approach to understanding violence risk: the structured professional judgement (SPJ) approach. In many respects, this book marks the 'coming of age' of SPJ. Developed by a group of people working at or affiliated with Simon Fraser University in the early 1990s, SPJ was intended to be an alternative both to unstructured professional judgement approaches to violence risk assessment and, importantly, to actuarial or non-discretionary risk assessment. The essential feature of the SPJ approach is that evaluators are provided with structure in the form of practice recommendations. These recommendations are evidence based in the true sense of the expression, that is, based on current views of the best available empirical evidence, scientific theory, and clinical experience.

As the evidence base on violence risk has grown, SPJ guidelines have evolved to address a number of basic steps in the process of risk assessment. SPJ guidelines now provide practice recommendations concerning such things as the sort of information that should be considered and how it should be gathered; which risk factors should be considered (at a minimum) in every evaluation; how to identify the most critical or relevant risk factors in a case and develop a coherent formulation of violence risk; how to develop scenario-based plans for managing violence risk; and how to communicate about violence risk. The assumption underlying the SPJ approach is that this sort of structure helps to mitigate the biases and errors that plague all decisions made under conditions of uncertainty.

SPJ will continue to evolve. Research groups around the world are findings ways that may help to give further structure and guidance to practitioners: how to take into account group differences such as age, gender, culture, or mental disorder; how to more systematically incorporate strengths and protective factors; how to formulate violence risk and develop management plans. Hopefully, in the coming years we will have more books of this sort (or more editions of this book!) that will incorporate the findings of these groups.

In the meantime, dear reader, use this book. I am pleased that you found the topic interesting enough to track down the book, and even more pleased you have perused the contents. But that is not enough. Let the contributions stimulate you, push you to think more deeply or differently about your practice and how you can improve it. Use this book.

Once again, Caroline and Lorraine, thanks and congratulations.

Professor Stephen Hart, PhD
Department of Psychology
Simon Fraser University
Canada

Index

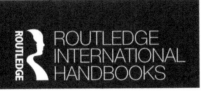
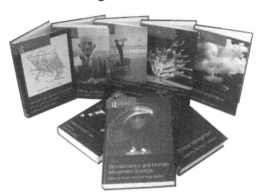
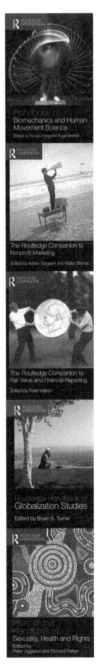

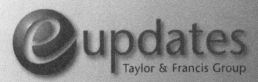
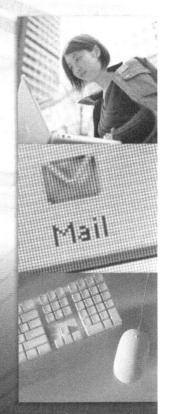